Tolley's
Guide to Man
Employee He

T0231359

Edited by

Dr Leslie Hawkins, Director of the Robens Centre for
Occupational Health and Safety, University of Surrey

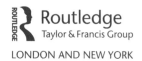

Routledge
Taylor & Francis Group

LONDON AND NEW YORK

First published by LexisNexis

This edition published 2011 by Routledge
2 Park Square, Milton Park, Abingdon, Oxon OX14 4RN
711 Third Avenue, New York, NY 10017, USA

Routledge is an imprint of the Taylor & Francis Group, an informa business

© Taylor & Francis 2002

A CIP Catalogue record for this book is available from the British Library.

ISBN 978-0-7545-1886-0

Preface

Physicians over the centuries, starting with Hippocrates, have realised that work caused disease. The birth of modern Occupational Medicine is usually attributed to a physician from Northern Italy, Bernadino Ramazzini, who published *De Morbis Atificum Diatriba* in 1713, a year before his death. In this book he described a wide range of diseases which he realised were associated with the work people were doing.

In the UK, as elsewhere in Europe, the industrial revolution marked the beginning of a wide-ranging change in work practices and working environments which were to have a huge impact on society. The advent of the factory took large numbers of people away from agriculture and into manufacturing. The demand for the raw material of manufacture and transport of industrial goods and materials meant large numbers of people moving to work in mines, road building, canal excavation and construction. The use of new forms of energy, such as coal, also brought with it increased atmospheric pollution and disease. Between 1760 and 1830 these major changes in society had brought with them a huge and growing epidemic of industrial diseases. Diseases such as pneumoconiosis (a fatal lung disease from breathing coal and other dusts), silicosis (another form of lung disease from breathing silica dust – common in the cast-iron industries), byssinosis (from breathing textile dusts and common in the Lancashire cotton mills), poisoning from lead (often from lead glazing in the potteries), infections such as anthrax (from infected animal hides), and deafness from industrial noise (first recognised in boiler-makers), became the 'classic' diseases of occupations.

Society moved very slowly to combat these physical, chemical and biological hazards associated with work, and as a result hundreds of thousands of people suffered appalling illness and had their lives shortened by the work they were engaged in. The first Health and Safety legislation was the *Health and Morals of Apprentices Act 1802* which limited working hours of 'parish apprentices' (pauper children who had been exploited by factory owners). The morals aspect probably came from the requirement in the Act for the factory owner to ensure that male and female apprentices slept in separate beds and that they were to be instructed in the principles of the Christian religion. The first *Factory Act* of 1819 was again aimed at protecting children, banning those under 9 from work in the cotton mills and limiting those between 9 and 16 to 12 hours per day! The first effective *Factory Act* (1833) provided proper enforcement inspectors but was again limited to fixing working times. The 1833 Act fixed a maximum working week of 48 hours for children aged 9 to 13 and a 68-hour week for those under 18. It also banned children under 9 from working in most textile mills. The *Factory Acts* of 1844 and 1847 limited the working day for women to 12 hours and for children aged 8 to 13 to a maximum of 6½ hours. Further *Factory Acts* in 1850, 1853, 1878, 1895, 1901 and 1937 extended these earlier Acts, which were mainly aimed at the cotton mills, to other industries, but they did little to protect workers from the hazards of their work, only to limit the time they were exposed to them.

The *Factories Act 1961* and later the *Health and Safety at Work etc Act 1974* were the first real attempts to put in place a legal framework that required an assessment of the risks of working with hazardous materials and processes. It took two hundred years from the beginning of the industrial revolution to arrive at a point when the law required employers to determine what risks to health they were exposing their workers to and ensure that these health risks were eliminated or reduced to a reasonably practicable level. Thankfully, the occupational diseases that were prevalent in the years following the industrial revolution are now largely eliminated, but there is no room for complacency. The classic diseases of occupations, with the exception of asbestos-related disease, are now replaced by modern occupational illnesses such as stress, upper-limb disorders and other musculoskeletal disorders. The 'old' hazards such as noise, chemicals, dust and infectious organisms are still with us but have changed with changes in the types of materials used in industry, changes in technology and the types of infectious diseases afflicting modern society. Nevertheless, they still pose a significant hazard in many occupations.

Modern occupational health is concerned not only with protecting the individual employee from work-related illness, but with protecting the organisation from the consequences of an employee who is ill or disabled, whether caused by work or not. Consequently, the focus in occupational health has shifted from statutory legal duties to common law compliance. The readiness in modern society for an employee to seek damages through the civil courts for ill-health caused by work has focussed attention sharply on the importance of preventing employees being adversely affected by their work.

This book is intended to give the manager of any enterprise, large or small, with the understanding of occupational health issues, some practical knowledge and an insight into when and how to seek expert help. Safeguarding your employees' health has at last become an essential rule of good business.

Dr Leslie Hawkins
December 2002

Contents

Preface   iii

Contributors   xiii

Acknowledgements   xvii

1   What is Employee Health? – *Leslie Hawkins*

Introduction   1
Health or safety?   1
What is health?   2
Why does an organisation need occupational health support?   3
Occupational health support provision   4
The interaction between work and home   5
Assessment of hazards and risk   5
Organising occupational health support   6
Fitness for work   7
Maintaining fitness for work   8

2   Legal Overview – *Gillian Howard*

Introduction   9
Statutory duties   10
Reporting of Injuries, Diseases and Dangerous Occurrences
    Regulations 1995   10
  Definitions   11
  Reportable diseases   12
  Method of notification   13
Corporate manslaughter   14
Recruitment   15
  Pre-employment assessments   15
  Data protection   16
  Disability Discrimination Act 1995   21
  Pre-employment warnings   21
  Negligence   21
  Lying   22
Managing short-term absence   22
  Identifying the problem   22
  Guidance   23
  Dismissal   23
Managing long-term or acute sickness absence   24
  Guidance   24
  Dismissal   25
  Conflicting medical evidence   25

Guidance for GPs   26
Consent   27
Dealing with 'malingerers'   27
  Including materials in the staff manual   28
  Covert surveillance   28
  Disciplinary procedures   34
Managing return to work   36
Disability discrimination   36
  Depression   38
  Employer responsibility   38
Medical confidentiality and human rights   39
Stress   39
Bullying   43
Violence   43

3   Managing Occupational Health – *Olivia Carlton*

Introduction – Aims and objectives of a company in managing
  occupational health   49
What should occupational health support achieve?   49
Occupational health management – the process   51
What kind of occupational health support is needed?   51
What occupational health services are available?   53
The occupational health team   54
  External health team   54
  In-house team   55
Role of different occupational health professionals   55
  Occupational physician   55
  Occupational health nurse   56
  Occupational hygienist   57
  Occupational therapist   57
  Ergonomist or human factors specialist   58
  Physiotherapist   58
  Counsellor   59
How to make a referral   59
  Sickness absence   60
  Work-related illness   61
  Fitness for work   61
The reply to a referral   62
Confidentiality   62
  Employee's consent   63
  Occupational health records   63
  Pre-employment occupational health questionnaires 64
The relationship between managers and occupational health
  practitioners   64
Ethical practice in occupational health management   65
Setting and monitoring standards   66
Enforcement   66
  Role of inspectors, the Health & Safety Executive and local
  authorities   66

Improvement notice 68
Prohibition notice 68
Employment Medical Advisory Service (EMAS) 69
Reporting of Injuries, Diseases and Dangerous
  Occurrences Regulations 69
Case studies 70

4   **Occupational Health Systems – *Denis D'Auria***

Introduction 72
Characteristics of service organisations 73
Setting up systems 74
First aid 75
  Minimum requirements 76
  Assessing the risks 77
  Employees working off site 78
  Members of the public 78
  Contents of the first aid kits 79
  Practical issues to be considered 79
Sickness absence 80
  Contributory factors 81
  Patterns of sickness absence 83
  Measurement 84
  Setting up the system 87
Case management 88
  Managing sickness absence – an integrated approach 89
Reporting workplace accidents and ill-health 90
Monitoring hazards and ill-health 91
  Stage 1 – Identifying the presence of hazards 92
  Stage 2 – Assessing risk 93
  Stage 3 – Controlling risk 93
  Stage 4 – Recovery 93
  Categorising risk 94
Health surveillance 96
  Individual health status 96
  Death in service 97
Safety representatives 98
Safety committees 99
Conclusion 100

5   **Biological Hazards – *Gail James***

Introduction 101
Legal requirements 101
  Control of Substances Hazardous to Health Regulations
    2002 101
  Management of Health and Safety at Work Regulations
    1999 102

Reporting of Injuries, Diseases and Dangerous
    Occurrences Regulations 1995   102
Public Health (Infectious Diseases) Regulations 1988   103
Respiratory and skin disorders   103
    Introduction   103
    Respiratory disorders   103
    What are they?   104
    Skin disorders   107
Blood borne viruses   112
    Introduction   112
    What are they?   112
    Assessing the risks   113
Zoonoses   116
    Introduction   116
    What are they?   117
    Assessing the risks   117
    Health surveillance   120
Travellers' health   122
    Introduction   122
    What are the risks?   123
    Food borne disease   126
Food health   127

6   Chemical Hazards – *Robin Howie*

Introduction   128
Legal requirements   129
    Health and Safety at Work etc Act 1974   129
    Chemicals (Hazard Information and Packaging for Supply)
        Regulations 2002   130
Chemical substances in the 'real world'   135
    Commercial confidentiality   136
    Chemical nomenclature   136
    Inadequate safety data sheets   136
    Proprietary or difficult to identify products   137
    EU hazard classifications may be less stringent than other
        authorities   138
Assessing the risks   138

7   Physical Hazards – *Leslie Hawkins*

Introduction – What are physical hazards?   141
Sound and noise   141
    Heath effects of noise   142
    Legal requirements   144
    Assessing the risks   144
    Health surveillance   145
Vibration   146
    Health effects of vibration   147
    Legal requirements   149

Assessing the risks 150
Health surveillance 152
Temperature 153
Working in hot environments 153
Working in cold environments 157
Thermal comfort 159
Light 165
A safe and pleasant environment 165
Performance of the task 166
General health and eyestrain 167
Legal requirements 168
Ergonomic aspects – *Margaret Hanson* 170
Health effects related to ergonomic risks 170
Ergonomic risk factors 172
Physical work environment 175
Psychosocial risk factors 176
Individual differences 177
Specific tasks 177
Legal requirements 178
Assessing the risks 178
The workplace environment 180
Sick building syndrome 181
What is it? 181
Legal requirements 182
Assessing the risks 183
Static electricity and non-ionising radiation 188
Static electricity 188
Non-ionising radiation 189
Ionising radiation – *Nick Lewis* 195
Legal requirements 196
Risk assessments 196
Radiation protection advisers 196
Health surveillance 197
Emergencies 197

8   Occupational Mental Health – *Graham Lucas*

Introduction 199
Mental health in the workplace 199
Prevalence of mental health problems 200
Risk as a cause of increased anxiety 202
Age and sex-related distribution 202
Legal requirements 202
Application of the Management of Health and Safety
at Work Regulations 1999 203
Disability Discrimination Act 1995 204
The organisation 204
Corporate social responsibility 205
Occupational health resources 206

Clinical management 207
    Identifying common mental ill-health triggers and
      symptoms 208
    Strategies in the training of occupational health
      professionals 208
    Destigmatisation and discrimination in the workplace 209
    Prescription drugs and over-the-counter medication 209
    Pharmacology of side effects of antidepressants 211
Factors affecting the individual 211
    Personality characteristics which are of occupational
      significance 212
    Physical health impairment 213
    Physical symptoms relating to psychiatric conditions 213
    Psychosomatic symptoms 214
Post-natal depression and female-specific anxieties 215
Stress 215
    Stress management 216
Post-traumatic stress disorder 217
    Clinical features 218
    Clinical management 218
Burnout 218
Alcohol and drug abuse 219
    Alcohol and drug policies 220
    Screening 220
Pre-employment medical examinations 221
Prolonged sickness absence 221
Sickness absence and ill-health retirement 222
Conclusions 222

9   Personal Protection – *Robin Howie*

Introduction 224
Legal requirements 225
    Control of Substances Hazardous to Health Regulations
      2002 225
    Noise at Work Regulations 1989 228
    Construction (Head Protection) Regulations 1989 230
    Personal Protective Equipment at Work Regulations
      1992 232
    Confined Spaces Regulations 1997 233
    Summary and comment on legislation 233
Role of personal protection 234
Setting up and running an effective personal protection
      programme 234
    Assess risks and identify where control is required 234
    Implement all reasonably practicable controls 234
    Identify who needs residual protection 234
    Inform wearers of consequences of exposure 235
    Select PPE adequate to control residual exposure 235
    Involve wearers in PPE selection process 235

Match PPE to each individual wearer   235
Carry out objective fit tests of PPE   236
Ensure that PPE does not create risk   236
Ensure PPE are mutually compatible   236
Train wearers in the correct use of their PPE   237
Minimise wear periods   237
Supervise wearers to ensure correct use of PPE   238
Provide suitable storage facilities for PPE   238
Maintain PPE in efficient and hygienic condition   238
Inspect PPE to ensure it is correctly maintained   238
Record usage and maintenance data   239
Monitor programme to ensure continuing effectiveness   239
Provide PPE free of charge   239
Types of PPE   239
Respiratory protective equipment   240
Personal hearing protectors   243
Protective clothing   247
Overall summary   249

10 Applying Risk Management and Risk Assessment in Occupational Health – *Lawrence Waterman*

Introduction   250
Benefits of a systematic occupational health risk management   251
What is risk assessment?   252
Legal requirements   252
Who can undertake health risk assessments?   254
What does 'competence' mean for occupational health risk assessments?   255
The role of staff   256
Specialist support   256
Practical risk assessment for health hazards   257
Stage 1 – Identifying the presence of hazards   259
Stage 2 – Identifying the controls already in place   260
Stage 3 – Evaluating risk   261
Stage 4 – Categorising risk   262
Stage 5 – Setting priorities   264
Stage 6 – Taking precautions: exercising control   265
Controls available include   267
Monitoring health risk exposures   269
Recording risk assessments   269
Keeping health risk assessment records   269
Review and audit   271
Case studies   272

11 Using External Expertise – *Leslie Hawkins*

Introduction   275
Is the need a real one?   275

Carefully consider the questions you want answered   276
Choose a consultant who has the right experience for the
    job   277
In-house versus external assistance   277
    The size of the organisation   278
    The nature of the organisation   278
    The occasional need   278
    Legal requirements   278
    Routine occupational health management   279
Where to get occupational health advice   280
    Direct employment   280
    Agencies   280
    Specialist service provider   281
    Sharing a service with others   281
    Local general practice   281
    HSE appointed doctor   282
Health and safety professionals   282
    Occupational physician   282
    Occupational health nurse   283
    Occupational hygienist   284
    Ergonomist   286
    Physiotherapist and chiropractor   287

Appendix: Further Sources of Information   288

Table of Cases   307

Table of Statutes   308

Table of Statutory Instruments   309

Table of European Legislation   311

Index   313

Contributors

General Editor

Dr Leslie Hawkins BSc PhD CBiol MIBiol MOISH

Leslie Hawkins trained as a Clinical Physiologist at St Bartholomew's Hospital in London, where he worked until he moved to the University of Surrey in 1970 as Lecturer and then Senior Lecturer in Human Biology. His research interests at Barts concerned the pathophysiology of chronic carbon monoxide exposure, which developed into a more general interest in Environmental Physiology after he joined the University of Surrey. In 1984 he was appointed to the Robens Institute to establish and Head an Occupational Health Unit; this has now become the Robens Centre for Occupational Health and Safety. Leslie now holds a Professorial grade post as University Director and Director of the Robens Centre. The Robens Centre undertakes consultancy and provides occupational health and safety services and runs postgraduate Diploma and Masters level courses in Occupational Health, Occupational Health Nursing, Hygiene and Safety. He is the University Vice-Chancellor's special advisor on occupational and environmental health. His research interests are mainly concerned with the health effects of working environments. He is a consultant to a number of companies and Government bodies on environmental and occupational health issues and on the management of health and safety at work. He is Law Society listed as an expert witness in the fields of health and safety and is involved in both civil litigation and public inquiry cases.

Authors

Dr Olivia Carlton MBBS DRCOG FFOM

Dr Olivia Carlton is an Occupational Physician. She has worked for London Transport and then London Underground for thirteen years and now advises the London Underground Board on occupational health policy and strategy and is also Head of their multidisciplinary Occupational Health Team. From 1997 she was seconded to the Department of Health for four years on a part-time basis to provide occupational health policy advice to the Minister for Public Health. She was closely involved in the development of the Government's Healthy Workplace initiative and led the Department of Health's input into the Government's occupational health strategy, 'Securing Health Together'. She was appointed to the position of Registrar of the Faculty of Occupational Medicine in May 2002.

Dr Denis D'Auria

Denis D'Auria is Consultant Occupational Physician and Director of Occupational Health Services at the Legge Hunter Centre, St Bartholomew's Hospital and the London NHS Trust. He is also Honorary Senior Lecturer in Occupation Medicine at Barts and the Royal London School of Medicine and the Department of Public Health Sciences at St George's Hospital Medical School. He is a Fellow of the Faculty of Occupational Medicine of the Royal College of Physicians and was recently elected an Honorary Member of the Society of Occupational Medicine. He is Honorary Editor emeritus of the journal 'Occupational Medicine'. He is also a member of the advisory board of 'Occupational Health Review'. Frequently instructed as an expert witness, he is also a writer and lecturer on occupational health and, in particular, related legal issues.

Margaret Hanson BSc(Hons) MErgS

Margaret Hanson is a Senior Consultant with Hu-Tech Associates Ltd and specialises in providing ergonomics advice and training, particularly on workplace design and musculoskeletal disorders. After graduating with a first class Honours Degree in Ergonomics in 1993 she spent eight years with the Institute of Occupational Medicine, where she undertook a wide range of ergonomics research. She is a guest lecturer at Heriot Watt and Loughborough Universities. Margaret is a registered member of the Ergonomics Society, and for a period was the Society's Annual Conference Programme Secretary (1998–2001). She is also a member of BSI Committee PH9/1 (Ergonomics of the Thermal Environment).

Gillian Howard LLB Dip Comp Law (CANTAB) Hon FFOM

Gillian Howard is an Employment Lawyer specialising in employment and medical negligence cases and is consultant to Gordon Dadds, Mayfair, Solicitors. She has both corporate and individual clients, and has a wide-ranging practice in contentious and non-contentious work. She represents clients at tribunals as well as advising and drafting on company policies and procedures. She has spoken at many public conferences over the years, and is the author of several books and publications, including Tolley's 'Drafting Contracts of Employment'.

Robin M Howie

Robin Howie joined the Institute of Occupational Medicine in Edinburgh in 1970. In 1974 he was made responsible for the Institute's Respirator Test Facility which originally tested respirators only for the then National Coal Board. Over the years he expanded the facility's scope by offering a service to respirator manufacturers and users and the Health & Safety Executive (HSE). From 1980 to 1995 he was responsible for developing new test methods for equipment such as protective clothing, disposable respirators, manual resuscitation devices and smoke hoods and for determining the performance of respirator filters and protective clothing against asbestos fibres. He also developed techniques and protocols for determining the reality of respirator performance in the workplace. During the period 1993–1995 he led an HSE-funded study to evaluate the effectiveness of respirators during asbestos removal. He was Senior Occupational Hygienist in an HSE-funded research project to develop noise exposure standards for divers and others working under hyperbaric conditions. He has recently led field studies to assess the performance of protective clothing during asbestos removal operations for a major multi-national clothing manufacturer and to assess the performance of respiratory protective equipment in the workplace.

Gail James

Qualifying as a Registered General Nurse in 1981, Gail James' first occupational health post was in 1987 with the Robens Centre for Occupational Health and Safety (University of Surrey) where she was responsible for setting up the travel vaccination clinic and gained experience in a variety of light and service industries. Gail has provided occupational health advice to flour mills, bakeries, depots and headquarters staff and set up an occupational health service for a large water utility company. In 1995 she gained a Masters degree in Occupational Health Nursing, investigating the health risks of working with sewage. Since 1999 Gail has been the Tutor at the University of Surrey responsible for the postgraduate Diploma and Masters courses in Occupational Health Nursing.

Dr Nick Lewis

Dr Nick Lewis trained in general practice and internal medicine. He trained in occupational medicine at London Transport, becoming a Specialist Occupational Physician in 1988. Since then he has worked for the Civil Service and British Rail. He is co-founder and company secretary of Trident Medical Services, an independent occupational health provider specialising in ionising radiation, in which capacity he is also Chief Medical Officer of the Atomic Weapons Establishment.

Dr Graham Lucas MB FRCP FRCPsych FFOM RCP D(Obst) RCOG

Graham Lucas is an Occupational and Aviation Psychiatrist. His current affiliations include: Priory Healthcare; Foreign & Commonwealth Office; Emeritus Consultant Psychiatrist at the Maudsley Hospital; Medical Member, the Mental Health Review Tribunal; Second Opinion Appointed Doctor to the Mental Health Act Commission; Visiting Professor at the Postgraduate Medical School, University of Surrey.

Formerly: Adviser in Mental Health to the Health & Safety Executive; Chief Consultant Psychiatrist, Ex-Services Mental Welfare Society; Medical

Member of Appeals Service; Consultant to British Airways and Civil Aviation Authority.

He also served as Major and Senior Specialist in Psychiatry in the Royal Army Medical Corps. His particular areas of interest include: work-related stress, post-traumatic stress disorder, anxiety, depression, alcohol and drug abuse.

Lawrence Waterman MSc MBIOH ROH FIOSH RSP FRSA

Lawrence Waterman is Managing Director of Sypol, one of the UK's leading health, safety and environmental consultancies operating across Europe, the Middle East and Africa. He is a Fellow of the Institution of Occupational Safety and Health (FIOSH), a Registered Safety Practitioner, a Member of the British Institute of Occupational Hygienists (MBIOH) and a Registered Occupational Hygienist. He is a member of the Council of IOSH, Council of the Parliamentary and Scientific Committee, 'Securing Health Together' Programme Action Group and HSC CONIAC Occupational Health Working Party. Recipient (jointly) of the 1995 Institution of Civil Engineers' medal for Safety in Construction, he reported to the Health & Safety Executive on Occupational Health Support for the construction industry. Lawrence is Occupational Health Advisor to the Heathrow Terminal 5 project, and led a team of 15 staff in providing health and safety support to the Department for the Environment, Food and Rural Affairs (DEFRA) during the 2001 foot and mouth epidemic.

Acknowledgements

Chapter 2 – we are grateful to Maybo Limited, Conflict Management Specialists, for permission to reproduce their Violence Checklist; and to AstraZeneca for permission to reproduce their Pre-employment Medical Questionnaire.

Chapter 7 – thanks go to Ellen Chapman, Clinical Director, the Robens Centre for Occupational Health and Safety, for checking the text, and Mr GCE Sallit, who helped Dr Nick Lewis with his section on Ionising Radiation.

Peter Kelly of the Health & Safety Executive provided invaluable help with references.

1   What is Employee Health?

Introduction

1.1   Taken at face value, the term *employee health* simply means the health of people who work for an organisation. But what is health, why should we be interested in the health of employees and what are the consequences of not having regard for the health of the people we employ? This book covers all these issues and provides those who have responsibility for people at work with the information and practical guidance necessary to ensure that employee health is firmly on the agenda of the organisation.

Apart from the moral point of taking care of our friends and colleagues, there is a strong legal obligation in the UK to ensure the 'health, safety and welfare' of employees and there are sound economic reasons why employee health matters. The fundamental legal duty is enshrined in the *Health and Safety at Work etc Act 1974, s 2(1)*. The statutory duty under health and safety law mirrors the common law that applies to everyone: whether at work or not, every person has a common law duty of 'reasonable care'. This applies where the consequences of a negligent act or omission could foreseeably result in harm.

The *Health and Safety at Work etc Act 1974* is strengthened by specific regulations and other Acts of Parliament, which together form a formidable array of legal obligation with which the modern employer is expected to comply. Many of these relate to safety whilst at work, ie the physical safety of people at work and the avoidance of accidents and injury. However, this book also deals with the equally important issue of occupational health support, ie the maintenance of health and the avoidance of illness and disease.

Health or safety?

1.2   We have a Health and Safety at Work Act, we write health and safety policies and we appoint health and safety advisors. Whenever we refer to the processes involved in ensuring that people are not harmed by their work, we use the term 'health *and* safety' as though they were synonymous terms: but, in practice, they are often taken to mean just safety. The large majority of enterprises interpret the requirement for health and safety as though all that it required is to assess and manage safety risks. For a variety of reasons, many organisations have a good understanding of the safety issues arising in their business, but have very little insight into what might cause their employees to become ill.

Adverse health outcomes are more difficult to envisage because they require greater technical understanding of which factors in the workplace may cause people to become ill. Hazard identification for health risks is not as easy as for safety risks. Health is also a more difficult issue to address because it lacks the immediacy or predictability of a safety risk. Failure to adequately guard a machine can fairly easily be identified as posing a risk of injury from exposure to moving parts. The consequences of failure to prevent exposure to a chemical that might cause dermatitis, however, can be harder to foresee: firstly there has to be an understanding that a particular substance can sensitise people to dermatitis; and, secondly, there has to be a realisation that this period of sensitisation might take many years before an ill-health episode occurs. Occupational health risks, therefore, require some understanding of what causes harm, how that harm might arise, what levels of exposure could be harmful, and the time it might take for effects to surface.

Crucially, the health risk assessment also has to recognise that existing medical conditions may predispose some people to further adverse health effects. The person with a history of back pain is likely to be vulnerable to back injury in a job requiring lifting and carrying; employees with a history of stress-related illness are likely to have a recurrence if they are subjected to the kind of pressures of work that have made them ill in the past.

There are distinctions to be made, therefore, between the practice of *occupational health* and *safety*, but in many ways the two are closely interrelated. If someone is injured at work, the effect on his or her subsequent health turns a safety issue into a health outcome; any distinction is therefore largely academic. In those organisations that have two distinct departments – one dealing with occupational health, and the other with safety – it is important that the two work closely together. Where, as is often the case, there is a safety provision but no in-house occupational health expertise, it is essential that any brought-in occupational health advisor works closely with the organisation's safety department.

What is health?

1.3   *Health* is defined in the World Health Organisation's Constitution as a state of complete physical, mental and social wellbeing and not merely the absence of disease or infirmity.

Employee health extends this definition to people in employment and suggests that people should expect that their work does not contribute to any adverse impact on their state of health. According to the principles of the United Nations, World Health Organisation and the International Labour Organisation, every citizen of the world has a right to healthy and safe work and to a work environment that enables him or her to live a socially and economically productive life.

Occupational health has no agreed definition but is often regarded as the means by which employee health is assured. It refers to the practical application of a very wide range of disciplines, which individually or collectively are used to investigate the conditions that create risks to the health of people at work. These include conditions in the work environment (physical, chemical and biological hazards), conditions relating to the psychological and social impact of work (psychosocial hazards) and factors associated with the vulnerabilities of individuals. Occupational health support is provided by a range of professions including doctors, nurses, psychologists, counsellors, occupational hygienists, toxicologists, epidemiologists, engineers, ergonomists and physiotherapists.

Why does an organisation need occupational health support?

1.4   The reasons why an organisation should have regard for the health of their employees are several and compelling. Employees are essential for the smooth and profitable running of any organisation. Employees who are ill are either absent, or working within limitations and below their best. This can have a severe impact on the efficiency of the organisation. In the commercial world, this in turn can impact on profits; and in the service and public sectors, this can affect efficiency and performance. Sickness absence can be a significant cost to any organisation.

An employer who allows an employee to develop an illness related to their work can be expected to be held liable. This liability can be criminal or can be pursued through a civil claim for damages, or both. Relevant statue law is enforced in the UK by the Health & Safety Executive (HSE) or in some cases by local authority environmental health officers. Enforcement is not normally punitive and enforcement officers in the UK have a reputation for encouraging improvement in health and safety practice before invoking their powers of prosecution. Blatant disregard for the law, however, or failure to take action over improvement and enforcement notices will result in prosecution and the punishment can be severe. Summary conviction in a magistrates' court carries a maximum fine of £20,000, but conviction on indictment in a higher court can carry an unlimited fine and for some types of offence can result in imprisonment.

The cost to the convicted organisation may not be calculated just from the level of fine and associated legal costs, but also from the major impact on its reputation. The HSE now make public a register of prosecutions and since April 2001 has also published a database of enforcement notices (see http://www.hse-databases.co.uk/prosecutions/ and http://www.hse-databases.co.uk/notices).

Equally damaging financially, and to the organisation's reputation, is the possibility of a successful civil claim for damages for illness caused by the negligence of the employer. As Gillian Howard examines more thoroughly

3

in CHAPTER 2, the test for such claims is one of reasonable foreseeability. Would it have been reasonable for the employer to have known that the claimant had a predisposition to asthma, for example, or would it have been reasonable for the employer to have known that exposure to glutaraldehyde can sensitise a person to asthma? Generally, it is no defence to claim ignorance: it is the employer's duty to make sure they know the risks of exposure to physical, chemical, biological and psychosocial hazards to which their employees might be exposed. It is also the employer's duty to know if an employee is vulnerable to any particular hazard by asking the appropriate questions and having the appropriate medical opinion. Only if the employee wilfully withholds relevant information might the courts decide on contributory negligence.

Occupational health support provision

1.5   There is a considerable inequality in the provision of occupational health support in the UK. Large enterprises (defined as having more than 250 employees) will tend to have more access to occupational health support than smaller organisations. Even so, occupational health in the large enterprises is very fragmentary with some having no provision at all, others having a minimal service and just a few providing full occupational health support. Small and medium-sized enterprises (employing fewer than 250 employees) account for 99% of private sector businesses, but only a few will have more than a basic occupational health service and many will have no access at all to occupational health advice.

In terms of need, there is little difference between the larger organisations and the small and medium-sized enterprises: both have equal need to protect their workers' health and both sectors will suffer the same type of consequence if they fail to do so. A MORI research study cited by the Occupational Health Advisory Committee ('Report and Recommendations on Improving Access to Occupational Health Support', Occupational Health Advisory Committee, HSC, 2000) revealed that small and medium-sized enterprises have a low awareness of occupational health issues, focusing mainly on safety rather than health and rarely using outside expertise to help with occupational health issues.

The Government has recognised the need to improve access to occupational health support and has backed a number of initiatives. For example, its 'Revitalising Health and Safety Strategy Statement' (Department of the Environment, Transport and the Regions, June 2000) contains targets to reduce the number of working days lost from injury and ill-health by 30% before 2010 and to reduce the incidence of cases of work-related ill-health by 20% before 2010; half of these targets are to be achieved by 2004. Additionally, the HSE's long-term occupational health strategy ('Securing health together: a long-term occupational health strategy for England, Scotland and Wales', HSC, July 2000) reiterates these targets and provides suggested programmes of work to ensure the targets are met.

The interaction between work and home

1.6   Occupational health practice has always faced the complexities of distinguishing hazards that people experience at work from the hazards they experience outside of work. Adults spend a quarter of their time at work and the conditions there are very often unique, exposing employees to hazards such as vibration or chemicals which they are very unlikely to encounter in their domestic lives. In these cases, diseases or ill-health, which are specific to a workplace risk, can sometimes be identified. It would be quite appropriate to term these *occupational diseases*, but in very many cases it is just not that simple. The disease or ill-health could be caused by the work, by the activities outside of work or by a combination of both. Musculoskeletal injury, for example, could be caused by lifting at work, or it could be caused by a sports injury or by gardening. A small initial back strain, caused by playing rugby, could result in a debilitating back injury when lifting an otherwise quite safe load at work. Is this an occupational disorder or a non-work-related injury? Stress is another good example of where factors in the person's domestic life often add significantly to the factors at work to create a level of stress that becomes unbearable and results in stress-related illness.

Trying to distinguish between work-related causes and non-work causes is curiously both important and unimportant. It can be important if there is any risk of litigation. The organisation must know to what extent it has caused the employee's illness or how it might have contributed to it. It needs to know this to defend any litigation and it needs to know in order to take remedial action to prevent a similar occurrence in the future. In terms of the effects on employee health and any impact on the organisation, it matters little whether the illness was caused by work, caused outside of work or aggravated by work. The effect is the same, ie the employee is likely to suffer reduced performance at work and there will be cost implications. Occupational health support is often said to be concerned with *the effects of work on health and the effects of health on work*. Whilst this is a rather well-worn concept, it nonetheless encapsulates the purpose of occupational health support.

Assessment of hazards and risk

1.7   All of the above makes it essential that the employer understands the hazards to which people are exposed and knows how to undertake a risk assessment. Modern health and safety law centres on the principles of risk assessment and risk management with the express aim of anticipating harm before it arises and taking remedial steps to prevent accidents and ill-health.

In CHAPTER 10, Lawrence Waterman examines risk assessment and explains how it works in practice. A properly-conducted risk assessment has many positive benefits to the employee and to the organisation:

- it complies with the law;

- it anticipates what might cause harm and under what circumstances; and

- it allows the development of 'reasonably practicable' risk reduction solutions.

To ensure that the risk assessment approach actually reduces the risk of a work-related illness, however, it must be more than a paper exercise. The risks which become apparent from a risk assessment have to be addressed and action taken to eliminate them or, at the very least, reduce them to the lowest 'reasonably practicable' level. This means that judgements, and sometimes difficult decisions, have to be made about what needs to done, whether such remedial action is feasible and how much can be spent on it: the risk assessment process becomes a meaningless exercise unless the threats to people's health are effectively removed.

Organising occupational health support

1.8   Occupational health support has the dual objectives of protecting the employee from illness caused by work and protecting the organisation from the liability that might arise if an employee is made ill by work.

There is potential here for occupational health practitioners to have a conflict of interests. On the one hand they are working in the best interest of the employees in helping them to establish the cause of their work-related illnesses and to help them recover and return to full work. On the other hand, they are working on behalf of the organisation, to limit losses caused by work-related ill-health, including any losses which might arise from sickness absence or from civil litigation or criminal proceedings. Sometimes these two objectives do not sit comfortably together but there is no real reason why they should not. In setting up in-house occupational health support, or when buying-in expertise, managers should ensure that they pursue a *proactive* occupational health service. Being proactive means being fully involved in the risk assessment approach and identifying and reducing the risks to the health of employees before they cause harm. A proactive occupational health service is a preventive service and this works in the best interest of both the employer and the employee. Too often, occupational health practice is *reactive*, ie responding to problems after they have arisen and when the threat of legal action creates a polarisation of interests.

Most organisations will have a safety policy and, if there are five or more employees, there is a legal requirement for this under the *Health and Safety at Work etc Act 1974, s 2(3)*, which requires employers to have in writing a statement of their general policy in respect to the health and safety at work of their employees and what the arrangements are for carrying out this policy. As highlighted earlier, often this is interpreted as requiring a 'safety policy' and the aims, objectives and arrangements for ensuring *employee health* are frequently overlooked. Organisations should ensure that they have an integrated health *and* safety policy, or have a separate occupational health policy. In this, the organisation should seek to show that it has the necessary arrangements in place to ensure a proactive approach to occupational health support.

In CHAPTER 3, Olivia Carlton examines some of the day-to-day issues involved in the management of occupational health support; and in CHAPTER 4, Denis D'Auria discusses management systems and provides practical information on what procedures should be in place to ensure successful occupational health management.

Fitness for work

1.9   Employee health should be a matter of concern from the time before an employee starts work with the organisation up until the employee leaves or retires. It is sound policy to ensure that prospective candidates are fit for the job for which they are applying.

In this context, fitness does not usually mean physical fitness, although that may be a requirement in some physically demanding jobs. Fitness for work usually means the absence of significant medical conditions which would limit the ability to undertake the work, be made worse by the job or make doing the job unsafe. In some industries, and in some jobs, there may be legal reasons for a pre-placement medical assessment and in some industries, such as offshore work, there may be industry standards for medical fitness. In many other organisations, there may be a policy to screen job applicants for fitness for the job. Pre-placement health screening is imperfect but it serves to ensure that new starters do not have medical conditions that may put themselves, or others, at risk by virtue of the nature of the work they will be expected to undertake or the conditions in which they will work. It also serves the purpose, in some cases, of making sure that any protection needed for the worker, such as vaccinations, are up to date and that any baseline medical conditions are documented. The latter may be particularly necessary for any worker in an industry where, for example, occupational deafness, respiratory disease or vibration white finger is a known risk: it is important to document the extent of any such condition at the start of employment so that any progression of the disease can be monitored and any potential claim that it was caused by the present employment can be countered.

The results of a pre-employment medical assessment are confidential and the organisation's management and human resources department will normally only be told either that the candidate is fit, is fit with certain restrictions, or is unfit for the job. Declining a person for a job because of a medical condition can fall foul of disability discrimination law. Gillian Howard discusses such legal issues in CHAPTER 2.

Maintaining fitness for work

1.10   Fitness for work is not just an issue at recruitment, but should extend for the whole period of employment. Maintaining employee fitness for the job they do is one of the important functions of an occupational health service. Fitness for work may change when a person suffers a medical condition. This may be temporary, during influenza, for example, but it may be long-term or permanent from a whole host of conditions such as injury, heart disease or severe mental illness. Fitness can also change with a change in job. Fitness for one job does not necessarily mean fitness for an entirely different job, even within the same organisation.

The occupational health service should be both supportive to the individual and to the organisation in coming to terms with change in fitness for work during employment. Helping the organisation deal with long-term absence and frequent short-term absences is another important role of the occupational health service. The legal pitfalls associated with managing sickness absence are discussed in the CHAPTER 2.

In maintaining fitness for work, occupational health support has the important role of health education. Employees have a legal duty under the *Health and Safety at Work etc Act 1974* to look after their own health and safety but the employer has a duty under *section 2(2)(c)* to provide such information and training as is necessary to ensure the health and safety of employees. Making sure that employees understand the risks to their health, how to protect themselves from harm, what symptoms to look for and what to do if symptoms arise, is an essential part of risk management.

This book aims to demystify occupational health support and give managers the tools and confidence to include health issues in their assessment of health and safety. The intention is to put the 'health' into health and safety. It aims to show how managing health issues, from recruitment to retirement, are as important to the success of any organisation as managing its finances, and how protecting it's most valuable asset, its employees, is as important as protecting the quality of its products and services. The HSE slogan 'Good Health is Good Business' is more than a slick cliché. The message it conveys is significant. Healthy workers do make a positive contribution to the success, efficiency and productivity of the organisation.

2   Legal Overview

Introduction

2.1   The rights and obligations of employers and employees concerning health and safety at work is derived from four main sources:

- the common law (ie law arising from decided cases);

- statute law;

- the employment contract; and

- the European Union.

In addition, occupational health physicians and nurses are required to comply with guidance and rules of conduct issued by their own professional bodies, for instance:

- the General Medical Council's 'Guidance on Good Practice' (available at http://www.gmc-uk.org/standards/default.htm);

- the Faculty of Occupational Medicine's 'Guidance on Ethics for Occupations Health Physicians' (5th edition); and

- the Nursing and Midwifery Council (formerly the UKCC) 'Code of Professional Conduct' (2002) (available at http://www.nmc-uk. org/cms/content/Publications/Code of professional conduct.pdf).

Managing employees' health at work is a complex but interesting issue, which some employers manage extremely well and others not so well!

Employers may understand their general statutory duties under the *Health and Safety at Work etc Act 1974, s 2*, but there are now many regulations imposing very specific and detailed obligations on employers in specific cases. For example, recently an employer was found to be in breach of its statutory obligations to carry out a risk assessment when employing pregnant women (*Mrs J B Hardman v Miss M Mallon (t/a Orchard Lodge Nursing Home) [2002] IRLR 516*). The *Management of Health and Safety at Work Regulations 1999 (SI 1999/3242), Reg 16* requires a risk assessment to be carried out of for pregnant women and women breastfeeding. None was done in this case. Failure to carry out such a risk assessment was regarded by the Employment Appeal Tribunal as direct sex discrimination. It is probably uncommon for an employer to carry out a risk assessment in such circumstances but it is a legal requirement and one which is vital, if, following the pregnancy, the woman alleges that either her health or that of her baby has been harmed by activities in the workplace.

Statutory duties

2.2 Employers have clear statutory duties imposed by under numerous Acts of Parliament. This title cannot cover in detail all the statutory duties imposed on employers; and other chapters in this book will consider the legal duties associated with specific hazards. However, the main duties we are concerned with in this book can be found in the *Health and Safety at Work etc Act 1974, s 2*.

Section 2(1) requires employers to take 'reasonable care' in the workplace, as far as is reasonably practicable. The remainder of that section places specific statutory duties on employers in the following ways:

- to provide and maintain a safe system of work;
- to ensure the safe use and transportation and storage of materials and substances;
- to provide adequate information, instruction, training and supervision;
- to provide adequate maintenance of buildings and premises; and
- to provide a safe working environment.

Whilst these duties are primarily focused on the responsibility of the employer to care for its own employees, employers will also owe a duty to ensure that other people's employees are adequately instructed and, in rare cases, trained before they are permitted to work on the client-employer premises (*R v Swan Hunter Shipbuilders Ltd and Telemeter Installations Ltd [1981] IRLR 403*).

Other statutory duties include undertaking regular risk assessments (under *the Management of Health and Safety at Work Regulations 1999 (SI 1999/3242)*, *Reg 3*, and see CHAPTER 10) and reporting accidents and incidents at work under the *Reporting of Injuries, Diseases and Dangerous Occurrences Regulations 1995 (SI 1995/3163)*).

Reporting of Injuries, Diseases and Dangerous Occurrences Regulations 1995

2.3 Employers, the self-employed and those in control of work premises are required under the *Reporting of Injuries, Diseases and Dangerous Occurrences Regulations 1995 (RIDDOR) (SI 1995/3163)* to report some work-related accidents, diseases and dangerous occurrences. Reporting accidents and ill-health at work is a legal requirement. The information enables the Health & Safety Executive (HSE) and local authorities to identify where, and how, risks arise and to investigate serious accidents.

The following must be reported:

- death or major injury;

- an over-three-day injury (that is when an employee or self-employed person has an accident at work and is unable to work for over three days, but does not have a major injury);

- a work-related disease; and

- a dangerous occurrence (this is when something happens that does not actually result in a reportable injury, but which clearly could have done).

Definitions

2.4   *Major injuries* are defined as:

- any fracture, other than to the fingers, thumbs or toes;

- any amputation;

- dislocation of the shoulder, hip, knee or spine;

- loss of sight (whether temporary or permanent);

- any chemical or hot metal burn to the eye, or any other penetrating injury to the eye;

- any injury caused by an electric shock or electric burn leading to unconsciousness or requiring resuscitation or admission to hospital for more than 24 hours;

- any other injury resulting in hypothermia, heat-induced illness leading to unconsciousness, requiring resuscitation or admission to hospital for more than 24 hours;

- loss of consciousness caused by asphyxia or by exposure to a harmful substance or biological agent;

- either of the following conditions which result from absorption of any substance or inhalation, ingestion or through the skin:

  o acute illness requiring medical treatment; or

  o loss of consciousness;

- acute illness which requires medical treatment where there is reason to believe that this has resulted from exposure to a biological agent or its toxins or infected materials.

Injuries reportable in respect of *members of the public* are confined to deaths, or major injuries which cause a person to be taken from the site of the accident to hospital.

Dangerous occurrences are those listed in *RIDDOR, Sch 2.*

Minor injuries are those which cause a person to be incapacitated for more than three consecutive days, other than those falling within the definition of a major injury.

Industrially linked diseases are set out in *RIDDOR, Sch 3*. This schedule lists forms of illness in Column 1, with, opposite each of these, a list of occupations or work processes in Column 2. If an employee contracts a Column 1 disease while working in a Column 2 process, it is notifiable. These include working with asbestos, hepatitis contracted while working with human blood products or body secretions or excretions, bone cancers or blood diseases while working with ionising radiations and hand arm vibration syndrome, while using various hand held tools or percussive drills or holding material being worked on by pounding machines in shoe manufacturing. (The reader is recommended to obtain a copy of *RIDDOR* to have as reference for the complete list of reportable diseases.)

Reportable diseases

2.5   The presence of a reportable disease is rarely, if ever, immediately related to a specific incident at work and so the employer's usual systems to identify reportable incidents will not pick up reportable diseases. The employer needs to be aware if their employees undertake work which is likely to put them at risk of developing such illnesses, and where risk assessment demonstrates the risk is more than low then they should have a system for picking up these diagnoses, even if health surveillance is not appropriate. They are, of course, also required to educate their employees about the risk, and so one of the elements of a system to pick up the presence of these can be the requirement that employees report problems.

If an occupational health practitioner becomes aware that an employee who undertakes relevant work has a reportable disease, the employer should be informed providing that the employee gives his or her consent. The employer should also be made aware of their requirement to report this under *RIDDOR*. There is currently no requirement on the GP or the occupational health practitioner to report the disease directly to the Health & Safety Executive (HSE) or local authority. If the employee refuses to allow the employer to be told, the occupational health practitioner must respect his or her right to confidentiality. If others are likely to be at risk, then the occupational health practitioner must consider their responsibilities to alert the employer to the presence of the hazard without identifying the relevant employee.

A case of disease in an employee *must* be reported *only* if written diagnosis has been received from a doctor, for example, on a medical certificate. Thus a manager who is in receipt of a medical certificate from a doctor about a member of staff, needs to scrutinise the certificate to ensure that they he or she understands the nature of the illness, the diagnosis of which is being certified and whether or not it is reportable. Doctors have received material from the HSE, asking them to use common descriptions of each disease set out in *RIDDOR*, so that employers can more easily recognise when a report under *RIDDOR* is required: this advice to GPs, which may also be of interest to employers, may be found on the HSE website at http://www.hse.gov.uk/pubns/hse32.htm. If there is any doubt about interpreting an employee's given diagnosis, the certifying doctor should be consulted. The obligation lies with the self-employed in respect of themselves; and with the training body in respect of trainees, who are injured during placement.

Managers often confuse reporting of a case of disease with admission of liability. Reporting under *RIDDOR* does not signify that it has been caused by work. Completion of such a report signifies only that a case of disease has occurred in an individual working on this process. It is no admission of liability and cannot be used as such.

Method of notification

2.6   In order to notify the relevant enforcing authority of incidents and diseases, there are specific procedures in place, as follows:

- Major injuries, deaths and dangerous occurrences must be notified by telephone, (see below) and followed by a written report (on Form F2508) within ten days.

- Minor injuries and industrially linked diseases are to be notified (on Form F2508) within ten days of the occurrence. The forms can now be filled in electronically on-line (see below).

- A diagnosed disease (which complies with those listed in *RIDDOR, Sch* 3) must be reported using Form F2508A within ten days of the doctor making the diagnosis known to the employer.

Records must be kept as the authorities may ask for further information of notified matters; and all forms can now be filed electronically on-line (see below).

Failure to provide this reporting system (and make the required reports) can attract criminal sanctions from the Health & Safety Executive (HSE). If, however, an employer can prove that all reasonable steps have been taken to have reportable events brought to his notice, but that he was not aware of a specific event or disease in question, he will not be found guilty of any such offence. For this reason, a robust reporting system is essential (see CHAPTER 4).

Reporting under *RIDDOR* may be completed in a number of ways. In addition to making reports to the local enforcing authority, the HSE has set up an Incident Contact Centre to which reports can be submitted. Consult the Incident Contact Centre website at http://www.riddor.gov.uk/. This site not only provides all the guidance and help you need in deciding if an incident or disease needs to be reported but the necessary forms are also there and can be filled in electronically. Alternatively you can download Form F2508 (for accidents and dangerous occurrences) or Form F2508A (for notifiable diseases) and these can be filled in manually and returned by post to:

The Incident Contact Centre
Caerphilly Business Park
Caerphilly
CF83 3GG.

You can also return the forms by fax to 0845 3009924. Where the incident needs to be reported verbally in the first instance, the telephone number is 0845 3009923.

There may be circumstances when it would be inappropriate to disclose information about an employee's condition or to pass it on to his or her employer. The reporting system introduced by *RIDDOR* contains nothing to alter this aspect of the normal ethical considerations of the doctor-patient relationship. However, in such circumstances the GP, with the patient's agreement, might be prepared to pass information to another practitioner either in an occupational health service (where one exists at the employee's place of work) or direct to HSE's Employment Medical Advisory Service.

Corporate manslaughter

2.7   In recent years there has been considerable government and media interest in the potential for introducing a new statutory offence of corporate manslaughter, to be introduced under the criminal law when deaths have occurred where the 'directing mind' (ie the directors of a company) have either known of the dangers or have closed their minds to the risks. Recent examples where such issues have been raised are the fatal accidents in the Clapham rail crash, the Piper Alpha oil platform explosion, the King's Cross fire and the 'Herald of Free Enterprise' ferry sinking.

The common law courts, however, have already considered this matter. In *A-G's Reference (No 2 of 1999) [2000] 2 Cr App R 207, [2000] 3 All ER 182*, following the Southall rail crash, a prosecution for corporate manslaughter and offences under the *Health and Safety at Work etc Act 1974* was brought against Great Western Trains. At trial, the train company was straightforwardly convicted for an offence under the Act.

The issue for that offence was simply one of determining whether, in the light of the facts revealed in investigations, the company had done all that was reasonably practicable to ensure the safety of passengers. The safety deficiencies revealed by the investigation disclosed that it had not. By contrast, the company was acquitted of corporate manslaughter after Scott Baker J ruled that liability for manslaughter could only be imposed on the company under the *principle of identification*. It was this ruling which came under the scrutiny of the Court of Appeal following a reference by the Attorney General.

The Court of Appeal affirmed that companies can be liable for the offence of manslaughter. In the context of this case, liability against the company required proof of grossly negligent corporate acts or omissions that caused the death of passengers. But how was *corporate* gross negligence to be established?

Rose LJ endorsed the trial judge's ruling that such a finding could only be made for this common law offence by satisfying the conditions of the identification doctrine. Accordingly, the negligence had to comprise acts or omissions perpetrated by corporate officers sufficiently senior to be identified with the company, ie persons whose conduct was the conduct of the company itself.

Recruitment

2.8   There is a clear duty at common law for employers to ensure that the job applicant is fit for the job in order to protect the applicant's health and safety and that of others. Carrying out an adequate pre-employment medical assessment will go a long way to ensure that this duty has been satisfied.

Pre-employment assessments

2.9   Many employers carry out some form of pre-employment medical assessment ranging from the use of medical questionnaires to full medical examinations by occupational health physicians or other doctors. Clearly the circumstances of the post and the potential post-holder will determine whether full medical examinations are required. In some cases the law will require them eg airline pilots under the Civil Aviation Authority rules, deep sea divers, etc and in other cases more detailed tests will be required, such as in employments where the employer has a drug or alcohol policy. What is important is that relevant questions are asked at pre-employment and that the answers are properly understood and the information obtained is processed lawfully.

Some employers may be advised by the occupational health physician to obtain the consent of the job applicant to seek disclosure of past medical records from the GP. This may be necessary where, for example, there is a declared medical condition which may have a serious impact on health and safety. In such a case the employer should seek the *informed written consent* for this procedure from the employee (see 2.23), ideally via its occupational health physician or occupational health nurse, and explain why in the particular case it is relevant. In *Surrey Police v Marshall (2002) EAT/774/01* such a procedure was followed where a job applicant for a very sensitive and responsible job, Fingerprint Recognition Officer, disclosed that she had bipolar affective disorder (manic depression).

In certain professions, such as for those working in the NHS and those in public transport, there are additional and higher duties on employment in relation to recruitment and that is the duty to safeguard members of the public.

The Clothier Report, ('The Allitt Inquiry: Independent Inquiry Relating to Deaths and Injuries on the Children's Ward at Grantham & Kestevern General Hospital', HMSO, 1994) examined the events surrounding the deaths and injuries caused by Beverley Allitt, a nurse at Grantham and Kestevan General Hospital. The Report put forward recommendations for the screening of people entering the nursing profession. The Report recommended that reasonable grounds for screening out applicants would include:

> 'excessive absence through sickness, excessive use of counselling or medical facilities, or self harm behaviour such as attempted suicide, self-laceration or eating disorder'.

The Report went on:

> 'Applicants should not be accepted for training until they have shown the ability to live an independent life without professional support and have been in employment for at least two years.'

The use of carefully designed medical questionnaires is essential in ensuring that good practice and compliance with the law is ensured. Astra Zeneca has kindly given their permission for an example of an excellent Pre-employment Medical Questionnaire to be published in this chapter (see pages 17–20 below). There is, of course, a need for each individual employer to tailor its own pre-employment medical questionnaire to suit the needs of the business, with its own organisation, products and risks in mind. For example, where the worker would work with known allergenic risks or with food or sterile products, additional health checks will be necessary and in some cases *required* by regulations.

Data protection

2.10   Under the *Data Protection Act 1998*, employers are required to obtain the employee's express written consent to obtain, process and disclose any sensitive data, which includes medical data (*section 2(e)* refers to any information relating to his physical or mental health or condition). There is a Data Protection Code of Practice which employers are required to follow. Part 1 concerns Recruitment and Selection. There is a section (at p 75 of the Code) concerning freely given consent. It states that the job applicant must be told clearly what information is being requested and what use will be

AstraZeneca

HEALTH QUESTIONNAIRE FOR JOB APPLICANTS

Part A – to be completed by HR or Recruiting Manager
Part B – Instructions for applicant

Check that the details in Part A above are correct.
Complete part C and D of the questionnaire on the following pages. Leave the rest of the form blank. The information given will be used by Occupational Health to decide whether a medical examination will be necessary before your offer of employment can be finalised.

Recruiting Manager Ext. No:		HR Officer Ext. No:	
Applicants Full Name		Maiden name	
Title	Male / Female	D.o.B.	
Address		Contact Telephone No.	
		Start date	
Proposed job			
Business / Department		Location	

Any requirements for regular health surveillance or occupational fitness assessment – please tick appropriate box

☐ Permanent position	☐ International Travel
☐ Temporary position	☐ Ionising radiation
☐ Work with pharmaceutical products in aseptic/sterile/clean areas	☐ Pharmaceutically active substances (e.g. agonists; steroids)
☐ Laboratory animals	☐ Respiratory Sensitisers
☐ Human tissue/Body fluids including waste	☐ Food handling
☐ Genetically Modified Organisms	☐ Driving on company business
☐ Use of Respiratory protection – BA	☐ Driving fork lift truck
☐ Noise >85Db	☐ Small print
☐ Skin irritants/Sensitisers	☐ Colour coding
☐ First Aid duties	☐ Other (please specify)**
☐ Working on regular nights between 22:00 and 06:00	☐ None of the above apply
**	

Part C – to be completed in full by applicant

1. If you have had a medical examination with this company before, when was it and where?
   Date: Place:

2. Sign and date the declaration.

3. **To ensure medical confidentiality, please return the questionnaire to Occupational Health in an envelope marked** *"Personal & Confidential"*

17

HEALTH QUESTIONNAIRE FOR JOB APPLICANTS

Details of GP
GP Name:
Address:
Telephone:

CONFIDENTIAL medical information on this form will remain confidential to the Occupational Health Service and will be held securely within the department. Human Resources and your Manager will be informed of your suitability for the job specified but no confidential medical information will be released without your informed consent. The purpose of this questionnaire is to allow the Company to fulfil their duty of care if you have any medical or health problems only. You can have access to your medical records held at any time.

OCCUPATIONAL HISTORY / PAST EMPLOYMENT

It is important to provide information if you have ever worked with or been in contact with any health hazards e.g. asbestos, dust, fumes, chemicals, pharmaceutical agents, and biological or physical hazards such as bacteria, viruses, genetically modified organisms and noise, lasers, radiation or laboratory animals.

Employers Name & Address	Dates from-to	Nature of your job and any significant health hazards

GENERAL MEDICAL HISTORY

Part D - To be completed in full by applicant

MEDICAL INFORMATION WILL REMAIN CONFIDENTIAL TO THE OCCUPATIONAL HEALTH SERVICE UNLESS OTHERWISE AGREED BY YOU

1. Do you or have you ever suffered from any of the following?
   Please tick if yes and give details of dates, severity, etc. in the space provided below.

		Fits, epilepsy, dizziness, vertigo, fainting, blackouts	☐
Depression, anxiety or 'nerves'	☐	Eczema, dermatitis or other skin condition	☐
Other Mental or Psychological Disorder (e.g. Phobias, Eating Disorders such as Anorexia/Bulimia etc.	☐	Kidney, bladder or urinary problems	☐
Eye/vision problems	☐	Heart trouble, high blood pressure, palpitations, angina, coronary thrombosis, rheumatic fever	☐
Ears or hearing problems	☐	Stomach or bowel trouble, persistent diarrhoea, ulcer, frequent indigestion, Crohns disease, colitis	☐
Allergies of any type, rhinitis, hayfever	☐	Any chronic virus infection, hepatitis jaundice	☐
Asthma, bronchitis, repeated infections, shortness of breath or lung disease	☐	Have you had any abnormal blood or other medical tests?	☐
Migraines or frequent headaches	☐	Have you been away from work or study due to ill health or injury during the last 2 years	☐
Diabetes or other endocrine (glandular) disorder (Thyroid, Adrenal etc.)	☐	Do you have or have had any permanent, recurring or persistent illness or disability of any type?	☐
Back, neck, shoulder, arm, hand, muscle or joint problems	☐	Are you regularly taking or using medication of any type	☐
Have you ever stayed in hospital or been to hospital or clinic as an out-patient, to casualty/emergency room or been sent for medical tests or other investigations?	☐	Is there anything else about your past or present health which you think Occupational Health ought to be aware of?	☐

Details:

_____

_____

_____

Have you ever smoked for as long as a year	☐ YES	☐ NO	If yes how much do you or did you smoke?
If an ex smoker when did you last stop?			
Alcohol How many drinks do you have in a week on average? (One drink is <u>half</u> a pint of beer, a glass of wine or a single short)			

MEDICAL INFORMATION WILL REMAIN CONFIDENTIAL TO THE OCCUPATIONAL HEALTH SERVICE UNLESS OTHERWISE AGREED BY YOU

Do you wear glasses or contact lenses?	☐ YES	☐ NO
Are you colour blind?	☐ YES	☐ NO
What is your height?		
What is your weight?		

Please give details of immunisations as below:

Immunisation	Dates Received
Hepatitis B	
Tetanus	
Other (Please specify)	

Please now sign the declaration below, and return to OCCUPATIONAL HEALTH marked "Personal & Confidential".

Declaration

I confirm that the information I have given on this form and questionnaire is true to the best of my knowledge.

Signed:	Dated:

FOR OCCUPATIONAL HEALTH SERVICE ONLY

Assessment and Action:

☐ Fit for proposed employment based on questionnaire alone

☐ Fit for proposed employment. Medical examination completed and satisfactory

☐ Referred to ....for opinion

☐ He/she should avoid..
A review is recommended in ....months

☐ Other remarks/advice regarding suitability and any accommodation.

Signed:_____ Date_____

Name:_____
(Block capitals)

made of it and a signature giving consent should be obtained. Other matters such as what is meant by 'consent freely given' is also explained. This can be obtained from visiting the website at http://www. dataprotection.gov.uk/dpr/dpdoc.nsf.

Part 4, still to be published, covers medical information.

Disability Discrimination Act 1995

2.11 Employers must now also be careful not to breach their obligations under the *Disability Discrimination Act 1995*. This requires employers not to discriminate against a person for any reason relating to their disability. 'Disability' is defined as a physical or mental impairment, lasting or likely to last for twelve months or more and which has a substantial and adverse effect upon one of the normal day day-to to-day activities defined in *Sch 1 para 4*.

If a job applicant has a disability then the employer is required to make reasonable adjustments to the workplace in order to accommodate that person and only if there is no reasonable adjustment that can be made and the employer can justify excluding that job candidate because of the disability or a reason relating to it, will the employer's duty be satisfied.

For further discussion of the *Disability Discrimination Act 1995*, see 2.31 *et seq*.

Pre-employment warnings

2.12 There is a common law duty on employers to warn prospective employees (and existing employees) of any potential risks to their health so that they can make an informed choice as to whether they wish to take up the employment. Such warnings should be in writing, setting out clearly what the risks are, what health effects there may be, what the employee should do if they have any health concerns and what measures the employer is taking to prevent or reduce those risks. (For an interesting discussion on some of these issues see *Mountenay v Bernard Mathews plc (1994) 5 Med LR 293*.)

Negligence

2.13 Failure to carry out a careful and thorough recruitment procedure could lead to claims for negligence from anyone who thereafter, and as a result of the negligent recruitment, suffers any loss through either physical harm or financial loss; and this could include loss as a result of a criminal act of another employee as well as a negligent (ie civil) act (*Nahhas v Pier House (Cheyne Walk) Management Ltd and Another, The Times, 10 February 1984*).

Lying

2.14   If a prospective job candidate lies about his health, then this can potentially give the employer a fair reason for dismissal, even after one year's successful employment. Whether the Employment Tribunal finds that such a lie justified dismissal will depend on the lie. Not disclosing medical information which is not asked for is not deemed to be a breach by the potential candidate and, therefore, would not justify dismissal if this omission was discovered at a later date (*O'Brien v The Prudential Assurance Co Ltd [1979] IRLR 140* and *Walton v TAC Construction Materials Ltd [1987] IRLR 351*).

It should be noted that various Employment Tribunals have taken the view that failing to offer up medical information (as opposed to deliberately concealing or lying about it) does not constitute any failure on the part of the job applicant to disclose relevant medical information. As it was put in the *Walton* case:

'Although there was no need for the purposes of this appeal to decide whether the appellant should have disclosed his addiction when applying for employment, it could not be said that there is any duty on the employee in the ordinary case, though there may be exceptions, to volunteer information about himself otherwise than in response to a direct question.'

Managing short-term absence

2.15   The case law has laid down clear guidelines for employers to dealing with persistent, short-term absence cases where the symptoms are transient, where there is no underlying medical condition and where the absences are frequent. In this scenario, there is no question about the genuineness of the symptoms: it is the number of absences, the unreliability of the employee and the commercial disruption to the employer's business that are the issues. Some employers have referred to such individuals as 'the walking virus'.

Identifying the problem

2.16   'Short-term' absence is defined in the Employee Absence Survey 2002, published by the Chartered Institute of Personnel Development (CIPD), as absences of five days per year or less. Medium-term absence is defined as absences of five days to four weeks, and long-term absence as anything over four weeks in a year.

Hence, it will be important for employers to have their own absence control management procedures in place for monitoring and managing absences problems: they should keep clear records, noting the reasons given for the absences on self-certification forms. Any employee with a worrying number of spells or days off for unrelated reasons (say four spells, each of ten days, in any twelve-month period) should be counselled by his or her supervisor in a private interview, asked for the reasons and, if necessary with their consent, their doctor may be asked to confirm whether there is an underlying reason for the absences. A model consent form is provided at 2.23.

Guidance

2.17   The Employment Tribunals have given helpful guidance on how to deal with short-term, persistent absence with unrelated symptoms and no underlying medical problem. In *International Sports Co Ltd v Thomson [1980] IRLR 340, Walpole v Rolls Royce Ltd [1980] IRLR 343* and *Lynock v Cereal Packaging Ltd [1988] IRLR 510*, employers were advised to:

- review the attendance record and investigate/seek reasons for the non-attendance;

- give warnings to the individual that their attendance must improve and the consequences if it does not; and

- hold a disciplinary hearing and consider what would be an appropriate penalty and then provide the opportunity to appeal.

A suggested action plan for supervisors is provided at 2.28.

If there is no underlying medical explanation for the absences, the employee should be warned or cautioned that, with the best will in the world, if attendance does not improve, the employee will lose his or her job as the employer is entitled to say 'enough is enough'.

The Employment Tribunals have not set a tariff of unacceptable absences. It is for the employer to determine when absence from work, even for genuine symptoms eg cold, 'flu, headaches, etc has become so commercially disruptive that they are entitled to say 'enough enough is enough'.

Dismissal

2.18   A subsequent dismissal would fall under the *Employment Rights Act 1996, s 98(1)(b)* namely 'some other substantial reason' – one of the five potentially fair reasons for dismissal.

The position has been clarified by the Employment Appeal Tribunal (EAT) in *Lynock v Cereal Packaging Ltd [1988] IRLR 510*, which held:

'What is important is that employers should treat each case individually where there is genuine illness with sympathy, understanding and compassion. The jargon of industrial relations in terms of warnings is not really the purpose of the system operated by the employer; it is to give a caution that the stage has been reached where with the best will in the world, it has become impossible to continue with the employment.'

On the issue of obtaining medical evidence, the same tribunal stated:

'Where one is dealing with intermittent periods of illness each of one is unconnected, it seems to us to be impossible to give a reasonable prognosis or projection of the possibility of what will happen in the future. Whilst an employer may make enquiries, it is in no way, in a situation such as the present, an obligation on the employer to do so because the results may produce nothing of assistance to him' ...

In *International Sports Co Ltd v Thomson [1980] IRLR 340* and *Walpole v Rolls Royce Ltd [1980] IRLR 343*, the EAT said:

'Where an employee has an unacceptable level of intermittent absences due to minor ailments, what is required is firstly that there should be a fairer view by the employer of the attendance record and the reasons for it; and secondly, the appropriate warnings after the employee has been given an opportunity to make representations. If there is then no adequate improvement in the attendance record, in most cases the employer will be justified in treating the persistent absences as a sufficient reason for dismissing the employee ... It will be placing too heavy a burden on an employer to require an employer to carry out a full medical investigation. Even if he did, such an investigation would rarely be fruitful because of the transient nature of the employee's symptoms and complaints.'

Finally, where an improvement *has* been made by the employee in attending work but that improvement is not 100%, it is appropriate for the employer to extend a final written warning and give the employee a further opportunity to attend work on a regular basis.

Managing long-term or acute sickness absence

Guidance

2.19   The Employment Tribunals have given useful guidance on how employers should deal with either acute and serious illness or long-term absence. Such cases are *East Lindsay District Council v Daubney [1977] IRLR 188* and *Spencer v Paragon Wallpapers [1976] IRLR 376*.

There are three main steps the employer *must* take:

* discover the true medical position by obtaining an up-to to-date medical report from the employee's GP or consultant (see 2.23);

- consult the employee or a member of his or her family to discuss the contents of that medical report and to ascertain from the employee their likelihood of return to work and preferred job and rehabilitation; and

- before taking any decision to dismiss, consider any suitable alternative employment including making reasonable adjustments to his or her original job or offering other duties such as 'light duties', either on a temporary or permanent basis.

A model letter of enquiry to the GP or consultant for these purposes is provided at 2.23.

Dismissal

2.20   Here any dismissal would fall under the heading of 'capability', as defined by the *Employment Rights Act 1996, s 98(2)(a)*, ie:

'the capability or qualifications of the employee for performing work of the kind which he was employed by the employer to do'.

Section 98(3) defines capability and qualifications in the following way:

- 'capability', in relation to an employee, means his capability assessed by reference to skill, aptitude, health or any other physical or mental quality; and

- 'qualifications', in relation to an employee, means any degree, diploma or other academic, technical or professional qualification relevant to the position which he held.

The timing of any dismissal will depend on many factors including the prognosis of the doctor, the length of service of the employee, the criticality of the job and needing to fill his or her position with a permanent replacement, whether sick pay has run out, etc.

Conflicting medical evidence

2.21   In the majority of cases, where a GP's prognosis that the employee is still unfit for work and the occupational health physician's assessment upon examining the employee is that they are fit for some duties, employers are entitled to rely upon their occupational health physician's assessment and should try to persuade the employee to be signed fit for some duties and/or light duties so that they can start the rehabilitation process.

Of course, this assumes that the employer will have recruited, or be contracted to use, a suitably experienced and qualified occupational health professional (see CHAPTER 4). Where this is not the case and where a doctor who is not an accredited specialist is acting in the capacity of a company advisor, the courts and Employment Tribunals will not regard that doctor as an expert; and indeed, they have on occasion criticised such doctors and their advice. This has become a particular issue now since the introduction of the *Disability Discrimination Act 1995*. In *Holmes v Whittington & Porter Ltd (unreported)* the Employment Tribunal held that the employers unlawfully discriminated against the Applicant when they were advised that no reasonable adjustments could be made for an employee who suffered petit mal attacks of epilepsy, because:

> 'that decision was made without knowing the full picture because it did not have sufficient information upon which to make those sorts of decisions in the absence of *specialist and the best medical advice*. It is not true to say that it is an enormous imposition on the employer, it just means the requirements of this Act are different from what has been required of employers before and that they just have to take more steps so that employees who are disabled persons are protected.'

For further discussion of the *Disability Discrimination Act 1995*, see 2.31 *et seq*.

Guidance for GPs

2.22   Some welcome advice to GPs about what action to take when signing employees off sick or unable to attend work, is available under the heading 'A Guide to Registered General Practitioners – Advice to patients regarding fitness for work' from the Department for Work and Pensions, part of which is reproduced below:

> 'Medical statements record the advice which you give to patients regarding the need to refrain from their usual occupation. Such advice is an everyday part of the management of clinical problems and you should always consider carefully whether advice to refrain from work represents the most appropriate clinical management. Doctors can often best help a patient of working age by taking action which will encourage and support work retention and rehabilitation.
>
> When providing advice to a patient about fitness for work you may wish to consider the following factors:
>
> • the nature of the patients medical condition and how long the condition is expected to last;
>
> • the functional limitations which result from the patients condition, particularly in relation to the type of tasks they actually perform at work;
>
> • any reasonable adjustments which might enable the patient to continue working – in relation to the workplace it is worth noting that

under the *Disability Discrimination Act 1995* an employer may be required to make reasonable adjustments for an employee with a long-term disability;

• any appropriate clinical guidelines – for example the Royal College of General Practitioners has produced clinical guidelines on the management of acute low back pain;

• clinical management of the condition which is in the patients best interest regarding work fitness;

As a certifying doctor you will also need to consider and manage your patient's expectations in relation to their ability to continue working.

In summary, you should always bear in mind that a patient may not be well served in the longer term by medical advice to refrain from work, if more appropriate clinical management would allow them to stay in work or return to work.' (Emphasis added.)

Consent

2.23   Any request for a medical report to a GP or consultant must be accompanied by the employee's *informed written consent* for disclosure of those medical details.

The need for 'informed' consent is crucial. Informed consent means that the patient has understood what has been told to him or her and in particular has understood any risks and benefits and has agreed to accept those risks. (There is a very useful discussion of informed consent in the Bristol Royal Infirmary's Inquiry Paper on Informed Consent, published in December 1999: see their website http://www.bristol-inquiry.org.uk/final_report/annex_b/images/CH_InformedConsent.pdf.)

See pages 28 and 29 for examples of model consent forms.

Dealing with 'malingerers'

2.24   There are two distinct categories of 'malingerers', ie the *lazy malingerer* and the *fraudulent malingerer*, and both can be dealt with under the employer's disciplinary procedure.

The fraudulent malingerer requires strong and clear management. The employer should begin investigations by obtaining the evidence, perhaps by use of covert video surveillance, and should then seek expert medical opinion as to whether the individual who has complained of a particular medical condition would be able to conduct himself as suspected or witnessed on the video.

Figure 1: Sample consent form 1

Authorisation form to GP

[To name of GP]

[Address]

[Date]

I authorise you to write a report on my current medical conditions and when I should be fit to return to some form of work and to release copies of all my medical records (including my consultant's reports and letters) relevant to my current medical conditions of stress and anxiety and my gynaecological condition(s) to Dr [A], the company's occupational physician, at [name of company].

I understand that these records will be kept strictly confidential and will be used by Dr [A] only for the purposes of making a prognosis and return to work recommendation and the litigation that I am currently bringing against [ABC Ltd].

SIGNED.. DATED....................

PRINT NAME ....

The lazy malingerer, however, has no dishonest intent nor is his or her conduct normally premeditated. With good management and motivation, therefore, it should be possible to persuade the lazy malingerer to attend work on a regular basis. The issues of management and motivation are outside the scope of this book, however.

Including materials in the staff manual

2.25 In order to pre-empt would-be malingerers, employers may wish to publish some guidance as to what an employee is *not* expected to be doing whilst off work in order to deal with some matters that may cause suspicion.

Covert surveillance

2.26 Covert surveillance, for example the use of private detectives or hidden cameras, should only be used where it is absolutely necessary and where the employer has a legitimate reason for doing so, eg to prevent or detect crime. Some useful guidance has been published, as follows:

Figure 2: Sample consent form 2

Authorisation form to company's occupational physician

[To Dr A, Occupational Physician to ABC Ltd]

[Address]

[Date]

I agree to undergo a medical examination by you and authorise you to provide a medical report on my psychiatric and mental health condition, your prognosis and when you assess that I will be fit to return to any form of employment with [ABC Ltd].

I understand you will be assessing my mental health condition in relation to my ability to return to work and what work and terms and conditions including hours and duties I will be fit for upon return to work and thereafter.

I understand that I have a right of access to this report before or after the report is prepared by you. I require a copy of the report before/after* it is sent to [ABC Ltd].

* Please delete as appropriate

I understand that this report will be kept strictly confidential and will be used only for the purposes of assessing my return to work and for the purposes of the litigation that I am currently bringing against [ABC Ltd] namely disability discrimination on the grounds of my syndrome and the stress that I say has been caused by my treatment by my employers.

The reasons for a medical assessment/examination have been fully explained to me.

SIGNED.. DATED....................

PRINT NAME..

- the draft Code of Practice, Part 3 on 'Monitoring at Work', under the *Data Protection Act 1998*, published by the Information Commissioner (see the website at http://www.dataprotection.gov.uk/dpr/dpdoc.nsf);

- the 'Use of CCTV' published by the Information Commissioner (www.dataprotection.gov.uk); and

- guidance from OFTEL on telephone surveillance 'Guidance on recording of telephone conversations' (Ref: 47/99, Date: 19 August 1999).

The use of private detectives and hidden cameras are now regulated by the *Regulation of Investigatory Powers Act 2000* and the *Telecommunications (Lawful Business Practice) (Interception of Communications) Regulations 2000 (SI 2000/2699).*

Figure 3: Sample sickness guidance

[issue on headed notepaper]

[Date]

Dear members of staff

Ref: Clarification of the sick pay scheme and sickness absence procedure

The Company operates its sickness absence and sick pay scheme on the Company and co-operation of its staff. For the vast majority of cases it works well. From time to time, however, cases are brought to light which cause the Company grave concern, as it appears that there may be serious abuse of the sick pay scheme.

In order to remind you, clarify and help you understand what is expected of you when or if you are off work, sick, and to understand what might raise doubts or queries in the mind of your Manager/Personnel Director concerning certain events and activities taking place during periods of sickness absence, the Company has drawn up some guidelines to all members of staff.

These guidelines form part of the Company's sick pay and absence authorisation procedure and thus form part of your terms and conditions of employment. It is therefore essential that you read and fully understand the following guidelines, since failure to follow the guidelines as set out below may lead to the non-payment of or the cessation of sick pay or recoupment from your future salary etc of any sick pay already paid in circumstances as described below.

Conduct during sickness absence

1   Authorisation for absence due to your own personal, genuine illness or injury is only made when that illness or injury prevents you from doing the work which you are employed to do. Paid sick leave cannot be granted for the illness of another member of the family or in cases where you need some time off for personal reasons. In these cases you are expected to ask for permission in advance, so

that alternative cover may be arranged. Such leave may be unpaid or may be taken out of annual leave.

2   In all cases of absence due to sickness or injury which necessitates taking time off work, it is expected that you will do your utmost to facilitate a speedy return to fitness and to work. In this regard, you are expected to act sensibly and honestly during the time that you are off work and to do nothing which is likely to aggravate your illness or injury or delay your recovery.

3   The Company therefore does not permit you to:

o   participate in any sports, hobbies or social or any other activities, attend and participate in religious or other meetings since these activities could aggravate the illness or injury or which could delay recovery. The exception to this rule would be where your doctor has prescribed exercise for you or where you have been granted prior written permission by your Manager to attend a meeting during your sick leave.

We expect you to be sensible. A gentle stroll to the local pub for a drink near the end of any period of sickness absence is acceptable. Going to the pub during the day or for the major part of the evening or most days/evenings will cause the Company to investigate the matter under the terms of its disciplinary procedure;

o   undertake *any other employment* whether paid or unpaid. If you declare yourself incapacitated from work in relation to your employment with the Company, it is deemed to be gross misconduct to undertake any other duties whilst off sick. Clearly the Company is your primary employer and if you are fit for any work activity at all, the Company expects you to report to work so that suitable work can be arranged should you not be fully fit for your normal duties;

o   engage in any work around the home or for a friend/third party in (engage in any work around the home or for a friend/third party in terms of home improvements, working on a car, etc. The Company expects you to seek to get better and recover from your illness or injury and will regard any such activity as gross misconduct warranting summary dismissal in an appropriate case;

o   engage in any activity which is inconsistent with the nature of your alleged illness or injuries (eg be seen walking round town with bags of shopping with an alleged injury);

NB: Where a depressive illness, anxiety, nerves or stress is involved, the Company will not pay any sick pay and reserves

(cont'd)

the right to deduct from future salary any sick pay already paid in circumstances where you are or have been involved in social activities such as singing in a band, competing in competitions, running another business, etc.

If you wish to become involved in any of these activities or any other activity, then you must clear this first in advance with the Personnel Director. He or she will then decide whether to grant you permission and whether sick pay should continue;

o take any holiday whether pre-booked or ad hoc during any period of sick leave except where this is authorised in writing by your doctor as convalescent leave after an operation.

This list is not exhaustive but merely contains examples of the kind of activities which the Company draws to your attention.

Finally I would like to thank you for your co-operation in making sure that our rules and sick pay scheme work well so that those who are genuinely in need of time off with pay receive just that.

The substance of this letter is incorporated into the Company's sick pay scheme.

Yours

[Director]

Other rules about sick leave

• Holidays/days of leave during periods of sickness absence

If you are off work due to illness or injury, whether this period is covered by a medical statement from your doctor, self-certification or otherwise, you are not expected to take any day(s) of leave whether pre-booked or not during your sick leave. If you should wish to honour any leave pre-booked or take (a) day(s) leave, you may do so only once this is approved by your Manager prior to the leave being taken. Please note that your Manager may at his or her discretion deem this day/these days as ordinary leave and as such sick pay will be suspended and days of normal leave taken (at the rate of pay paid for holiday leave).

Any employee who takes any such days, whether this be holiday or attending conferences, meetings, sports or leisure activities and the like, without prior authorisation, will be deemed to have breached the rules of this Company and as such will become liable to disciplinary action. This may include but not be limited to the suspension of sick pay for all or part of the sickness absence, suspension without pay as a disciplinary measure and a formal written warning. In any serious case, the Company may deem this to be an offence of gross misconduct which may result in summary dismissal.

Normally any holidays or attendance at any outside activity or location during sick leave will only be authorised as still counting as sick leave if it is convalescent leave specifically authorised in writing by your own doctor.

Status of self-certificates and medical certificates

Evidence of illness or injury

- Self-certification (for seven calendar days or less)

  Should your absence last less than seven calendar days (counting Saturday and Sunday) you will be required to report to your Manager immediately you return to duty and complete a self-certification form. The reasons given by you for your absence must satisfy your Manager before they will authorise your absence and counter-sign the self-certification form. Should your Manager have any doubts about the reasons given by you or for any other reason, they may not counter-sign the self-certification form. This may result in either non-payment of sick pay or a delay in payment until a Manager has reviewed your case. Until your self-certification form is counter-signed by a Manager no sick pay can be authorised.

  In such a case, the position will be discussed with you, first in the context of an informal counselling interview. Depending on the outcome of that meeting, you may be formally warned should the circumstances warrant it.

  When your self-certificate has been counter-signed by your Manager, it will then be forwarded to Payroll and Human Resources.

- Medical certificates (for more than seven calendar days)

  If you are absent for more than seven calendar days (including Saturdays and Sundays) or as soon as you know that you will be away from work for more than seven calendar days, you must get a medical statement from your own doctor. This must be sent immediately to your Manager who will forward a copy to the Wages department. You will be required to let your Manager know when you will be fit to return to work.

  Your Manager will send a copy of any self-certificates to the relevant Manager if necessary.

  All medical statements obtained from your doctor covering the total absence save for the first seven days must be sent straight to your Manager.

(cont'd)

You should ensure that your absence is covered by a current medical statement at all times. Failure to do so may result in a delay in paying you sick pay.

Please note that all medical statements submitted must satisfy your Manager and whilst medical statements normally provide adequate evidence of unfitness for work, they may not be conclusive evidence for sick pay purposes, depending upon other factors and the circumstances surrounding your particular case.

For example, any member of staff with a medical statement from his doctor certifying 'Back pain' may be suspended from the sick pay scheme and disciplined if he/she is seen marching on a rally or conducting him/herself in any way which is inconsistent with such a diagnosis.

Should there be any query or problem regarding any medical statements submitted, this will be discussed with you and the matter may be referred to senior management for investigation and further action may be taken if necessary.

Disciplinary procedures

2.27 In the case of the fraudulent malingerer, the following procedures may be adopted.

Asking for leave and it is declined

2.28 Employees who ask for leave and it is declined may still feel that they are entitled to take it or may have already booked the holiday and therefore decide to take it anyway. The following procedure is suggested:

- Manager to call the employee in to the office the afternoon before the first day of the leave requested.

- Make opening remarks such as: 'You are looking very well today,' etc.

- Remind employee of the refused leave application and produce the form with the refusal marked, dated and signed.

- Ask the employee to confirm that they have understood that the leave has been refused, why it has been refused and to confirm that they will be at work on ....day.

- Explain how the company views going absent in breach of an express instruction not to take the leave ie that it is regarded as gross misconduct. Explain why it is gross misconduct.

- Confirm that if in the unlikely event they are unfit for work, the manager will require medical evidence which is acceptable to him or her and self-certification forms may not suffice.

- Confirm the conversation in writing, date and sign it and give the employee a copy.

Employee fails to attend work

2.29   If the employee fails to attend work on a day that he or she is expected at work, the following procedure is suggested:

- Ring the telephone number and note down the number of times the telephone rings, the times of the day the number is tried and confirm with the operator there is no fault on the line.

- Keep careful dated notes of this procedure.

- If the employee telephones the manager, return the call immediately to validate that the employee has rung from home.

- If the answer phone is on, leave an urgent message that you require a conversation with the employee as soon as he or she feels fit enough to speak.

- State on the answer phone (if there is one) that you are so concerned at the non-appearance at work, that you intend to visit the employee at home and can the employee confirm when such a visit would be convenient.

- Visit and search for the individual. Make a note if the house is locked up. Visit any neighbours and explain that the individual has not been seen at work and enquire if they know where the employee is.

- Leave a note that you called (you will have written one in advance and taken a copy). This note will state that you called, that there was no-one in and that you require an immediate telephone call to explain where the employee is and why they are not at work.

- You may also require that the employee has an immediate medical examination (during or after) the absence, to be carried out by the occupational health practitioner.

- You are entitled to treat going on holiday whilst claiming sickness as gross misconduct as:

    o   this is regarded as fraud (making a fraudulent claim on sick pay);

    o   there has been a breach of mutual trust and confidence (lying on the self-certification form); and

    o   there has been a flagrant breach of an express instruction not to take holiday.

- You are entitled to investigate the circumstances surrounding a medical certificate if you have evidence of conduct inconsistent with the illness or injuries, eg a man signed off with 'sciatica' seen marching on a TUC rally!

- A full disciplinary hearing should follow with all the evidence presented and the employee asked for an explanation.

- Decide whether or not to take disciplinary action and, if so, what form it should take.

- The employee should be given an opportunity to appeal should be given.

Managing return to work

2.30   It is very important for employers to plan and manage a return to work following any significant absence due to illness or injury, etc. This means ensuring that a properly thought out and agreed staged return may be appropriate, in some cases with modified or alternative duties, reduced hours, less onerous targets and objectives, etc.

In *Young v The Post Office [2002] IRLR 660*, the Court of Appeal held as follows:

'The employers were in breach of their duty of care in failing to ensure that the arrangements made for the claimant's return to work after an absence of four months due to a nervous breakdown brought on by stress at work were adhered to, with the result that, within seven weeks of returning to work, the claimant again found himself under stress and suffered a recurrence of his psychiatric illness. The judge was entitled to reject the submission that it was up to the claimant to speak out if he felt that he was under stress.

Where an employee has already suffered from psychiatric illness resulting from occupational stress, it is plainly foreseeable that there might be a recurrence if appropriate steps are not taken when the employee returns to work. The employer owes the employee a duty to take such steps and to see that the arrangements made are carried through.

In the present case, despite arrangements made to ensure that the claimant could return to work at his own pace, two weeks after his return he had been sent on a week-long residential course and within seven weeks he was back doing the same job which had originally caused him to suffer stress. Promises that he would be visited regularly by members of management and that his capacity for work would be assessed were not kept. The employers were therefore in breach of duty.'

Disability discrimination

2.31   It many cases of acute or long-term sickness absence, employers and occupational health physicians must be aware of their duties under the

Disability Discrimination Act 1995 as such absences are often caused by what the Act defines as a 'disability'. The definition of disability, as defined by the Act, has already been discussed at 2.9. Recent case law has given guidance to Employment Tribunals on how to *interpret* the meaning of 'disability' under the Act (see *Rugamer (Appellant) v Sony Music Entertainment UK Ltd (Respondents); McNicol (Appellant) v Balfour Beatty Rail Maintenance Ltd (Respondents) [2001] IRLR 644*, and *College of Ripon & York St John (Appellants) v Hobbs (Respondent) [2002] IRLR 185*).

In the joint appeal by Rugamer and McNicol, the Employment Appeal Tribunal (EAT) held that it may not be possible to establish either a physical or mental impairment where the 'physical' impairment is psychosomatic in nature. In addition, if this psychosomatic condition is not a clinically well-recognised illness, then no mental impairment will be established.

The EAT held that:

'The employment tribunals did not err in finding that functional or psychological overlay, which appeared to be the only explanation for the restriction of the applicants' movements and activities, was not a physical impairment within the meaning of the definition of disability in the *Disability Discrimination Act*.

The dividing line between physical and mental impairment depends on whether the nature of the impairment itself is physical or mental, rather than on whether a physical or mental function or activity is affected (since a physical impairment may affect mental activities as well as physical ones, and vice versa). Direct assistance in considering the line between physical and mental impairments can be obtained from the distinction drawn by the Court of Appeal in the context of certain mobility and disability benefits between a physical disablement which is a manifestation of a person's physical condition, and a 'functional disablement which is not, even though it may have the effect that they are unable to carry out physical activities.

In each of the present cases, there was evidence before the tribunal making it proper to conclude that whatever impairment or restriction the applicant might have had was not physical but a manifestation of his psychological make-up, and on that basis that no physical impairment had been established.

The employment tribunals did not err in finding that the applicants did not have mental impairments within the meaning of the definition of disability, since there was no clear evidence in either case that the applicant had a clinically well-recognised illness.'

In the second appeal, the Hobbs case, the EAT held that the tribunal was entitled to hold that Ms Hobbs had a 'physical impairment' when she had symptoms describable as physical. There was no statutory definition of 'impairment' and nothing in the Act or Guidance that prevents a tribunal from finding that an impairment can be something that results from an illness as opposed to itself being an illness. It can thus be cause and effect.

Depression

2.32 Take 'depression' as an example of a disability. The employee must show that the kind of depression that they have falls within ICD 10 of the World Health Organisation's 'International Classification of Diseases' and that the condition has a substantial effect upon one of the day-to-day activities. These are listed in the *Disability Discrimination Act 1995, Sch 1 para 4*:

- mobility;
- manual dexterity;
- physical co-ordination;
- ability to lift or move everyday objects;
- hearing, speech or eyesight;
- continence;
- memory, ability to learn or concentrate; and
- ability to perceive the risk of danger.

Both a Code of Practice and Guidance Notes have been published to assist employers in understanding their obligations under the Act. These can be found and can be downloaded at the following website: http://www.drc-gb.org/drc/Documents/defdisability.doc.

The Guidance Notes gives some useful examples of what would be regarded as having a substantial effect upon someone with depression such as to bring them within the scope of the Act. These examples are:

- intermittent loss of consciousness and associated confused behaviour;
- persistent inability to remember the names of familiar people such as family or friends;
- inability to adapt after a reasonable period to minor change in work routine;
- inability to write a cheque without assistance;
- considerable difficulty in following a short sequence such as a simple recipe or a brief list of domestic tasks.

The type of depressive illness that is therefore likely to fall under the Act would be serious.

Employer responsibility

2.33 Under the *Disability Discrimination Act 1995* the employer discriminates against a person for a reason relating to his or her disability if the employer refuses to recruit, dismisses or otherwise subjects that person to a detriment during employment (*section s 5(1)*). Further, the employer discriminates if he fails to make reasonable adjustments for that person (*section 5(2)*). The employer's defence is justification on both counts (*section 5(3)*).

The disabled person does not have to compare himself or herself with someone able-bodied to show discrimination (*Clark v TDG Ltd t/a Novacold [1999] IRLR 318*) and the employer does not have to have actual knowledge of the disability to become liable under the Act (*section 6(6)*; and see *HJ Heinz v Kenrick [2000] IRLR 144*).

The Act lists examples of the kinds of reasonable adjustments that employers are required to consider making and what factors the Employment Tribunals will take into account in determining whether it was reasonably practicable for the employer to make the adjustment sought (*section 6(2)–(4)*; and *Kenny v Hampshire Constabulary [1999] IRLR 76*).

Medical confidentiality and human rights

2.34   Doctors and nurses are bound by their respective governing bodies (General Medical Council (GMC) and Nursing and Midwifery Council (NMC)) to keep clinical details strictly confidential (save in certain exceptional and well-known cases). The most obvious exceptions are where the patient has given his or her informed consent to disclosure or where there is an over-riding duty to society to disclose the clinical details (see *W v Egdell [1990] 1 All ER 835* and the US case of *Tarasoff v Regents of the University of California, 551 P 2d 334 (Cal 1976)*).

Under the *Human Rights Act 1998, s 8(1)* everyone has a 'right to respect for their privacy, family life and correspondence' subject to certain exceptions in *section 8(2)*.

There has been some controversy concerning employers making home visits to absent employees: some unions have suggested that this might breach *section 8*. It is unlikely. If an employer first makes an appointment and does not arrive unexpectedly, there can be no breach of the right to respect for privacy or family life. If the employee has been unresponsive and has failed to communicate or contact the employer, then it may be reasonable and justifiable for the employer to make a home visit to ensure the welfare of that employee.

Stress

2.35   Stress-related illness is becoming a serious problem for employers. The Court of Appeal recently heard four appeals on whether employers were negligent for stress-related illness suffered by their employees (see

Sutherland (Chairman of The Governors of St Thomas Becket RC High School) (Defendant/Appellant) v Hatton (Claimant/Respondent); Somerset County Council (Defendants/Appellants) v Barber (Claimant/Respondent); Sandwell Metropolitan Borough Council (Defendants/Appellants) v Jones (Claimant/Respondent) Baker Refractories Ltd (Defendants/Appellants) v Bishop (Claimant/Respondent) [2002] IRLR 263).

The Court of Appeal gave guidance on how the courts should treat future stress claims, summarised below.

- There are no special control mechanisms applying to claims for psychiatric (or physical) illness or injury arising from the stress of doing the work the employee is required to do. The ordinary principles of employer's liability apply.

- The threshold question is whether this kind of harm to this particular employee was reasonably foreseeable. This has two components:

  o an injury to health (as distinct from occupational stress) which

  o is attributable to stress at work (as distinct from other factors).

- Foreseeability depends upon what the employer knows (or ought reasonably to know) about the individual employee.

  Because of the nature of mental disorder, it is harder to foresee than physical injury, but may be easier to foresee in a known individual than in the population at large.

  An employer is usually entitled to assume that the employee can withstand the normal pressures of the job unless he knows of some particular problem or vulnerability (ie staff who feel under stress at work should tell their employers and give them a chance to do something about it).

- The test is the same whatever the employment: there are no occupations which should be regarded as intrinsically dangerous to mental health.

- Factors likely to be relevant in answering the threshold question include:

  o The nature and extent of the work done by the employee:

    – Is the workload much more than is normal for the particular job?

    – Is the work particularly intellectually or emotionally demanding for this employee?

    – Are demands being made of this employee unreasonable when compared with the demands made of others in the same or comparable jobs?

- Or are there signs that others doing this job are suffering harmful levels of stress?

- Is there an abnormal level of sickness or absenteeism in the same job or the same department?

o Signs from the employee of impending harm to health:

- Has he a particular problem or vulnerability?

- Has he already suffered from illness attributable to stress at work?

- Have there recently been frequent or prolonged absences which are uncharacteristic of him?

- Is there reason to think that these are attributable to stress at work, for example because of complaints or warnings from him or others?

• The employer is generally entitled to take what he is told by his employee at face value, unless he has good reason to think to the contrary. *He does not generally have to make searching enquiries of the employee or seek permission to make further enquiries of his medical advisors.*

• To trigger a duty to take steps, the indications of impending harm to health arising from stress at work must be plain enough for any reasonable employer to realise that he should do something about it.

• The employer is only in breach of duty if he has failed to take the steps which are reasonable in the circumstances, bearing in mind the magnitude of the risk of harm occurring, the gravity of the harm which may occur, the costs and practicability of preventing it, and the justifications for running the risk.

• The size and scope of the employer's operation, its resources and the demands it faces are relevant in deciding what is reasonable; these include the interests of other employees and the need to treat them fairly, for example, in any redistribution of duties.

• An employer can only reasonably be expected to take steps which are likely to do some good: the court is likely to need expert evidence on this.

• An employer who offers a confidential advice service, with referral to appropriate counselling or treatment services, is unlikely to be found in breach of duty.

• If the only reasonable and effective step would have been to dismiss or demote the employee, the employer will not be in breach of duty in allowing a willing employee to continue in the job.

(cont'd)

- In all cases, therefore, it is necessary to identify the steps which the employer both could and should have taken before finding him in breach of his duty of care.

- The claimant must show that that breach of duty has caused or materially contributed to the harm suffered. It is not enough to show that occupational stress has caused the harm.

- Where the harm suffered has more than one cause, the employer should only pay for that proportion of the harm suffered which is attributable to his wrongdoing, unless the harm is truly indivisible.

- The assessment of damages will take account of any pre-existing disorder or vulnerability and of the chance that the claimant would have succumbed to a stress-related disorder in any event.

As far as disability discrimination claims are concerned, the Employment Appeal Tribunal (EAT) recently gave guidance (*Morgan v University of Staffordshire [2002] IRLR 190*). Here Ms Morgan claimed she had become depressed as a result of her treatment at work and eventually resigned and claimed constructive dismissal and disability discrimination. Her GP had written only 'depression, anxiety and stress' on her medical statements and his notes contained no other details.

In a 'stress' case, in order to rely upon the *Disability Discrimination Act 1995*, the employee must establish that they have a clinically well-recognised illness and as such the EAT will normally require a medical report from a psychiatrist with a diagnosis that falls within the ICD 10 Classifications. They include both 'Mood [affective] disorders F30-F39' and 'Neurotic, stress related and somatoform disorders F40-F48'. So, for example, F43 lists the following disorders:

'F43 Reaction to severe stress, and adjustment disorders

F43.0 Acute stress reaction

F43.1 Post-traumatic stress disorder

F43.2 Adjustment disorders

.20   Brief depressive reaction

.21   Prolonged depressive reaction

.22   Mixed anxiety and depressive reaction

.23   With predominant disturbance of other emotions

.24   With predominant disturbance of conduct

.25   With mixed disturbance of emotions and conduct

.28   With other specified predominant symptoms

F43.8 Other reactions to severe stress.'

The EAT held that such terms as 'stress', 'anxiety' and 'depression' used on their own without any supporting medical explanation will not suffice in establishing a clinically well-recognised mental illness. The EAT suggested that qualified psychiatrists should in many cases be called by the employee to give evidence of the mental illness that they are claiming.

Excellent summaries on stress can be found in 'Hunter's Diseases of Occupations' (9th edition) and in Chapter 7 of the book 'Fitness for Work – The Medical Aspects' (Cox, R et al (eds), 3rd edition).

Bullying

2.36   Any form of bullying could amount to harassment and if the employer fails to take adequate steps to protect or prevent bullying in the workplace, the employee may have a claim for constructive dismissal, personal injuries and possibly discrimination on grounds of race, sex or disability.

Well-drafted and published policies, training of managers and the encouragement of employees not to initiate or condone a bullying and hostile working environment, will go a long way to protect employers from such claims.

Violence

2.37   Statistics show that violent attacks at work are increasing. Employers have both a statutory and common law duty to protect their workers from such risks. The duty is to take reasonable care to guard against reasonably foreseeable risks of injury.

Risk assessments should highlight specific occupations where the risk of violence is high. The *Management of Health and Safety at Work Regulations 1999 (SI 1999/3242), Reg 3(1)* specifically concerns the duty of employers to carry out risk assessments, and states:

'Every employer shall make a suitable and sufficient assessment of–

(a)   the risks to the health and safety of his employees to which they are exposed whilst they are at work; and

(b)   the risks to the health and safety of persons not in his employment arising out of or in connection with the conduct by him of his undertaking,

for the purpose of identifying the measures he needs to take to comply with the requirements and prohibitions imposed upon him by or under the relevant statutory provisions'.

Workers in both the public and private sectors are at risk. This includes local authority workers such as social workers, teachers, housing officers and benefits staff. Police officers are at risk as are many NHS staff working in hospitals, ambulances and community care. In the private sector, transport and retail workers can be vulnerable, as are security staff and those working in licensed premises, banks and building societies.

Injuries resulting from acts of (non-consensual) violence against an employee are reportable under the *Reporting of Injuries, Diseases and Dangerous Occurrences Regulations 1995 (SI 1995/3163)*.

There are two useful websites to assist employers in dealing with workplace violence:

http://www.workplaceviolence.co.uk/ and http://www.hse.gov.uk/pubns/indg69.pdf.

Conflict management specialists Maybo Limited has produced a useful checklist for employers, which is reproduced below.

Figure 3: Checklist for employers

Prevention

Recognition

❑ Have you undertaken a comprehensive review of violence towards staff?

❑ Have you specifically assessed the risk of violence to staff in each area of work?

❑ Is the review/risk assessment process repeated at specific intervals?

❑ Have you examined key flashpoints and the underlying causes of conflict and violence?

❑ Do you have an effective classification and recording system for violent incidents?

❑ Are you aware as to the extent to which risk reduction measures are applied?

❑ Do you know which measures are effective and which are not?

❑ Have you undertaken a formal analysis of training and support needs for each role performed?

❑   Have employees been consulted in the above areas?

Policy

❑   Do you have a policy that specifically addresses violence towards staff?

❑   Does the policy demonstrate commitment of the management of this issue?

❑   Have front line staff been involved in the development and review of the policy?

❑   Does the policy state how risk will be assessed and controlled?

❑   Does the policy identify whom it affects, and outline the responsibilities of management and staff?

❑   Does the policy address the management of the media?

❑   Are clear objectives and performance indicators set?

❑   Is it clear how transgressions will be dealt with?

❑   Does the policy have a communication strategy?

❑   Is there a process in place for the evaluation of each element of the policy?

❑   Is there a periodic review and update of the policy?

Best practice

❑   Do you have safe practice guidance for your lone and team workers?

❑   Have front line staff been involved in the development of this?

❑   What method do you have for measuring the extent to which this guidance is followed?

❑   Do your line managers actively promote and monitor best practice?

❑   How is best practice identified, updated and communicated across the organisation?

Service delivery

❑   Have you identified sources of frustration for staff and customers/service users?

❑   Have you sought feedback from each of these groups in this?

(cont'd)

❏ Have steps been taken to address the root causes of frustration and dissatisfaction?

Design

❏ To what extent does the working environment contribute to the quality of service delivery?

❏ Has the personal safety of staff been specifically considered in the design and layout?

❏ What risk reduction measures have been incorporated into design and layout?

Security personnel

❏ Is the role and responsibilities of security staff clearly defined within your violence strategy?

❏ Have security staff received comprehensive training to deal with violent behaviour/incidents?

❏ To what extent do your security staff value, and contribute to service delivery?

❏ Are they clear as to the policy on physical interventions and trained in accordance with this?

❏ Have they been consulted in the violence management process?

❏ Do they possess the equipment necessary to perform their role effectively?

Security measures

❏ How effective is your access control?

❏ Is CCTV used effectively in both the prevention and management of violent incidents?

❏ Are panic alarms utilised and placed effectively in risk areas?

❏ Are staff aware of how to respond to these?

❏ Are lone workers provided with the means to secure assistance?

Response

Incident management

❏ Do you have clear incident management procedures?

❏ Are managers and staff aware of their roles and responsibilities should an incident occur?

❑ Have these procedures been tested and rehearsed by staff?

❑ Do secure areas exist that provide a 'place of safety' for staff – and an emergency exit for staff?

❑ Has the role of other agencies been established and planned for?

❑ Is there operational resilience and contingency plans?

❑ Do you have a clear plan for managing media interest?

❑ Do you have clear post incident procedures and support processes (see below)?

Reporting

❑ Do you have an effective reporting system?

❑ Do managers and staff understand reporting requirements within RIDDOR?

❑ Are staff taught how to write up an incident and account for their actions?

❑ Do staff clearly understand the importance of, and personal benefits of reporting?

❑ Are incident reports followed up and staff kept informed?

❑ How do line managers support and reinforce this process?

❑ How is the information managed and utilised by the organisation?

Training

❑ Have you conducted a training needs analysis concerning violence at work?

❑ Is training tailored to meet the specific context and challenges within each job role performed?

❑ Is training delivered by expert trainers, with credibility in the subject area?

❑ Do you evaluate the effectiveness of training in the workplace post-course?

❑ How is training followed up and reinforced in the workplace?

❑ Is refresher training built in?

❑ Do you train frontline staff in personal safety awareness and interpersonal skills for:

   ❑ Preventing conflict and reducing risk?

(cont'd)

❑ Dealing with conflict and risk situations that do arise?

❑ Are physical interventions taught to staff whose job may require them to lay hands on another person?

Support

Employee support and post-incident procedure

❑ Are managers aware of the increase in legal cases surrounding stress and psychiatric injury?

❑ Do you have clear post incident procedures?

❑ Is there an educative process that helps prepare and equip staff to deal with stress and traumatic events?

❑ Are line managers equipped to assess and respond to immediate and longer term staff support needs?

❑ Do line managers demonstrate this support for staff in the workplace, and follow up incidents?

❑ Can line managers and staff access additional support including counselling where appropriate?

❑ How does the organisation ensure that learning is drawn from incidents and fed back?

❑ Do you have a skilled response team which can respond to a difficult incident?

❑ Do you provide legal advice and support to staff when appropriate?

3 Managing Occupational Health

Introduction – aims and objectives of a company in managing occupational health

3.1   To state it simply, most companies, however large or small, wish to minimise the harm they do to their employees – if possible, by preventing harm completely – and to treat their employees in such a way as to maximise their employees' commitment and hard work. Companies also usually wish to obey the law.

Companies where public safety is of key importance (eg public transport, nuclear power generation, food preparation, etc) also need to prevent their employees' ill-health adversely affecting public safety. This will form a part of their approach to occupational health management and will lead to some method of assessing fitness to work.

Managing occupational health effectively will allow a company to improve its risk profile and improve its productivity. These, then, are the underlying aims of a company in introducing systems and services that will have an impact on occupational health. It is fairly unusual for a company to spell out its aims and objectives in this way but can be very helpful in assessing what systems and services are needed.

What should occupational health support achieve?

3.2   In order to decide what occupational health support should be achieving for a company, the company needs to decide what it wants, how much it can achieve through its own systems and what specialised support it needs. So the company will require some kind of *needs assessment*.

For small and medium-sized enterprises, the needs for occupational health support have been described in a report known as the OHAC Report ('Report and recommendations on improving access to occupational health support', Occupational Health Advisory Committee, HSE, 2000). In brief, OHAC identified many employers as having the following needs:

- The need to be educated on and their awareness raised of the following issues:
  - o the existence of health problems for which competent advice may be required;

      o how to obtain that advice;

      o how to ensure that competent persons appointed from within the workforce are working within their knowledge and experience and when to seek further help;

      o an integrated approach to risk management;

      o ways of using occupational health support and advice to create a healthy working environment;

      o ways of complying with legislation;

      o ways of involving workers in the control of risks.

- The need for help with hazard identification, risk assessment and implementation of controls (eg ergonomic measures, process and system design) that is simple, focused and preferably sector specific.

- The need for practical help with prevention of ill-health through the use of management tools such as monitoring of sickness absence, health surveillance, and systems that allow a balanced flow of work.

- The need for help with human resource issues, good management skills, flexible working policies, and healthy living issues.

- The need for advice on fitness for work issues, redeployment, rehabilitation and employing the disabled.

- The need for help with setting up first aid and, where appropriate, other treatment services (eg stabilisation of injuries and acute ill-health, helping disabled workers stay at work, preventive medicine and vaccinations for employees travelling abroad, helping to manage addictions).

- The provision of a local 'one-stop shop' approach to business advice, including occupational health and safety.

At a conference considering how primary care could help in occupational health, one manager of a small company described his 'wish list' as including a desire for employers, employees and occupational health specialists to work together more profitably, almost like an annual 'health check' of the business, as follows:

- access to a helpline;

- a health kit/guidance pack for employers;

- medical consultation for staff who want extra medical help;

- published statistics to help drive the right decisions;

- closer consultation between employers and the medics looking after our staff; and

- maybe introduce a recognition standard to encourage good practice.

(See 'Staying Fit for Work: a report of a conference on 8th March 2001', DH/DSS, 2001.)

Occupational health management – the process

3.3 To assess how to improve a company's risk profile, the company will need to assess the risks to employees, agency workers and contractors to health at work. The requirement for workplace risk assessment (see CHAPTER 10) will assist in this. It is worth remembering that in general, paid work contributes to improved health, but work can be harmful to health. It is naive to believe that we can achieve a situation where work will never be harmful to people, but such harm should be prevented where possible and identified when it occurs.

The assessment of workplace risks to health will lead to a consideration of how these can be minimised, controlled and managed to be as low as is reasonably practicable, what training is required in the understanding of the risks, what (if any) health surveillance is required and what (if any) support will be required for those who are made ill by their work despite all the preventative measures in place. This should lead to an understanding of what (if any) specialist occupational health support the company needs. Even to undertake the assessment of risks, the company may need to get some specialised occupational health advice (see CHAPTER 11).

To assess how to improve a company's productivity in relation to managing occupational health the company will need to consider its approach to sickness absence and its attitude to employee morale. Absence attributed to sickness can cause major reductions in productivity. The management of such absence includes decisions considered to be in the human resource management arena, such as whether to continue to pay people during periods of absence, but will also include issues that occupational health professionals would be expected to advise on or deliver. These include:

- pre-employment medical assessments, which can identify conditions for which the person may need workplace adjustments (which if they don't get may have a deleterious impact on their health);

- assessments when an individual is off sick to advise on likely return to work and any adjustments made;

- arrangements for fast track to treatment services such as physiotherapy; and

- arrangements for private health care provision usually through insurance.

What kind of occupational health support is needed?

3.4 There are several different types of help that may be needed, for example:

- help with individual people who have problems relating to illness and their work;

- help with workplace risk assessments;

- help with specific problems, such as:

  o compliance with the *Health and Safety (Display Screen Equipment) Regulations 1992 (SI 1992/2792)*;

  o the need for health surveillance for employees who are exposed to certain chemicals; and

- help with policy advice.

The OHAC report (HSE, 2000) gives a model for occupational health support. This is shown in FIGURE 1. It shows the user having three levels of need for advice:

Figure 1: Model of tiered approach to delivery of occupational health support

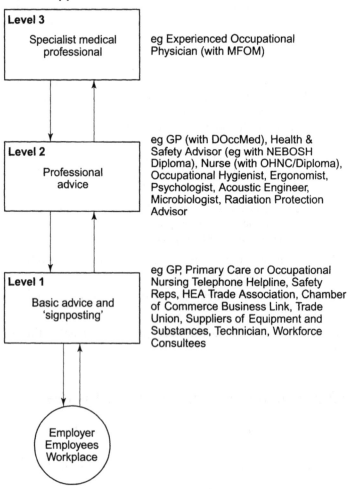

- the first level of support will answer general problems;
- the second level of support deals with specific problems; and
- the third level of support is the specialist occupational physician.

This is a useful model, but it doesn't always work this way round. Sometimes it will be the occupational health nurse or the occupational health physician who recognises the need for other levels of help. The third tier level of help is not necessarily always the physician: it may be an ergonomist, an occupational hygienist or other specialist.

The company needs to consider how it will meet the first level requirement, which is basic advice and signposting towards more specialist help. Large companies can expect to meet this wholly from within. Smaller companies may need access to external help, even for the most basic advice, such as finding out what the law requires of them in relation to occupational health. Several telephone help lines are currently being provided and evaluated and this may prove the most useful form of first line occupational health support for small and medium-sized enterprises.

For larger companies, it may be appropriate to use an in-house service or an external specialist occupational health provider. The decision will relate to the needs assessment and the level of need. For example, large organisations which have considerable issues relating to the impact of health on work/work on health will require regular access to an occupational health nurse and physician, whereas smaller companies may need considerable advice about controlling workplace risks, but only rarely need access to medical or nursing advice about an individual. (For further information on buying in external expertise, see CHAPTER 11.)

What occupational health services are available?

3.5   The following is a list of the types of services that occupational health service providers are likely to offer:

- advice on workplace risk assessment;
- advice on managing sickness absence, which may include medical assessments;
- advice on rehabilitation of employee after injury or illness;
- advice on reasonable adjustments made in the workplace relating to someone's illness or disability;
- pre employment medical assessments;
- advice about employees whose health may be affecting their work, or whose work may be affecting their health;
- health surveillance for exposure to known harmful agents;
- advice on human resource and occupational health policy;

- health promotion;

- treatment services such as physiotherapy; and

- drug and alcohol testing.

Other types of help are available, and information on occupational health professionals (at 3.9 *et seq*) gives more details of which specialists are likely to be able to help with different types of problems. For further discussion of these health professionals, see CHAPTER 11.

The occupational health team

3.6   The occupational health team is usually a 'virtual' team. If there is *an* actual team, there will be some elements of virtuality about it, because the skills needed to manage occupational health are so broad that the team will call on other people to advise in certain circumstances. The make up of the team (where there is one) is likely to depend on the focus of occupational health care in the company that the team is serving.

External health team

3.7   Private occupational health companies offering services to many different organisations are likely to have large teams and their make up is likely to reflect the needs of the companies and organisations they serve. Other providers of occupational health advice include occupational health projects, which exist in some cities in the UK. Some of them work directly with individuals, either through their GP practice or by direct referral. Some work with employers. They tend to be staffed by non-professional people (not doctors or nurses) who nevertheless usually have extensive experience of workplace health and safety issues. They often work to assist the GP in identifying and managing workplace health issues.

In industries where there are high legislative requirements for safety, the occupational health team is likely be made up predominantly of doctors and nurses. Where productivity and/or prevention of a specific work-related problem are the key issues, the team may have health care professionals such as physiotherapists or counsellors. Where there are many physical, biological or chemical workplace hazards then the team will need an occupational hygienist. In some companies there is a focus on wellbeing and, thus, the emphasis may be on providing more nurses and psychologists. Increasingly companies also call on the expertise of ergonomists and 'human factors specialists'.

The underlying point is that there is a range of specialist skills that a company will consider useful in managing the health and, in particular, the occupational health of their employees.

In-house team

3.8   In companies large enough to have an occupational health team, it is common for the safety team to be managerially separate from the occupational health team, and there will inevitably be some areas of overlap between the two. For example, the implementation of the *Manual Handling Operations Regulations 1992 (SI 1992/2793)* and the *Health and Safety (Display Screen Equipment) Regulations 1992 (SI 1992/2792)* may be the responsibility of either the safety or the occupational health teams. Hence, where there are two teams, good management requires close communication between them.

Each professional group has a particular focus for their work in occupational health, but there is considerable crossover of skills. In some companies a nurse may be advising on a problem that a doctor would advise on in another company and that an occupational therapist would be advising on in a third company. These specialists can be expected to understand the limits of their own competence and to whom they can turn for competent advice when they have reached those limits. Managers who use these specialists will also benefit from some understanding of the strengths of each type of specialist.

Role of different occupational health professionals

Occupational physician

3.9   Occupational physicians can advise on the medical conditions that people have and the implications for their work. They are skilled in diagnosis and can advise about the implications of both diagnosis and treatment on work capability. They are skilled in advising in complicated situations where many parameters need consideration. Specialists in occupational medicine are trained to advise on all aspects of occupational health and to know when professional advice other than medical advice is needed. Specialists in occupational medicine will be on the General Medical Council specialist register and usually have the qualification of Member (MFOM) or Fellow of the Faculty of Occupational Medicine (FFOM). The Faculty of Occupational Medicine can advise on relevant qualifications; whereas the Society of Occupational Medicine can advise in the location of a suitable physician (for contact details of both bodies, see APPENDIX: FURTHER SOURCES OF INFORMATION).

Doctors who are not specialists in occupational medicine (although they may be specialists in other disciplines) who work in occupational health should have some qualification in occupational medicine or be working towards qualification under the supervision of a specialist. The exception to this rule is where a specialist in another discipline is being asked to advise within their area of competence. For example, if a consultant dermatologist has expertise in occupational dermatology then their advice on a case of occupational dermatitis will be very valuable in terms of the disease, its treatment and prevention of deterioration.

General practitioners have a role in occupational health management via their certification of illness requiring absence from work. There is training in this provided by the Department for Work and Pensions. GPs are not automatically trained in other areas of occupational health but are very often the only form of medical advice immediately available to small and medium-sized enterprises. General practitioners with an interest in occupational health are expected to obtain the Diploma of Occupational Medicine.

For further discussion of occupational physicians, see 11.19.

Occupational health nurse

3.10   There are currently between 6,000–7,000 nurses working in occupational health nursing. Of these approximately 3,250 hold the Nursing and Midwifery Council (NMC – formerly UKCC) recordable qualification of Occupational Health Specialist with diplomas and/or degrees. For contact details for the NMC, see APPENDIX: FURTHER SOURCES OF INFORMATION.

Occupational health nurses work in a variety of locations: within the private sector of industry, businesses and trade/services and the NHS. The core elements of their work include:

- provision of care, promotion of health, health surveillance and assessment;

- risk assessment and risk reduction, promotion of health and safety;

- prevention of ill-health, and environmental monitoring;

- in some cases management of the occupational health service, research, practice development, evaluation of interventions;

- measuring of outcomes;

- advising employers and working closely with other members in occupational health services such as medical colleagues and safety officers; and

- linking and liaising with primary care trusts.

In addition the occupational health nurse must be able to interpret, advise on and implement a wide-ranging area of health and safety legislation. Where medical diagnosis or complicated medical advice is needed, they will usually refer the case to a doctor.

For further discussion of occupational health nurses, see 11.20.

Occupational hygienist

3.11   An occupational hygienist is trained to look at workplace hazards and assess the level of risk. This is exactly the same process that every health and safety professional should undertake. However, because of their training and experience an occupational hygienist is better at assessing some hazards than other health and safety professionals and these are usually considered to be the physical, biological and chemical workplace hazards. In pure terms the training is biology, chemistry, engineering, mathematics and physics. However because of the need to relate to the workforce in order to obtain meaningful exposure data there is also a large element of psychology in the training in order to understand the implications and impact of proposed actions on the workforce. This is called the *psychosocial element* of an occupational hygienist's work.

Armed with this training the occupational hygienist looks at hazards in the workplace, decides if they are competent to assess the level of risk or whether they need assistance. Once the level of risk has been evaluated a decision has to be made as to whether the risk is as low as is reasonably practicable. If further control measures are required, whether they are engineering controls or administrative controls, an occupational hygienist has received the training to advise on the controls, and on the cost effectiveness of the control options.

Occupational hygienists are registered with the British Institute of Occupational Hygiene (BIOH), which will be merging with the British Occupational Hygiene Society (BOHS) by the end of 2002. For contact details, see APPENDIX: FURTHER SOURCES OF INFORMATION.

For further discussion of occupational hygienists, see 11.21.

Occupational therapist

3.12   Occupational therapists assess an individual's physical and psychological functioning within a given environment and use the principles of activity analysis to problem solve any dysfunction. In the UK they are little used in occupational health, but they have the potential to be extremely useful because of their skills. They are used in other countries to advise on the 'fit' between work and people, especially at an individual level and their advice may include recommendations about workplace adjustments.

The overall aim of an occupational therapy intervention is to enable an individual to retain employment, return to employment following illness or injury or to be able to access work particularly within the remit of the *Disability Discrimination Act 1995*.

Access to occupational therapists working in the occupational health field is limited. A few are employed by companies specifically to assist in the occupational health management of their employees, whilst others can be found in independent consultancies.

Ergonomist or human factors specialist

3.13 Ergonomists also advise on the fitness between work and people, but usually in the context of workplace design. Their work not only includes physical design of workstations and equipment but also extends to the design of software in order to make it easy to use. In the USA they are often called 'human factors specialists', and that name is becoming more common in the UK. They can help by the application of a range of techniques, combined with an understanding of the human capabilities to ensure efficiency, health and safety, etc. Their areas of expertise include:

- workplace layout;
- task design;
- control layout;
- software design;
- lighting;
- job design; and
- procedures design.

For contact details, see APPENDIX: FURTHER SOURCES OF INFORMATION. For further discussion of ergonomists, see 11.22.

Physiotherapist

3.14 Physiotherapists treat more than musculoskeletal problems: other areas that might be relevant are pain management, usually for chronic pain problems, neurology (strokes, damaged nerves, neuropathies, etc), respiratory (chronic airway obstructions, asthma), burns and mental ill-health (relaxation).

Physiotherapists who operate in the workplace are likely to develop expertise in postural assessment and in manual handling training. Other activities that occupational physiotherapists get involved in are work-station assessments, pre-employment screening, work hardening, functional capacity evaluations, return to work programmes, a variety of training, etc. Although there is not a specific speciality within physiotherapy related to occupational health practice, the Association of Chartered Physiotherapists in Occupational Health and Ergonomics (ACPOHE) is the particular interest group. For contact details, see APPENDIX: FURTHER SOURCES OF INFORMATION.

Counsellor

3.15   Counsellors work with their clients to help them identify what is troubling them and how to address it. They use different techniques according to their training. For many companies counselling is offered through an employee assistance programme. This can be part of occupational health or employee health provision. Counsellors should have formal arrangements for supervision as this is part of the requirement for professional conduct. A qualification at Postgraduate Diploma level is usually considered the minimum qualification. Accreditation is usually with the British Association of Counselling and Psychotherapy (BACP) but can be with the British Psychological Society (BPS), the United Kingdom Council for Psychotherapy (UKCP) or the Association of Humanistic Psychotherapists and Practitioners (AHPP). For contact details, see APPENDIX: FURTHER SOURCES OF INFORMATION.

How to make a referral

3.16   This section discusses how to refer an individual to an occupational health physician or nurse with a request for advice.

It is important to describe what the problem is, what you need to know and what the work is that the person does. The referral should be discussed with the individual before they are referred. In an ideal world, the individual would be given a copy of the manager's referral and of the advice that the occupational health practitioner gives. FIGURE 2 provides an example of a checklist for a referral for a case of sickness absence.

It helps if the person making the referral understands the areas of competence and the limitations of their advisor. Occupational health physicians and nurses should be able to advise on the impact that illness can have on a person's work and the impact that a person's work can have on their health. The doctors will be skilled in diagnosis.

Sometimes managers use their occupational health practitioner to take the blame for unpalatable decisions but this is not good practice. For example, if someone is not performing properly and they have a medical condition, it can be tempting to assume that the medical condition is the problem. Where the medical condition is not the problem then the poor performance should be dealt with through disciplinary procedures. It is better to use the occupational health practitioner to advise on whether or not there is a medical problem. If the problem is seen not to be medical then deal with it through the other available channels.

The following gives some tips on the types of questions to ask for particular types of cases. In all referrals it is important that as much information as possible is given about the case to the occupational health practitioner, as indicated in the checklist below.

Figure 2: Sample checklist for sickness absence referral

Please forward as much information as you can. This will help us deal with your case as quickly as possible and avoid delays in entering into correspondence to obtain background information from you. Please enclose any other information or concerns that you feel may be relevant or useful.

1	Employee's name and employee number.
2	Occupation and work location.
3	Dates of current sickness (from – to).
4	Diagnosis or cause of sickness.
5	(If diagnosis not known) Copy of GP's certificate and outcome of discussions with GP regarding treatment plan, and indication when may return to some work.
6	Details of medication (name, dose, when started). Details of any other treatment. Length of course prescribed.
7	Interview notes, home visits, etc.
8	Details of previous sickness absence with dates and reasons, if relevant (eg repeated sickness absence due to the same reason).
9	Return to work date if one has been indicated.
10	Signed consent form if one has been provided already.
11	Your own (managers) observations, comments, problems.
12	Questions you would like addressed.
13	Any other information which may be relevant.
14	Confirmation that manager's concerns have been fully discussed with employee.
15	Occupation and work location.

Sickness absence

3.17

- Given the employee's current (and previous) medical condition, treatment, progress etc when are they likely to be returning to work?

- Are they likely to be able to return to work within the next month/6 months/12 months?

- When they return are they likely to be able to commence full duties?

- Can they get back to work sooner if adjustments are made?

- If so, what adjustments are recommended?

- If not, when they can get back to work, will they require a period of adjustments to their work initially and if so, what type of adjustments and for how long?

- Will they require a medical examination on return to work?

- Will the employee's medication restrict them at work and, if so, what restrictions are likely to be applied?

- What is the likelihood of further problems?

- Is there anything that can be done at work to minimise this?

- Is there anything the individual can do to minimise further problems?

Work-related illness

3.18   The information you should give:

- What the problem is.

- Has the person seen their GP, if so what has the GP said?

- What the work is.

- Have there ever been any similar cases?

The questions you are likely to want to ask are:

- Is this condition likely to be work-related?

- What if anything can be done to improve the design of work

- Can the person continue in the work and, if so, are there any reasonable adjustments which are required?

- What is the long-term outlook?

- If the person cannot continue in their work what can the person do?

- Is there anything the company can do to assist the person?

Fitness for work

3.19   Again, it is important to describe what is wrong with the person, whether or not they have seen their GP or specialist and, if so, what has been said and what the job is. The questions to be asked are:

- Will this condition affect the person's work and, if so, for how long?

- Are there any regulations relating to this condition in this particular work (eg driving)? If not, ask what the level of risk is.

It is the manager who should decide whether or not they can tolerate the level of risk described to them for a person who has developed an illness which may affect their fitness to do their job, unless there is legal regulation (eg professional drivers are not allowed to drive if they have insulin diabetes mellitus). Having said that, very often the occupational physician or occupational health nurse will be delegated management responsibility to advise the managers on whether or not someone is fit for a job. This is because the occupational physician or nurse sees a great many cases whereas each individual manager may only deal with one or two. It is worth remembering, however, that the physician or nurse is using their delegated management responsibility here. The manager can challenge the advice but if the manager decides to overrule the occupational health practitioner they should fully document the basis on which they have made that decision.

The reply to a referral

3.20   When a referral has been made to an occupational health practitioner, it should contain answers to the questions asked about the length of illness, the modifications needed and the future prognosis. The physician or nurse may need more information from the manager, the GP and the specialist in order to make a full reply.

The rules of confidentiality will apply and any details of the illness, or indeed the name of the illness, will not be mentioned unless it is known that the manager knows what this is.

Where the occupational health practitioner advises on workplace adjustments, they may well be able to describe some adjustments that can be made but the manager may be better placed to consider what workplace adjustments are appropriate. For example, an occupational health practitioner may advise that a reduction in working hours for a period of time would be appropriate, but only the manager can decide whether, and how, this can be introduced.

Confidentiality

3.21   A manager can expect to receive advice from their occupational health advisor on the implications for work of someone's medical condition but they do not have the right to know what is wrong with their employee. There is a tension here, because good management practice teaches managers to ask their employees about what is wrong and to get all the information about the programme for medical investigations and treatment. The checklist given at 3.16 asks for all this information. Managers *do not have a right* to obtain this information, but it is good practice to ask and most employees are happy to provide the information.

An occupational health practitioner who is a doctor or nurse must abide by the standards of medical confidentiality and these are specific and demanding. Occupational health practitioners from the professions allied to medicine (such as physiotherapy and occupational therapy) are also expected to apply similar standards of confidentiality. If the professional advisors do not abide by these standards they not only run the risk of losing the trust of the individual who has been referred for consultation but also of being in breach of their professional standards. This could lead to disciplinary action from their professional body or even, in extremis, removal from the professional register.

Employee's consent

3.22   An occupational health practitioner will, therefore, limit their advice about an individual to information about the impact on work of that person's medical condition unless they have the written consent of the individual to reveal information about the medical condition. If the manager has made it clear that they already know what is wrong with the person, then the occupational health practitioner may refer to this in their advice but will not give any new information about the medical condition. The advice is likely to be related to fitness for work, the likelihood of return to work, with timescales, and adjustments to work that may be suitable

If the employee does give their written consent to the occupational health practitioner to reveal the nature of their condition then this can be communicated, but there are several caveats to this. The occupational health practitioner or employer must not put any pressure on the individual to give their consent. If consent is given it must be informed consent; that is to say that the person must understand what information is being released, to whom, the purposes for which it will be used and the possible consequences of that use. Consent must be given freely, under no duress or threat and applies only for the time and event for which it is given. (See further CHAPTER 2.)

The employee's right for medical information to be kept confidential can be overruled, if a court serves a subpoena requiring the information to be made available to a court or if the occupational health practitioner considers that there is an over-riding public interest for breaching confidentiality. The occupational health practitioner will have access to professional advice and will only breach confidentiality in extreme cases.

Occupational health records

3.23   The occupational health practitioner also has a responsibility to keep their records secure and confidential. The employer should agree with them how long these records should be kept after an employee has left the company. Six to ten years is the usual timescale for this, although there may be legal provisions that require that they are kept for longer. The occupational health practitioner will advise on this.

There are interesting legal provisions about who *owns* the occupational health records. If the occupational health practitioner is external to the company the records belong to the occupational health practitioner. If the occupational health practitioner is in-house, the physical records belong to the employer but the information entered in them belongs to the occupational health practitioner. Hence, in this situation, the employer owns the physical record but does not have the right to read it.

The employer will receive written advice from their occupational health practitioner and will need to consider how to store this, usually in the personnel record. They should make arrangements to keep this information reasonably confidential.

Moves towards increasing openness in the UK have given people the right to see their records. Employees have the right to see both their personnel files and their occupational health records (*Access to Medical Reports Act 1988* and *Access to Health Records Act 1990*). Managers should be aware that the employee has the right to see what is written in a referral for occupational health advice. It is good practice to give the employee a copy of the referral letter and the occupational health practitioner's reply.

Pre-employment occupational health questionnaires

3.24   These are often used as a form of pre-employment assessment and are given or sent to a person who has been offered a job by the employer. Once they have been completed the arrangements should be such that the employer does not see them. They should be sealed and sent to the occupational health practitioner. They should not be filed on the staff record.

The relationship between managers and occupational health practitioners

3.25   The occupational health practitioner is sometimes accused of being 'a tool of management' or, conversely, of only seeing the employees' points of view. Developing and maintaining good relationships between the occupational health practitioner and managers, human resources specialists, employees and their representatives will increase the effectiveness of company's occupational health management.

The work of the occupational health practitioner is often achieved through persuasion and negotiation. This is because it so often operates at the interface between manager and employee, influencing return to work arrangements, changes in work environment, adjustments to work, etc. People working in the occupational health field often have considerable opportunity to understand organisational issues through their access to employees and managers on issues that are sensitive. They can use this understanding to positively influence the occupational health of employees by proposing changes and improvements. In order to achieve any influence, the trust and respect of both sides is needed. Such trust can be nurtured by the following means:

- by supporting the work of the occupational health practitioner from 'the top';

- by utilising only professional and knowledgeable occupational health practitioners;

- by understanding of the business priorities and business processes;

- by confidentiality issues being clearly defined;

- by regular communications between all parties;

- by having a clear understanding of the roles played by each party;

- by a fair process for giving advice and making decisions.

Most of these are self-explanatory or have been covered elsewhere. It is important that there is a fair process for giving advice and making decisions because the advice given by an occupational health practitioner can have a major effect on an individual's employment status. For example, the occupational health practitioner's advice may result in someone losing his or her job. It is therefore important that the process for giving advice is seen to be fair. This can be achieved through explaining what the process is, what criteria are used and what influences the practitioner when formulating this advice. In large companies this can be provided through written standards and protocols. For small companies it is less likely that there will be agreed processes. The occupational health practitioner will be able to advise on the criteria that they use.

Ethical practice in occupational health management

3.26 There are ethical dilemmas in the management of occupational health because the interests of all parties are not always aligned. An example of an ethical dilemma is where an employee's ill-health is having a negative impact on their productivity and their contribution to the business they work for. The employer may wish to discontinue their employment. For the employee this may have a deleterious effect on their long-term physical and mental health because of the effects of unemployment. The occupational health practitioner will often operate at this interface. Their role will be to recommend interventions to make it easier for the employee to achieve productivity levels acceptable to the employer, including perhaps advice on workplace adjustment and some negotiation with the employer about what those levels are. In some cases, however, the employee's job will be withdrawn, to their disadvantage, but to the advantage of the business.

Another example of an ethical dilemma is where the occupational health practitioner considers that the work, or something about the workplace environment, is contributing to an individual's illness, but the person refuses to give their consent for their manager to be told. The decision on how to act in this case will depend on the likelihood of others being harmed.

Managers need to be aware that occupational health practitioners:

• will see such issues as having an ethical dimension;

• will have access to professional guidance on ethical issues; and

• are encouraged to discuss ethical dilemmas with their professional colleagues.

The importance of maintaining confidentiality is discussed at 3.21 *et seq.*

Setting and monitoring standards

3.27   Standards are set to assist in delivering consistency of a service or product. There is emphasis in health care services on standards relating to clinical practice being based on evidence. This can be difficult to achieve, but some kind of effort should be made to base practice in evidence. It is easier to do this if there is a system in place for peer benchmarking and audit. There are standards relating to professional practice developed and published by the professional groups listed in the section on the occupational health team.

A good example of the standards that can be helpful in managing occupational health services are the standards relating to NHS Plus. The NHS offers occupational health services to external clients through an agency called NHS Plus. There are standards for NHS Plus applying to fundamental principles, delivery of services, facilities, people working for NHS Plus, business arrangements and professional conduct. These top-level standards are given below, at FIGURE 3. The more detailed requirements can be seen on the NHS Plus website (see http://www.nhsplus/). Even small companies may find these useful as they indicate the principles that should underpin occupational health service delivery on any scale.

An important principle in occupational health is that the person providing advice to an employer about an individual understands the nature of the work that the individual does. It is therefore important that the standards both of managing service delivery and of professional conduct include the requirement that occupational health practitioners keep up to date with the working conditions of the people they serve, and that they are enabled to do so.

Enforcement

Role of inspectors, the Health & Safety Executive and local authorities

3.28   Any workplace can be inspected by an inspector from either the Health & Safety Executive (HSE) or the Local Authority, to assess

Figure 3: Top level standards for NHS Plus service providers

Introduction

This document sets out the standards for NHS Plus service providers. The first part sets out the basic requirements and the second part provides amplification and further information. These standards will be subject to review.

Fundamental Principles
- NHS Plus providers must be able to demonstrate that they provide an adequate service to their NHS client.
- Each NHS Plus provider has documentary evidence that it has the full support of the employer (usually the Trust) to undertake external commercial work.

Services Provided
- NHS Plus providers publish a list of the services offered.
- Where standards exist relating to delivery of a service, they should be used.

People
- Each NHS Plus provider uses people who have the necessary qualifications and competencies to undertake their work.
- People in training are properly supervised.
- Sufficient support is available, either from the NHS Plus staff or from the employing Trust, to manage contracts and provide administrative support.

Facilities
- Facilities are appropriate to the service offered.
- All equipment is adequately maintained.
- Facilities are accessible to all, or the NHS Plus provider can demonstrate that it is working to meet this.

Business arrangements
- NHS Plus providers will have a written agreement about the services to be provided with each customer.
- There are arrangements for indemnification for all NHS Plus staff and contractors working on their behalf.
- NHS Plus providers can reject work.

Professional Standards
- Professional ethical codes are followed.
- Commercial confidentiality is maintained.
- NHS Plus providers have evidence that the business and professional practice complies with the requirement of clinical governance.
- NHS Plus service providers will, within a year of inception, take part in a local or regional audit group.

compliance with health and safety law. The responsibilities and powers to do this are bestowed by the *Health and Safety at Work etc Act 1974*. The nature of the inspector who calls depends on the type of workplace. There are many HSE inspectorates including those of Factories, Agriculture, Mines and Quarries, Printing, Construction, Nuclear Installations and Railways.

Local authorities have responsibility for inspection for all food preparation covered by food hygiene regulations, so even in workplaces usually inspected by an HSE inspector, the local authority environmental health inspectors can inspect if there is any food handling. The local authority is responsible for inspection of any HSE premises, and the HSE is responsible for inspections of local authority premises regardless of the nature of work undertaken. Local authorities also enforce in low-risk premises such as offices.

Inspections will tend to focus on the *Health and Safety at Work etc Act 1974, ss 2, 3 and 6*, namely:

- the general provision that risks are managed as low as reasonably practicable;

- that the risks to any people who may be affected by work activity are properly managed; and

- that work equipment is adequate and fit for purpose.

Inspectors have powers to enter premises, to examine and investigate as appropriate, to take measurements and photographs and make recordings, and to take samples of articles and substances. They can also seize and render harmless (by destroying or otherwise) any article or substance, they can require information to be provided to them and they can give evidence in legal proceedings.

Inspectors can give verbal advice, written advice, an *improvement notice*, a *prohibition notice* (which can be delayed or immediate) and they can prosecute. Where there has been a death, the crown prosecution service may prosecute.

Improvement notice

3.29   If an inspector considers that a person is contravening a relevant statutory provision or has done so and is likely to continue or repeat the contravention, he or she can serve an improvement notice directing that such action be remedied within a specified time.

Prohibition notice

3.30   If the inspector considers that an activity involves or will involve a risk of serious personal injury, he or she can serve a prohibition notice directing that the activity should not be carried on unless matters are remedied.

A person served with an improvement or a prohibition notice has a right of appeal. It is an offence to contravene any requirement or prohibition imposed by an improvement or a prohibition notice.

Employment Medical Advisory Service (EMAS)

3.31   The Employment Medical Advisory Service (EMAS) is part of the Health & Safety Executive (HSE) field operations directorate. It is regionally located and consists of qualified occupational physicians (medical inspectors) and occupational health nurses (occupational health inspectors). They have the same powers as regulatory inspectors and are involved in the investigation and inspection of premises. EMAS doctors act as expert witnesses for the HSE, Local authorities and Crown Prosecution Service (CPS) cases.

Reporting of Injuries, Diseases and Dangerous Occurrences Regulations

3.32   Employers, the self-employed and those in control of premises have a legal duty to report certain work-related injuries, diseases and dangerous occurrences under the *Reporting of Injuries, Diseases and Dangerous Occurrences Regulations (RIDDOR) (SI 1995/3163)*. In terms of managing occupational health it is important to have in place a mechanism whereby this legal duty can be met (the mechanism for reporting such events is detailed at 2.6).

One or more persons within the organisation should have responsibility for making any necessary reports and have the knowledge and understanding of the Regulations to know what to report and how to make the report. It is important to recognise that it is the employer's responsibility to report under *RIDDOR* and not that of the GP or Occupational Health department. The employer (or self-employed person) or a person in control of premises is the 'responsible person' who has the legal duty to report under the regulations. In practice, it is probably best for someone in the Human Resources or Personnel department to have the delegated authority to make the report as this is likely to be the central point within the organisation where it becomes apparent that someone is absent for a reason that requires reporting (including reporting under the three-day absence rule (see 2.3). However, if someone in the Human Resources or Personnel department is nominated with this responsibility then it is important that a mechanism exists within the organisation for accident and incident reports to be submitted to that person so as to report dangerous occurrences and acts of violence which may not have caused absence from work.

Case studies

3.33

Case study 1 – the bad company

John was 47 years old; he worked in an engineering workshop and had been off sick with depression for two months. His manager contacted him to say he wanted him to see the company's occupational health practitioner who worked in the company for one day each week. John had never attended for such a consultation before and wasn't at all sure what to expect. When he got there he found that although his manager had made the appointment he had not sent any referral information. John himself explained what was wrong, that he was taking anti-depressants, that he thought the depression had been precipitated by the death of his mother four months earlier and that he was feeling a little bit better but did not think he could cope with all aspects of his job yet.

John left the consultation without being clear what advice his manager was going to be given and didn't hear from his manager for another three weeks. In the mean time he saw his GP who gave him a certificate to remain absent from work for another four weeks. His manager then rang him to say that he'd received advice from the occupational health practitioner that John might be able to get back to work with some temporary modifications to his working hours and no need to supervise others until he felt well enough. John agreed to give this a try but wondered why it had taken three weeks to sort this out. He wasn't sure where he stood in terms of returning to work when the GP certificate was still advising him to refrain from work.

Comment

In this simple example the importance of communication is highlighted. Ideally John should have had a copy of the referral that his manager has made to the occupational health practitioner, but even if not he should understand what his manager is going to say. John may well have been able to get back to some aspects of his work at the time of his consultation. The occupational health practitioner would be expected to tell John what advice he or she was intending to give the manager. John himself could have rung his manager after the appointment; it can be useful to ask the employee to do this, rather than leaving all the responsibility to the manager. If someone feels well enough they can return to work before the GP certificate expires, but it is courteous to let the GP know.

Case study 2 – the good company

Amanda worked for a company of solicitors. She was coming up to her thirtieth birthday. Having worked for two partners, she had recently been working for three of the partners, typing up their reports. She discussed the implications for her workload with her manager and was confident that she could cope with this. After several weeks she noticed she was developing wrist pain each evening at the end of a hard day's work. A year earlier she had read the information her employer provided on how to set up her workstation and manage her work and had made some alterations to her workstation as a result. She had also been subject to a formal workstation assessment (under the *Health and Safety (Display Screen Equipment) Regulations 1992 (SI 1992/2792)*) as her employer had identified her as a heavy user of computer equipment. This assessment was satisfactory.

She checked with the office health and safety representative about what she should do about the wrist pain. The representative told her to tell her manager and ask for an immediate referral to the occupational health practitioner. This was arranged within a week; she attended for assessment and examination. She was reminded of the need for short but regular breaks from typing and was able to negotiate with her manager some temporary changes of work, swapping some typing with another colleague for photocopying. The occupational health practitioner gave her a note for her GP to put the GP in the picture. Her wrist pain got better but returned as soon as she reverted to the previous levels of typing at work. At her review appointment with the occupational health practitioner she mentioned that she had been also doing a lot of typing at home because she was doing a dissertation for a Masters degree. She hadn't mentioned this at the first appointment because it was very important to her and she didn't want to be told she should stop doing this.

The occupational health advisor obtained her permission to discuss the case with the manager and the three of them talked it through together. Following that discussion her manager was able to agree a distribution of typing between the office staff that took some of the typing load from Amanda and she made sure she stopped typing every hour for a few minutes. She asked the health and safety representative to remind her to do this. She remains well and now she has finished her Masters dissertation she is looking for a more demanding job.

Comment

Even this 'ideal' case illustrates the problems that can arise. This company not only has good management arrangements for DSE assessment, but apparently good relationships between managers and staff, a well-informed health and safety representative and fast access to specialist occupational health advice. Nevertheless, it isn't until the second appointment that Amanda admits she is doing things at home that are contributing to her symptoms.

4 Occupational Health Systems

Introduction

4.1   Some years ago an editorial in the British Medical Journal commenced with the statement that occupational health is like Paris: it means different things to different people. Therein lies the difficulty in writing this chapter on occupational health systems, for without agreement about what we are seeking to achieve, it is difficult to write about what is required.

It is acknowledged that less than 50% of UK employees are covered by occupational health services with any degree of specialist expertise. Some organisations do not require external professional expertise and rely on management input and experience to achieve its objectives. In certain situations, however, professional resources may need to be bought in, to deal with specific areas. Care, however, must be exercised in ensuring that the correct resources are selected.

The needs of the organisation will depend on many factors, and these may include:

- size of the concern;
- nature of the business;
- culture of the organisation;
- aims and objectives of the occupational health service;
- the occupational health services avalable.

This list is, by no means, exhaustive, as there is a host of additional influences on system requirements. At a more general level, the systems that are put in place are driven by three, clear, strategic influences:

- the legal requirements;
- professional advice; and
- business issues.

This chapter outlines a systems view of service organisations, such as an occupational health service. This is an essential pre-requisite to understanding how occupational health systems interface with the business and, more particularly, the workforce. The chapter then highlights some characteristics of service organisations, which are crucial to designing systems, and lastly reviews some examples of systems required as a result of the drivers identified above. The chapter concludes with a discussion of the considerations in setting systems up and utilising them for the mutual benefit of working men and women and their employers.

Characteristics of service organisations

4.2   Management experiences in manufacturing sectors cannot be translated simply to the service organisation. Service organisations are sufficiently unique in their characteristics to require quite separate and distinct management approaches.

The client/customer needs to be seen as a participant in the service process. The situation is quite different from, say, the output of a manufacturing system and thus, enlarges the concept of the system. The client/customer becomes an input, transformed by the service process into an output. A degree of satisfaction is usually associated with the transformation.

Service managers become responsible for both production and marketing in this open-systems view, with the client/customer as a participant. In manufacturing, production, marketing and finished-goods inventory roles are quite separate. Such an interface would neither be possible, nor appropriate.

Marketing performs two important functions in daily service operations. First, the consumer/service user is educated to play a role as an active participant in the service process. Second, it helps promote demand-smoothing, so that the service user and customer needs can more closely match service capacity. Marketing activity must be co-ordinated with scheduling staff levels and continual evaluation of the service process.

For services, the process is the product. The involvement of the customer in the service process makes the closed system approach of manufacturing impractical. The pace is, no longer, determined by the machine and the output cannot easily be measured to ensure compliance with the contract specification. Therefore, in service organisations, operations and marketing functions are usually more closely integrated.

Customers may arrive with differing demands. Hence, multiple measures of performance are necessary in any reasonable performance management system. Service employees interact directly with customers, in a manner that leaves little scope or opportunity for management intervention. Thus, services require extensive training and employee empowerment to act appropriately in the absence of direct supervision.

Furthermore, customer impressions are based on their total experience of the service, not just on the explicit service performed. Concern therefore, for employee attitudes and training is a necessity in service organisations, to ensure that quality is maintained. The customer's view of the service experience can include such matters from service facility design to the availability of tea/coffee and up-to-date magazines in the waiting areas. In the open-system concept, recognising the client/customer as a resource encourages active customer participation in the service process, which will increase productivity and in turn, create a competitive edge.

These comments are relevant to occupational health services. Firstly, in any occupational health service, the customer is not always the person who walks through the door. We need, perhaps, to distinguish the 'service user' or 'client' and the 'customer', who is more likely to be the employer. Second, the effective use of an occupational health service can only be possible with extensive education of both management and employees. Third, effective use of occupational health services will depend on recognition that personnel, whether they are physicians or nurses, need to adhere to their own professional codes of practice. Failure to accept that essential prerequisite will result in damage to the credibility of the occupational health service with the employees and possibly difficulty in retaining professional occupational health staff. Fourth, occupational health services are often benchmarked against other services and they are no exception in their requirement for multiple performance indicators. It is easy to monitor inputs and services provided. It is easy to monitor compliance in certain regulated areas or with service-level agreements expressed in terms of time and volume. It is not easy to monitor outcomes and effectiveness. This has serious effects when attempting to evaluate the use and benefits of an occupational health service to the company and for this, different and more complex approaches are necessary. The provision of an effective occupational health service, therefore, takes place, not exactly in the department premises, but throughout the company, at all levels. This situation is exceptionally difficult to monitor.

The unique characteristics of the occupational health service introduce special challenges for its providers: their product is intangible, time-sensitive and simultaneously provided and consumed. These actions, coupled with the client/customer access, discussed above, suggest that it is time to materially alter the view of the 'product' most appropriate to the occupational health service. Their unique selling point is advice and the provision of first-class advice to the business that is timely, relevant and practical remains the most valuable 'product' that an occupational health service can make available to its employers or, indeed, increasingly, to customers in occupational health services which have a multiple client portfolio.

Setting up systems

4.3   Setting up systems for occupational health practice is no different from the establishment of any other project within a business. Many managers, however, find that the involvement of health issues makes the process intimidating and their lack of knowledge and familiarity with this area may prevent them reaching decisions calmly and rationally.

To begin with, one should be clear about the need which has to be fulfilled. Is it a legal obligation? If so, under what Act or regulation does this arise? Before making any decision, ensure that the appropriate, Approved Code of Practice or other Health & Safety Executive (HSE) advice has been taken into account. If it is not a legal requirement, what are the benefits to the company of the output from this system? If it is aimed at reducing, say, sickness absence, then the benefits are clear. If it is just a matter of convenience, it is equally necessary to be clear, always ensuring that priority is give to those systems that fulfil legal obligations before those that are simply 'nice to have'.

Thus, systems must have clear aims and objectives. Within these, there must be a clear understanding of how the system will work. Thus, for instance, how will staff actually receive their first aid training? How will the sickness absence information be collected throughout the company? More particularly then, what will be done with the information? Will it be used to close the feed-back loop and lead to a programme of continuous quality improvement? Or will it simply be there to rest on file?

In order to manage a new system, resources will be needed. It will be necessary for the decision-maker to make an explicit assessment before deciding whether or not the additional work in implementing and maintaining the system can be absorbed within existing resources.

Lastly, the system should be capable of measurement. The HSE has produced a guide ('Successful Health and Safety Management', HSE, 1997) aimed at those organisations that understand the principles of occupational health and safety management and wish to improve their existing approach to performance management. The framework considers how to measure performance, in such a manner which goes beyond reliance on injury and ill-health data alone. The guide can be found at http://www.hse.gov.uk/opsunit/perfmeas.htm.

First aid

4.4   Since the *Factories Act 1961*, an employer has been required to make provision for the management of sudden illness and injury at work. Despite occupational health being a protective and preventive discipline, the business will naturally turn to this function for professional advice in an area where relatively few line managers will feel at ease.

First aid requirements are now set out in the *Health and Safety (First Aid) Regulations 1981 (SI1981/917)* (as amended 1997). The requirements contained in these regulations should not be confused with enforced altruism. Employers may be required to demonstrate compliance during enforcement visits or inspections from the Health & Safety Executive (HSE).

First aid is defined in *Regulation 2* and covers the management of injury or illness, pending the arrival of definitive medical care. It also includes the treatment of minor injuries that do not require the intervention of a doctor or nurse.

The first aider must hold a valid certificate of competence in first aid at work, issued by an organisation whose training and qualifications are approved by the HSE. These are not restricted to the voluntary aid societies, such as St John's Ambulance. In-house courses may be possible, to be provided by the occupational health service and subject to certain restrictions and prior approval by the HSE. A number of commercial courses are also available, provided both in-house and off site.

An employer is required, under *Regulation 3(1)* to provide appropriate equipment and facilities to be rendered when necessary. Contrary to popular belief, this does not extend to provision of a first aid room. Under *Regulation 3(2)*, the employer has an obligation also to provide suitable and sufficient numbers of first aiders, trained and qualified to standards approved by the HSE. Lastly, by virtue of *Regulation 4*, the employer must inform the employees of the arrangements for first aid, including the locations of equipment, facilities and personnel.

Minimum requirements

4.5   First aid sets out to reduce the effects of injury and sudden illness at work. Provision must be adequate and appropriate for 'all the circumstances'. First aid personnel and facilities should therefore be available:

- to give immediate assistance with both common injuries and illness or those likely to occur from specific hazards encountered whilst at work; and

- to summon an ambulance or other professional help as necessary.

There is no fixed level of provision prescribed in the *Health and Safety (First Aid) Regulations 1981(SI 1981/917)*. The exact level of provision depends on the circumstances in each workplace. However, it is recommended that the minimum first aid provision for each work site is as follows:

- a suitably-stocked first aid container;

- an appointed person to take charge of first aid arrangements; and

- information for employees on first aid arrangements, most usually by way of a first aid notice.

The manager is in the best position to assess the department's needs. This may require consideration of the following factors:

- workplace hazards and risks;

- size of the workforce for which the manager is responsible;

- the accident history of the workforce in that location;

- the nature and distribution of the employees;

- the remoteness of work locations from emergency medical services;

- the accessibility of the work location to the emergency medical services;

- the needs of peripatetic workers and others who work alone; and

- annual leave and other absences of those with responsibilities of the provision of first aid.

The risk assessments carried out under the *Management of Health and Safety at Work Regulations 1999 (SI 1999/3242)* are particularly relevant here. Information gleaned from these sources may help by informing management of the consequences of, and first aid needs of, failing control measures. For carrying out risk assessments, see further CHAPTER 10.

Whenever staff are working on the employer's premises, either first aiders or 'appointed persons' will need to be present. Two or three persons will need to be trained for these roles and all shifts must be covered. *SI 1981/917* does not go so far as *requiring* a formal written assessment of first aid provision; however, it is always important to record the basis for a decision, not least in case managers need to justify their provision of first aid in the future.

Assessing the risks

4.6   Clearly there are a number of issues to consider in assessing first aid. Principal amongst these are identification of the risks of injury and ill-health arising from work, as has been identified at 4.5. First aiders will be required, if these risks are in any way significant.

One would also need to consider any specific risks arising from work that is carried out in the department in question. For example, handling of hazardous substances, dangerous tools, dangerous machinery, loads or animals. Under these circumstances, first aiders may require specific training. There may be a need for extra first aid equipment, precise siting of first aid equipment, or informing emergency services. Under some circumstances, a first aid room may, indeed, be an appropriate facility to put in place, although it is recalled that this is not a legal requirement. The department itself may have varying levels of risk, in which case, these will need to be identified. Therefore, the provision of first aid may be different throughout the department. If there are large numbers of people employed in the location in question and the accident risk is high, then first aid may well be required.

Managers, in assessing these needs, will need to consider accidents or cases of ill-health that have occurred over the previous twelve months. They should take into account their nature and location where they happened. First aid may need to be located in certain areas, or indeed, the contents of the first aid box may need to be considered. Similarly, consideration must also be given to any inexperienced employees, employees with disabilities or those with special health problems.

If the premises for which the assessment is being carried out is spread over several buildings on the site or multi-floor occupancy, provision will need to be considered for every building location or each floor. It is not sufficient to have first aid provision in a nearby building. Similarly, if there is shift work, or out-of-hours working, first aid provision will be required for all shifts and at all times.

If the workplace location is remote from the Emergency Services, they (both Fire and Ambulance Services) should be informed of the business' concerns and any special arrangements considered jointly. Members of the public, work-experience trainees or employees with reading or language difficulties will need to be considered in the provision of first aid.

Employees working off site

4.7 Managers frequently forget their obligations to meet the first aid needs of employees who work away from their main employment base; and those who travel regularly or travel elsewhere, eg those staff who are involved in, say, inter-site transportation. Employers vehicles should carry first aid kits and drivers should be trained in the basic principles of first aid, if not required to have a full in-date certificate. Consideration should also be given to personal communications facilities for them.

Members of the public

4.8 Although not specifically required to do so by the *Health and Safety (First Aid) Regulations 1981 (SI 1981/917)*, managers should also consider the public in making their assessment of need and consequent provision for them. This is unlikely to be covered by employers' liability insurance cover, but will usually be incorporated into public liability policies. This has two important consequences. First, both public and employees are included in first aid provision, it is essential that the standard is not allowed to fall below that required by the Regulations. Second, where public provision is included, account needs to be taken of other legislation and guidance, such as the *Road Traffic Act 1988*.

Contents of the first aid kits

4.9   A minimum stock of first aid items normally include:

- A leaflet giving general guidance on first aid.

- Twenty individually wrapped, sterile adhesive dressings of assorted sizes, appropriate to the type of work. This should be of detectable blue colour type for food handlers where appropriate.

- Two sterile eye-pads.

- Four, individually wrapped, triangular bandages, preferably sterile.

- Six safety pins.

- Six medium-sized, individually wrapped, sterile, un-medicated wound dressings (12 × 12cms).

- Two large, sterile, individually wrapped, un-medicated wound dressings (18 × 18cms).

- One pair of sterile gloves.

The contents of the first aid container should be modified only on the advice of an occupational health service.

Typically, travelling first aid kits, for staff who are mobile, should contain the following:

- A leaflet giving general advice on first aid.

- Six individually wrapped, sterile adhesive dressings.

- One large, sterile, individually wrapped, un-medicated wound dressing (18 × 18cms).

- Two triangular bandages.

- Two safety pins.

- Individually wrapped, moist, cleaning wipes.

- One pair of disposable gloves.

Practical issues to be considered

4.10   The following is an outline implementation plan:

- Carry out needs assessment.

- Draw up first aid policy and agree with appropriate committee, usually Health and Safety Committee.

- Decide on role and function of the 'competent person'. Normally they are required to summon an ambulance. Some organisations find it worthwhile to train them in basic life-support as an aide to the first aider.

- Decide on who should co-ordinate these arrangements. If an occupational health service is available, this would seem appropriate.

- Decide on first-aid requirements of those who travel, or are away from site. Special attention should be give to those who travel overseas or in remote areas. This needs to be seen as a fundamental part of their pre-trip briefing.

- Identify a supplier of suitable first aid supplies and decide on a means of distribution.

- Arrange a process for replacing used items in the kit and decide whether or not it is worthwhile identifying the circumstances of their use as a means of feed-back.

- Implement the system as agreed with safety representatives and the workforce.

- Provide a process to ensure training is kept up-to-date. First aid skills that are not often exercised are known to be lost in two to three years.

- Ensure arrangements for reporting events and reasons for their use are being implemented. Such follow-up may have implications for improving training, as well as overall occupational health and safety in the business facility.

- Consider formation of first aid group to provide mutual support and feed-back for those with limited experience. This need not be elaborate, but an employer might consider an annual training day or even just a simple newsletter to encourage communication and sharing of experience.

Sickness absence

4.11   The control of sickness absence is the responsibility of management, not the occupational health service. The presence of a mild or moderate degree of ill-health, however, should not automatically mean that the affected person will take time off work. Other factors of which managers should be aware may make significant contribution to absence levels. TABLE 1 sets out the business case for taking a serious interest in controlling sickness absence.

A small reduction in the level of absence attributed to sickness can contribute considerable value to the organisation or business. Thus, in this hypothetical company, a small reduction of 2% in overall sickness has a pay-back in the order of £3.4 million.

It is important to distinguish between the persistent, intermittent, short-term

Table 1 – Benefits of reducing sickness absence: a hypothetical case study

Assumptions:			
Number of staff	12,475		
Number of working days per annum	230		
Pay bill		£1,722 million	
Value of working day (average) = £1,722 million / (12,475 × 230) = £60			

	Absence level		
	Actual 6%	*Target 4%*	*Saving*
Estimated loss due to absence (days) = 6% × ??	172,155	114,770	
Estimated total costs of absence	£10.3 million	£6.9 million	
Therefore, savings from achieving sickness absence target ie reducing sickness level from 6% to 4% = £10.3 million – £6.9 million			= £3.4 million

absences, which are not linked with a consistent medical condition and where an employer may argue 'substantial reason' for dismissal and genuine, long-term, acute or chronic sickness absence. There is a duty on management in respect of the latter, to seek alternative employment where a return to the original job is impossible.

Where there is residual disability, minor modifications to the original job may aid an employee to return to work, particularly where occupational injury or disease is responsible. In these cases, decisions must be demonstrably based on reasonable actions. Managers must have sought appropriate medical advice including that of the occupational health service. Employers are not expected to create a vacancy. Equally, it should not be assumed that an employee would or should be prepared to take any job on offer.

Contributory factors

4.12   The reasons for sick leave are often highly complex and usually influenced by non-medical factors. The level of absenteeism may be associated with such factors as age, gender, personality, domicile, working conditions and sickness benefits.

Sickness absence increases with age, but the patterns will be different. Below 20 years of age, an employee is likely to have a higher frequency of short-duration absence, particularly in their first five years of employment, a difficult transition period from home and school. Absence becomes a coping mechanism for stress which is probably related to difficulties encountered in integrating into the team, living by new rules and the necessity of learning new techniques, processes and procedures. With increasing age, any absences tend to be longer in duration, reflecting the possible onset of more serious ill-health.

Absence rates are consistently greater in females than in males, related to social and domestic responsibilities, rather than illness. Department of Social Security statistics suggest that there is a higher number of claimants for sickness and invalidity benefit amongst women under 30 years of age, compared to men of the same age group. This usually correlates with the ages of starting a family.

Matching personality to a job has become an important issue. Psychological assessment, aptitude tests and even more speculative techniques, such as handwriting analysis and astrological forecasts, have been employed to fit 'round pegs into round holes'. There is now a major industry built around training and accrediting non-psychologists in certain psychometric tests. A mismatch between job requirements and personality, particularly where team work is involved, can lead to dissatisfaction and eventual sickness absence.

Working conditions may be more important than social and demographic factors in influencing absenteeism. Dull, unrewarding employment, with low status, or work which may be hazardous, stressful and physically demanding are all relevant. Unskilled workers have three times the sickness rates of that for managerial grades.

The size of the work group has been shown to be important. The larger the group, the more anonymous each individual becomes. Reorganisation into small groups, where each worker has responsibility for a particular component of the end product has been shown to raise morale and self-awareness and reduce absenteeism. The downside of this approach to organisation of work is that it does raise costs. However, the message is clear. The feeling of being welcomed and needed is important, and the attitude of the manager may play a part in how quickly a sick employee decides he or she is ready to go back to work.

The length of sickness absence is often related to factors including the company sick pay scheme, the length of employment and the number of hours worked per week. Organisations, providing fully-paid sick leave for six months, followed by half-paid leave for six months, may know from experience that employees often return when their fully-paid sick leave entitlement expires, independent of their health status. Part-time, low paid workers may even be financially better off on sick leave as their statutory sick pay may open the door to individual additional benefits, increasing their income to greater than when at work.

Patterns of sickness absence

4.13   In very general terms, sickness absence can be broadly split into two types, long-term and short-term. Neither has a clear definition. Long-term absence includes absences of several weeks or more. Short-term absences, on the other hand, relate to single days or spells of absences, or absences lasting less than a few weeks. However, where organisational policies are concerned, it is essential that a difference is defined in explicit terms, as referral and management actions will be triggered by the type of absence that is recorded and the definition within the policy.

The importance of trigger points in policy formulation is considerable. Organisations which have a policy of six months' paid sick leave, might, for example, benefit from a trigger point of three months. However, many would consider three months to be too long a period of time before investigation and referral. Thus, 14 or 28 days is frequently taken as the threshold for the beginning of an investigation.

Clearly, not all cases warrant investigation, particularly where an outcome is more easily forecast: for example, somebody who has been off because of a hospital admission due to acute appendicitis, will be returning in due course. Herein lies a downside of using definitive trigger points for investigation. Obviously, a balance has to be struck and, hence, to avoid unwarranted demand on the limited resources of an occupational health service, there is much to be gained from maintaining a system of initial discussion between, say, the Human Resources manager and individual line managers before triggering investigations by the occupational health service. Even though the likelihood of a return to work is often improved by early intervention of the occupational health service, this is most likely only where there is sufficient management flexibility in arranging alternative and more appropriate forms of work.

Short-term sickness absence is more often associated with self-limiting conditions. The question of substance abuse and problem drinking may also need to be considered. Long-term sickness absence, on the other hand, will be more often associated with significant medical problems. Short-term absenteeism, which becomes frequent is usually unpredictable and, therefore, more disruptive to production or service delivery. Most people regard it as more amenable to management control than long-term sickness absence might be.

There remains, however, the possibility that short-term sickness absence may mask a significant medical problem. Hence, discussion with the occupational health service or a referral of the employee to their GP might be of value. Repeated short-term sickness absences may well be due to factors in the workplace. Studying sickness absence patterns, therefore, will be of assistance to managers, who are increasingly responsible for assessing workplace risks. Identification of such factors will be far more important than a mechanistic and disciplinary approach to managing sickness absence.

Sickness absence is too often regarded as a disciplinary issue and little interest is paid to it as a symptom, worthy of investigation. For these reasons, sickness absence is not solely an occupational health issue. An approach that combines perspectives of human resources, line managers and occupational health, including the collection, collation and analysis of sickness absence data can be extraordinarily productive.

Measurement

4.14   Comparatively few companies regularly collate sickness absence data; fewer identify the causes; and still fewer identify specific diagnoses in any formal way. Nonetheless, sickness absence is repetitive and requires measurement of both the duration and frequency. Both measurements need to be compared in order to decide on the most appropriate management response.

Two core concepts

4.15   In the measurement of sickness absence, there are two essential elements which lie at the heart of this activity. First, there is the notion of *incidence*. The incidence is the number of new cases arising during a defined period, usually one year. Second, there is the *prevalence*, which is the number of cases that exist in the community at any one time. If the period is limited to, say, one day as a sickness absence measurement, this is known as *point prevalence*. If it is over a longer period, it becomes known as *period prevalence*.

The difference is minimal when dealing with acute cases which are usually of short duration. In chronic diseases, the duration of illness is increased reflecting a wider difference between point and period prevalence.

Mean number of spells per person

4.16   A spell of absence is usually defined as an uninterrupted period of absence, irrespective of its duration. All spells of sickness absence should be included in any calculation or system aimed at systematic data collection; indeed, if a system is designed for absence management, then *all* absences, of whatever nature, should be recorded. Any subsequent analysis could be based on those absences which did not have prior authorisation. The measure is also known as the *spell inception rate*. It is a measure of the frequency of an employee taking spells of sickness absence during the period in question, usually one calendar year. The mean number of spells per person in the period under analysis, is calculated as the total number of new spells of absence, commencing in the period as numerator and the average population at risk during the period as denominator.

Mean number of spells per person =

$$\text{Mean number of spells per person} = \frac{\text{Total number of new spells per person in calendar year}}{\text{Population at risk}}$$

Severity

4.17 The severity of a disease is expressed by the duration of sickness absence. It is expressed as the mean number of days of absence attributed to sickness per person in the period, again normally one year. The rate is calculated as the total number of days' absence attributed to sickness in the period, expressed as the numerator and the average population at risk during the period as the denominator.

$$\text{Severity rate} = \frac{\text{Total number of days sickness absence per annum}}{\text{Population at risk}}$$

These rates are usually calculated for a twelve-month period and during this time, the population will vary as there will be new recruits and others will leave. Thus the population will vary in size over the course of the year and this must be taken into account in calculating the average: see 4.19 for the methods to be adopted in making this calculation.

The duration of absence is normally counted from the first or substantial part of a day that the person is absent. The final day is counted as the day preceding the day of return to work, or the day preceding the day the employee is retired/dismissed/dies. In quoting these rates, it must be clear whether or not one is counting calendar days or actual working days or hours lost, as comparison would not otherwise be justified.

Prevalence rates

4.18 Prevalence rates of sickness absence can be calculated for defined periods and is known as the point prevalence rate. It is calculated from the number of persons absent on a day as numerator and the population at risk on that day as denominator. These rates are particularly useful when attempting to identify the progress of epidemics or days or periods in a business when absenteeism is particularly high or low.

The rate can be calculated thus:

$$\text{Prevalence rate} = \frac{\text{Number of persons absent on the day}}{\text{Population at risk}}$$

Population at risk

4.19   In calculating these rates, there is a need to estimate the population 'at risk'. This means the number of people at risk of taking absence in an organisation throughout a defined year. It is actually a head-count and should include part-time staff as well as full-timers but it also includes people leaving the organisation or joining it during the year under consideration. There are three options for arriving at an estimate of the population at risk.

If the working population is stable, a mid-year census would suffice. A second option might be a mean of four, quarterly population figures. A third, and indeed the preferred, option would be a mean annual population, taken from a computerised payroll, which would be derived from person, months or days for salaried and weekly-paid staff, for every individual employed, for some or all of the twelve months under study.

Frequency distribution

4.20   It should be readily apparent to the more numerate reader that the distribution of both the number of spells per person and their severity (duration) will be highly skewed, a pattern repeated in most organisations. The following breakdown is now widely accepted as a rule of thumb for any one year:

- roughly one-third of the staff will take no absence at all;

- roughly one-third will take a few short-term spells, usually self-certificated; and

- roughly one-third of employees in an organisation will take a longer absence, usually medically-certificated.

As a result of these distributions of absence, it is found in most organisations that about half the total absence is caused by less than one-tenth of the workforce. For these reasons, sickness absence policies need a commitment to record information about absences, so that the problem can be managed effectively, without being excessively intrusive to the individual, or time-consuming for the management.

Instead of imposing a single threshold for referral arbitrarily identified for universal application throughout the company, the distributions can be used to determine appropriate standards for attendance and trigger points for management interviews and referral for occupational health advice. It is relatively easy to calculate the median number of days and spells and the number exceeded by 5, 10 or 20% of the employees with the worst absence records, thus informing any decision about setting manageable trigger points for action. Other companies devise scoring systems which relate to thresholds for management action. The best known of these is the Bradford score. This is calculated as n^2D where n is the number of spells and D is their total duration. The score is heavily influenced by short-term sickness absence, which is more disruptive than long-term. Some organisations investigate those with a defined level of score – say 1,000.

The usual tests of statistical significance rely on the so-called 'normal distribution' and therefore cannot be used in sickness absence data, being generally highly skewed. It may be possible to compare proportions of individuals with particular absence characteristics, such as high or low-absence duration or frequency, using techniques such as the chi-square tests or other non-parametric statistical tests.

Percentage working time lost

4.21   Calculating the number of those absent on a given day as a percentage of those who are scheduled to attend is a common statistic measured by managers. Another variant is the total number of scheduled hours lost, attributed to sickness as a percentage of the total number of hours scheduled to be worked. Daily rates are often averaged over any period to give a picture of the trend in absence and the severity. The data can be used to set targets and compare performance amongst units. They can be useful in budgeting for the costs of sickness absence and setting management improvement targets. They are *not* helpful in identifying short and long-term sickness absence or in defining causes, whether medical or organisational. Nevertheless, the figure is often encountered in managerial workforce reports.

Setting up the system

4.22   Companies setting up measurement systems for absence management must decide whether they will record calendar or working days lost. The loss of calendar days method is more representative of true incapacity rather than absence from work, which it tends to over-estimate because of the inclusion of weekends. The working days lost method reflects more accurately the direct financial losses to the business and potential impact on production and service provision. When comparing a company's sickness absence experience with either published studies or that of another organisation, it is necessary to ensure that one is comparing like with like. It may be necessary to apply a small correction factor to a rate derived from a study based on calendar days to apply it to a company which measures working days.

Age, gender and occupational status needs to be included in any systematic measurement of sickness absence if the data is to be of any use.

Many organisations believe that the extra hassle from attempting to classify the reasons for absence should be avoided. This is a bad mistake. It is not too difficult to devise a classification system which will need to accommodate all authorised absences, lateness, self-certificated sickness absence and medically-certificated absences.

Recording the medically certified absences may appear intimidating to many, but it is not too difficult to perform with the aid of a medical dictionary. However, there are more complex classification systems available, where medical advice is to hand, such as the World Heath Organisation's International Classification of Diseases ('ICD-10').

Case management

4.23   The role of the occupational health service in case management is first, to determine whether the absence is associated with a specific medical condition and, secondly, to obtain an accurate diagnosis. Frequently, this requires contact with the individual's own GP, as well as the occupational health service.

The individual must give a written, informed consent, when the occupational health service is seeking a report from their GP in relation to their health status. There are some who argue that written, informed consent is also necessary when individuals are referred formally to the occupational health service. This is particularly important to avoid any misunderstanding, should circumstances become contentious at a later stage. It also ensures that individuals come to the occupational health service fully informed of the reasons for their referral and likely implications. All that is needed is a consent for the referral to take place and for a report, based on that consultation, to be made available to the manager.

In seeking consent for a report from his or her GP, an employee needs to be understand the implication of the consent and the use made of the information contained in the report. This must include the fact that it will serve as the basis for a report to their manager, which may result in work modification, medical retirement or other consequence. (See also 2.23 and 3.21 *et seq.*)

In no other area of occupational health practice is the difficulty of an occupational health service more amply illustrated. Many companies take the view that they who 'pay the piper, call the tune'. Occupational health professionals, irrespective of whether they are doctors or nurses, see their role differently. The occupational health service can be most effective if there is a climate within the company in which many referrals are informal, at the request of an individual employee, rather than mandatory referrals from management. For these reasons, the self-referral rate is frequently regarded as a representative figure of the standing and credibility of the occupational health service within the workforce. Clearly, the role of work in the origin and pathogenesis of these conditions becomes quite important and can become embroiled in any subsequent litigation. It is essential for the occupational health service to ensure that any statements made in clinical records and in reports to management concerning conditions that are work-related, can be fully substantiated on clinical grounds.

Managing sickness absence – an integrated approach

4.24   Once a system has been set up and quarterly reports created, covering incidence, severity and prevalence rates, causes, the worst 5% (or other percentile such as 10 or 20%), median duration of sickness absence, pay lost, etc, these can be distributed to unit managers. In addition, monitoring the unit's position in the hierarchy of the company in terms of absence management control can often be helpful in spurring managers on towards a more effective approach.

These quarterly reports should help establish the size of the problem and where the problem units lie within the organisation. As the percentage of working time lost increases and the mean spells per person rates go down, this would be regarded as sufficient evidence of an increase in long-term sick leave. This should prompt an early case-conference with the occupational health service to identify causes and agree an action plan.

Having determined the size of the problem, its concentration in specific units, areas or occupational groups needs to be assessed. Summarising the severity of sickness absence in frequency terms by individual operational units will give an idea of a problem in any given location. A similar analysis across units by occupational category might contribute to identifying the cause.

That units or occupational groups categories have such peaks of sickness absence may be due to the health of individuals, their system of work, their working environment, or their relationship with the organisation. Appropriate investigations should always begin with discussions with the occupational health service. These help determine whether or not there are any factors relevant to the situation under discussion. Thus, for example, a change in the working system of a group of data entry operators, such as the introduction of new equipment, may result in an increase incidence of work-related upper limb disorder. It is not necessarily the introduction of new equipment; simply a subtle change in practice may have a similar effect. A factory used to making light, summer dresses may have similar experiences, if the employees are suddenly required to work on heavy denim.

Appropriate interventions need to be decided jointly in discussion with line managers, human resource specialists, the occupational health service and any other stakeholders. Once the agreed action plan and measures have been introduced, the impact needs to be evaluated and a reduction of sickness absence in the target groups needs to be clearly identified.

In the design and delivery of *absence control action plan*, the occupational health service may contribute by, for example, having more frequent case conferences to deal with an anticipated increase in numbers of referrals from one particular work location found to have excessive sick leave patterns. Occupational health professionals may help in establishing measurement systems to check that the response is timely and appropriate. Support and advice to management may be provided to enable appropriate questions to be asked at relevant management interviews to ensure as effective a solution as possible.

Combining the talents and perspectives of line management, occupational health services and the human resources department is, perhaps, the most effective means of dealing with absence problems in working units. It is simply not acceptable to pass 'sickness absence cases' to the occupational health service in the mistaken belief that the occupational health service has the appropriate solution. The occupational health service uses other means to deal with absence problems, including presentations (ie 'tool-box' talks) on personal health or health promotion issues. Where joint approaches have been used involving all interested parties, reductions of over 50% in sickness absences burdens have been achieved. This writer believes that this has as much to do with the unified involvement of all stakeholders as it has with the actual measures introduced.

Occupational health professionals may have some difficulty with the notion of case conferences, raising as it does a tension between advice and confidentiality. Liaison is vital between the occupational health team and line managers in managing absence and is a fundamental necessity in its effective control. At such liaison meetings, actions can be agreed and progress in individual cases monitored. A case conference approach is an obvious response to the situation, where progress of cases can be discussed on a regular, say monthly, basis. However, participants should realise that such conferences must be undertaken without revealing clinical details. The emphasis in discussions will need to concentrate on functional and temporal interpretation of clinical assessments. By bringing all disciplines together, much can be done to agree individual responsibilities and actions in each case of absence. Involving managers from different functions within the organisation may facilitate cross-functional placement of those with temporarily or permanently impaired health and help to maximise appropriate placement of individuals and minimise appropriate re-training and recruitment costs.

Reporting workplace accidents and ill-health

4.25   Laws have been in place for many years requiring the notification of accidents in the workplace. It was not until 1980, however, that a set of regulations was introduced which applied to all premises where people were employed, requiring notification either to the local authority or the Health & Safety Executive, and not only of major incidents, but also of dangerous occurrences. Subsequently, in 1983, the statutory sick pay scheme was introduced, which shifted the burden of short-term sick pay from the Department of Social Security to the employer, effectively removing the automatic procedure for notifying the Government of minor injuries at work. Identification of occupational risks of contracting disease was also essential for the informing of subsequent occupational health policy. Further regulations were made in 1985 and were again up-dated in 1995, replaced by the current regulations, the *Reporting of Injuries, Diseases and Dangerous Occurrences Regulations 1995 (RIDDOR) (SI 1995/3163)*. These current regulations place a duty on the employer or other person in control of work premises to report accidents in the workplace. *RIDDOR* is more fully-discussed in CHAPTER 2.

The legal duties under *RIDDOR* make it essential that there is a robust system for reporting of diseases, accidents and dangerous occurrences within the organisation. The system is likely to be less than sufficient unless there is 'buy in' from senior management within the company. It is, for example, most likely to be effective if all reports are to be incorporated into quarterly performance reports, required by divisional or senior management within the company. That is to say, reporting is made a part of the management line and not something that is peculiar to the health and safety system to be reported routinely to the health and safety committee. A reliable and comprehensive reporting system is essential.

Those companies, ie those which have health and safety officers, are likely to have robust systems in place for the reporting of accidents. Relatively few will have similar systems of sufficient character and efficiency to report diseases. Collation of reportable events not only contributes nationally to the proper informing of policy, but also constitutes a means of surveying and maintaining health surveillance of the workforce as a whole.

Occupational health services are often asked to accept responsibility for reporting accidents and disease. It is often argued that this may bring the duty of confidentiality of each health professional towards the workers into conflict with their duty to the employer. Others will, instead, follow the view that it is in the interests of both the employer and the employee to comply with legal obligations and inform national policy.

Monitoring hazards and ill-health

4.26   Today's worker is more likely to carry out a greater variety of tasks which involve potential or actual exposure to a greater variety of hazards to health, than, say, 30 years ago. Attempting to identify a likely cause of an adverse effect has, therefore, become a significantly more complex task. Appropriate action to prevent further injury has, equally, become more difficult. Preventing ill-health in the workforce rests on an identification of workplace hazards and control of subsequent exposures to levels which are deemed to be as low as reasonably practicable. The sheer complexity of many workplaces demands a systematic and integrated approach to avoid wastage of resources and inappropriate action.

More particularly, within the UK, chemical hazards are controlled by the *Control of Substances Hazardous to Health Regulations 2002 (SI 2002/2677) (COSHH)*. Other hazards, such as noise, manual handling and ionising radiation are covered by specific legislation. All other workplace hazards are covered by the *Management of Heath and Safety at Work Regulations 1999 (SI 1999/3242)*, the *Health and Safety at Work etc Act 1974* and by the common law duty of care. These constitute significant pressures on employers, who have no option but to respond with a system that encourages regular and thorough in-depth review.

The management of hazard, therefore, can be broken down into several stages; and in this model we break it down into four stages:

Identify ➜ Assess ➜ Control ➜ Recover

Such an approach should be applied by line managers to locations or activities within location, under their responsibility. It will require professional input from many other disciplines associated with occupational health and safety. In order that line managers can be assisted with delivery of an action plan with clearly assigned priorities, ie what needs to be done to comply with legal obligations and the company objective of preserving the health of their workforce. Staff involved in this operation should become part of the risk management process not only for the information they can provide and education they received but also so that there is a sense of shared ownership over the activities.

For further discussion of the risk assessment process, see CHAPTER 10.

Stage 1 – Identifying the presence of hazards

4.27 Identifying hazards requires a thorough knowledge of the workplace activity. Precisely how this is achieved will depend very much on the nature and scale of the operations involved. A 'walk-through' survey may be all that is required but on occasions, more detailed techniques will be necessary. Essentially in this stage, the manager is required to consider what can happen. It may be useful to know the history of the workplace; perhaps, such matters as sickness absence, accident experience or dangerous occurrences that have taken place. When considering the nature of the operation, it is also important to consider the nature of the tasks being carried out by individuals. For this analysis to be reliable, it is not sufficient to rely on job descriptions, which have a habit of not actually reflecting what goes on in the workplace. The phenomenon is known as 'job creep'. Thus, any systematic investigation of hazards on the shop floor should involve a task analysis of individual workers, to reflect the present situation, in essence, a risk assessment as required by the *Management of Heath and Safety at Work Regulations 1999 (SI 1999/3242)*.

Stage 2 – Assessing risk

4.28   The second stage requires an assessment of risks. Here, the manager is required to consider the likelihood of harm and the consequences of exposure. Again, this is likely to require professional input, in terms of probability and a description of the consequential damage.

Stage 3 – Controlling risk

4.29   The third stage requires control of the risks. Professional input may be required from occupational health staff, particularly including toxicologists and occupational hygienists to ensure that the risks are adequately controlled. Control measures include:

- elimination of hazard;

- substitution of hazard;

- enclosure of source;

- local exhaust ventilation;

- general ventilation;

- isolation or segregation of source;

- reorganisation of work procedures;

- personal hygiene; and

- personal protective equipment.

Thus, this third stage is aimed at the prevention or minimisation of exposure. It is a management decision whether exposure needs to measured before control philosophy is adopted. However, many hygienists would say, if there are limited funds, the funds should be directed towards control, rather than exposure surveys. It is acknowledged, however, that this is very much a personal decision to be made by the individual manager at the specific time, depending on the circumstances with which they are confronted.

Stage 4 – Recovery

4.30   Similarly, in the fourth and last stage, recovery, professional input will be needed, particularly from occupational hygienists and a medical professional as well as engineers and production specialists. The aim of this part of the system would be to limit the consequences of exposure, with a view to mitigating adverse effects. The engineers and production specialists would need to assist in reinstatement of operations procedure.

This sort of approach should be applicable to both current and new activities. In enlightened companies, an occupational health opinion will be sought at a design stage for any new facilities, thus maximising the value of experience and minimising the need for potentially expensive 'retro-fitting' in the event of later problems.

Categorising risk

4.31   Assessment of workplace risks to health is arguably best achieved by considering the significant tasks involved in a given work activity, identifying the acute and chronic hazards to health posed by all chemical, physical, biological and ergonomic agents or stressors present and estimating the likely exposures involved in each task. Thus, enabling the appropriate choice of control measures to be made. Other procedures are possible, such as those based on the review of individual hazards, but the task-based health risk assessment has a widest applicability and the least chance of overlooking a significant hazard and thus, a potentially significant risk to health. Also, experience has shown that it is the most efficient approach in the majority of circumstances. The focus should not only be on the process associated with the task, but also on any associated ancillary tasks, such as preparation and clearing up afterwards. Account will also need to be taken about other tasks being taken out in the vicinity and deciding the impact, if any, they will have on the operator of the particular task under investigation.

After this, the probability of occurrence needs to be determined to decide the degree of risk and therefore, the need for control measures. Such measures should include, not only those to prevent over-exposure, but also controls to mitigate the consequence of any that might occur.

Several methods are available to determine risk and thus, the need for control, but the use of some form of risk matrix has become increasingly popular as a screening technique. Thus, adverse health effects can be rated in Categories from I–IV, as follows:

- I = Potentially fatal as a result of either acute or chronic exposures.
- II = Irreversible health effects.
- III = Reversible effects, but with temporary consequences of concern.
- IV = Reversible effects.

Where insufficient or no data are available the default rating II is usually used.

Exposures are rated from A to E.

- A = Exposures likely to exceed the relevant occupational exposure limit.

- B = 50–100% of the occupational exposure limit

- C = 10%–50%.

- D = 1%–10%.

- E = Exposures unlikely to exceed 1% of the limit.

Again, a default rating B is recommended if adequate information is unavailable.

The hazard rating is then plotted against the exposure rating in a risk matrix, with action priorities depicted in the matrix as:

- Category 1 – requiring intervention.

- Category 2 – requiring improvement of existing systems.

- Category 3 – requiring existing systems to be maintained.

The following matrix is derived from a hypothetical case study:

Table 2: Risk matrix

	Health effect				
Exposure rating	A	B	C	D	E
I	1	1	1	1	1
II	1	1	2	2	2
II	1	2	2	2	2
IV	2	2	3	3	3

The decision to improve or simply maintain control measures is of course, dependant on the nature of the exposure and many other influences besides. However, the matrix is an aid to decision-making and assists in the assignment of priorities. More sophisticated analyses and more complex ratings can be devised at will. What is needed, however, is a system that shows progressive improvement in exposure control.

Risk management processes will require access to information on the probabilities of specific events and the nature and severity of the likely consequences. Depending on the complexity of the activities under review, such information may be available within the organisation, using the knowledge and experience of managers and the workforce. In most cases, however, specialist occupational health advice will be needed and may require significant access to information systems. Small and medium-sized enterprises may well need to 'buy in' external resources.

It is a well-recognised experience that situations change with the passage of time and such formal hazard and risk assessment need to be regularly carried out to ensure that any system devised is maintained up to date. However, it should be recalled that identification of risks requires action. In the event of a personal injury claim arising within the factory of concern, formal risk assessment need to be disclosed as part of the pre-trial discovery process. Failure to act or demonstrate an intention to act on these risk assessments can be held to be negligent. Risk assessments are for action, not for filing.

Health surveillance

4.32 The legal obligation of an employer is to provide a safe place of work. The relevance of this to accidents is well established and the management of accidents within workplaces is well known. Difficulties, however, come with managing ill-health, because the relationship to the workplace is often not as clear-cut as that of workplace accidents. More particularly, it becomes less clear when the effects are not so acute as otherwise one might expect.

Individual health status

4.33 One of the easiest ways of monitoring the impact of ill-health is to assign a health status to every member of staff. Assuming that an occupational health service is available, most members of staff, who are at work, will be considered fully fit for their role, but others will have certain work restrictions applied to them, eg, no heavy lifting, etc. This situation can be summarised in a simple classification scheme, amended to meet the needs of any workplace.

A simple example might include:

- fit for work, without restriction (F_1);

- suitable for work, but subject to work restrictions as listed (F_2);

- temporarily unfit, but to be reviewed in a specified period of time (U_1); and

- permanently unfit (U_2).

A term needs to be assigned to each of these classes such as that introduced in parentheses. It is a simple matter to collate information along these lines in a spreadsheet. Thus, as a performance indicator and report to management, the percentage of people in each category over the period in question would be an index of 'the impact of' ill-health within the business.

More closely related to performance will be the changes in status within the period in question, and the percentage of people transferring from one state to another would be an indication of the performance of the occupational health service, depicting a change in the level and health status of the individual. The approach is very much that taken in the Armed Forces.

Where records of sickness absence, which are diagnosis-specific are maintained, it is not too difficult to derive some information from such systems, relating to ill-health. However, at all times, one must be clear that sickness absence is a complex phenomenon, which is only partly due to ill-health. In a computerised system, it is not too difficult to derive a report for all absences in excess of one week or else all absences medically certified and thus obtain an analysis by occupation or job/work category and unit within the company. In the event of the system being based on working days, a correction will need to be applied to the rates in order to give a closer estimate of morbidity (see 4.34). The method depends on a computerised system being available and of course, every attention being paid to its limitations.

The system can be improved by following the incidence of conditions, particularly relevant to the occupations followed by the workforce in the business. There are a number of well-known lists of such sentinel health events classified by their degree of prevention, which may be useful in this respect. Reportable diseases and their associated working conditions would be a useful source for the identification of such conditions.

Medical retirements are a management procedure, which reflect the impact of ill-health on working capacity. A file of medical retirements can provide useful information on the nature of ill-health that affects working capacity. Thus, the incidence of medical conditions that result in ill health retirement can be benchmarked against other organisations carrying out similar activities and the general population from whence the workforce is drawn. This may give important clues about working conditions and their impact on the business.

Thus, a simple, descriptive analysis of the future years lost by disease-category may help assign priorities to future control strategies. Future years lost can be computed simply by subtracting the age at retirement from the normal retirement age. Thus, this simplified analysis consisting of incidence and future years lost by disease category, when presented to a board, can do a great deal to focus the mind in relation to the impact of ill-health on working capacity. It is even amenable to financial impact analysis.

Death in service

4.34 The last level of ill-health monitoring is the so-called 'deaths in service' file. Death certificates are often needed for pension schemes and identifying the cause of death should be a relatively easy exercise concerning those who die whilst in service. Nonetheless, this may well represent further evidence of the impact of working conditions on the ill-health of the workforce and monitoring the deaths in service is appropriate. Ideally, this will be easiest where an occupational health service is in existence. However, this is not absolutely necessary. Maintaining a 'death in service' file is a relatively simply exercise, which can be compared to the population at risk as identified above and the resulting rate monitored on an annual basis. Fluctuations that are not paralleled in the local community, where it is likely that most of the workforce is recruited, should raise suspicions among senior management, there being a problem in the workplace that warrants investigation.

A combination of deaths in service and sickness absence is often termed 'medical wastage'. This is particularly found in older literature. This should not, therefore, be taken literally for the reasons outlined above. But, the use of a death file has much to commend it, since the occurrence of death is a clear and explicit event, without the uncertainty surrounding morbidity episodes. It also allows the cause to be verifiable.

Safety representatives

4.35   The Robens Committee in 1972 recommended that worker-participation in health and safety should be put on a statutory footing ensuring that good practices are disseminated widely and not restricted to a few enlightened employers.

The *Health and Safety at Work etc Act 1974, s 2(4)* provides that regulations be made for the provision of appointment by recognised trades unions of safety representatives from among the employees and that those representatives shall represent the employees in consultation with the employers. The *Safety Representatives and Safety Committees Regulations 1977 (SI 1977/500)* and Approved Code of Practice 1977 finally came into force in 1978. New, general provisions were added to the 1977 Regulations by a Schedule to the *Management of Health and Safety at Work Regulations 1999 (SI 1999/3242)*.

Every employer must consult safety representatives in good time about the introduction of changes in the workplace, health and safety information, training and so on. He must also provide them with reasonable facilities and assistance. The employer must not dismiss or discriminate against a safety representative who is doing his job in good faith.

In a case before the European Court of Justice, *Commission of the European Communities v United Kingdom [1994] ECR 1–02435*, the European Court held that a law that imposed an obligation to consult workers, but excluded a large percentage of the workforce, was contrary to EU law. The Government's response was the *Health and Safety (Consultation with Employees) Regulations 1996 (SI 1996/1513)*, which now provides that where there are employees who are *not* represented by safety representatives, the employer shall consult those employees in good time on matters of health and safety, either directly or through elected representatives for each group. Each representative must be consulted, given information and provided with training in the same way as a trade union representative. Clearly however, such representatives will not have the benefits of a trade union behind them and it calls into question whether or not they can be as effective as the union-backed representatives. They are protected against victimisation by the *Employment Rights Act 1996*.

Union-appointed safety representatives should be notified in writing to their employers and should normally be employees with at least two' years service. Numbers will depend on the nature of the workplace and the levels of risk. It is the duty of the employer to consult them on matters of health and safety. They also have a right to reasonable time off, with pay, for training.

They have the powers to investigate potential hazards and dangerous occurrences and to routinely inspect the workplace or part of it on giving reasonable notice in writing to the employer of their intention to do so, usually every three months. This can be more often if there have been substantial changes in the working conditions or new information. In the event of a notifiable disease or accident, they have the right to inspect the scene as long as it is safe to do so.

Statutory regulations provide that a safety representative, although liable to prosecution as an employee, under the *Health and Safety at Work etc Act 1974, ss 7* and *8*, shall not be under any additional legal duty by virtue of exercising his functions as a safety representative. A representative who forgot to mention to the manager dangerous fumes reported to him by an employee, will not be legally liable for that failure. A safety officer would have no such immunity.

Safety committees

4.36 Every employer, if requested to do so by at least two safety representatives, must establish a Safety Committee. Safety committees should be concerned with relevant aspects of health and safety and welfare of employees at work in relation to their working environment. The functions of a safety committee could include:

- study of accidents, diseases, statistics and trends, so that reports can be made to management, with recommendations for improvement;

- liaison with HSE inspectors or similar;

- discussion of reports from safety representatives;

- development of work safety rules and safe systems of work;

- monitoring the effectiveness of safety training; and

- monitoring the adequacy of safety and health communications in the workplace.

Occupational health and safety personnel should be ex-officio members of the committee. However, the active participation and membership of the committee should involve both worker and management representatives.

Employers and safety committees alike would be well-advised to take into account that health and safety is a concern of everyone associated with the business, employer and employee alike. There is, therefore, little value in confrontation or in not sharing information with one's partners. Failure to do so clearly places one side or the other at a disadvantage, instead of leading to co-operation and speedy resolution of the issue under discussion, to the benefit of the workforce. Both will lose.

Bringing in a consultant and not involving safety representatives, staff or their representatives will of course, be counter-productive. Co-operation in these matters will be extended to the benefit of all concerned.

Where there is a regular programme of safety inspection, they are often led by safety officers. Involving line managers and safety representatives and other members of the safety committee has several distinct benefits. First, it increases the chances of detecting any likely problems. Second, it sends a message to workers of the concern expressed by everybody involved in the business. Third, it ensures shared ownership of the problems confronted. With strong, professional leadership, a mutual concern for both the business and employees, health and safety need not be an issue for collective bargaining, but an issue that brings together employers and employees alike.

Conclusion

4.37   This chapter has looked at the nature and characteristics of a service organisation and how these apply to an occupational health service. An occupational health service sits at the interface between employer and employee. As health professionals, their prime concern remains with people, whilst taking into consideration the needs of the business. Their ethical standards ensure that the occupational health service maintains credibility and integrity amongst the workforce, without whose co-operation they would fail in providing value to their employers. Employers, equally, have an interest in maintaining that unfettered communication channel, because without an occupational health service and the provision of high-quality health advice, managers would make decisions, which were less informed, often impractical and may well have adverse outcomes.

Occupational health systems need clear aims and objectives, related to the *purpose* of the occupational health system and the needs of the company. Without these being explicitly put in place, it is likely that the implementation and maintenance of systems, examples of which have been included in this chapter, will be nothing but meaningless activity.

5 Biological Hazards

Introduction

5.1   Biological hazards are those which arise from exposure to materials of a biological origin. Sometimes these are viable pathogenic organisms, and in the case of bacteria and viruses the risk of exposure is therefore one of infection. Frequently biological hazards arise from exposure to substances which originate from living organisms and cause ill-health most often because of an allergic reaction to the substance. In the working environment we are exposed to a wide range of such materials depending on the nature of the work but including animal dander, plants, fish and crustaceans, moulds, wood dusts and pollens. All materials of biological origin, including infectious micro-organisms, come within the definition of 'substances', under the *Control of Substances Hazardous to Health Regulations 2002 (SI 2002/2677) (COSHH)*, and therefore require a risk assessment to be undertaken (see CHAPTER 10).

This chapter deals with a range of hazards of a biological nature and explains how these substances can affect employees and what needs to be done to recognise and control the risk to health.

Legal requirements
Control of Substances Hazardous to Health Regulations 2002

5.2   Under the *Control of Substances Hazardous to Health Regulations 2002 (SI 2002/2677)* the employer is required to assess the risk to employees and others affected by the work (*Regulation 6*) and identify and instigate protection measures, such as safe work practices, safe equipment, immunisation to protect their health (*Regulations 8* and *9*). As with all health and safety matters, employees must be given adequate information, instruction and training on any risks to their health and the measures required to protect them (*Regulation 12*). Employees are expected to adhere to any control measures implemented to protect their health.

Under *Regulation 11* employers are required to undertake health surveillance when there is a reasonable likelihood that the disease or effect may occur under the particular conditions of the work and there are valid techniques for detecting indications of disease or the effect. In some circumstances a health record may be all that is required, in others, the health surveillance will need to be carried out by a medical professional (occupational health physician or nurse).

Management of Health and Safety at Work Regulations 1999

5.3   Employers are responsible under the *Health and Safety at Work etc Act 1974* and the *Management of Health and Safety at Work Regulations 1999 (Management Regulations) (SI 1999/3242)* for the protection of employees, the public and anyone affected by the organisation's work. In order to comply with the legislation employers must, in consultation with their employees and safety representatives, undertake an assessment of the risk, identify the measures required to control the risk, communicate their findings to all relevant parties and review the effectiveness of the control measures on a regular basis.

Employer's duties under the *Management Regulations* overlap with those under the *Control of Substances Hazardous to Health Regulations 2002 (SI 2002/2677) (COSHH)* with regards to the need to undertake risk assessment and implement controls. Risk assessment is not required twice and would only be expected under the requirements laid down in *COSHH* and its Approved Codes of Practice.

There is a requirement, however, under the *Management Regulations* to provide local safety policies and codes of practice covering accident/incident reporting procedures and safe working practices.

Reporting of Injuries, Diseases and Dangerous Occurrences Regulations 1995

5.4   The employer is required to report to the Health & Safety Executive (HSE) any diseases cited as 'reportable' under the *Reporting of Injuries, Diseases and Dangerous Occurrences Regulations 1995 (SI 1995/3163), Sch 3* in order to provide a national record of occupational diseases. The following biological (and in some cases chemical) hazards referred to in this section are reportable to the HSE on Form F2508A:

- occupational asthma from a range of stated agents;

- extrinsic alveolitis;

- occupational dermatitis from a range of stated chemical agents;

- skin cancer;

- folliculitis;

- acne (from mineral oil, tar, pitch or arsenic);

- any accidental contact (ie puncture by a contaminated needle) with a blood borne virus that is likely to cause severe human illness must be reported as a 'dangerous occurrence';

- hepatitis (A, B, C or D) due to their work;

- legionellosis;

- anthrax;

- brucellosis;

- avian chlamydiosis;

- ovine chlamydiosis;

- leptospirosis;

- lyme disease;

- Q fever;

- rabies;

- streptococcus suis;

- tuberculosis; and

- any infection attributed to work with animals or potentially infected material from animals.

For method of notification, see 2.6.

Public Health (Infectious Diseases) Regulations 1988

5.5   Under the *Public Health (Infectious Diseases) Regulations 1988 (SI 1988/1546)* any diagnosed cases of anthrax, leptospirosis and rabies must be notified to the local authority.

Respiratory and skin disorders

Introduction

5.6   Although not always biological in nature, this section will consider respiratory and skin irritants and sensitisers, respiratory and skin infections. All of these conditions could require permanent redeployment of the affected individual, lead to chronic ill-health and may even be fatal if uncontrolled or unnoticed. The following guidance will provide information on what respiratory and skin disorders are relevant in the work setting, risk assessment, the legal duties of the employer and employee and where to seek further information.

Respiratory disorders

5.7   A *respiratory irritant* is a substance that can cause irritation at the site of exposure if exposed in sufficient concentration and/or over a sufficient period of time. Common respiratory irritants are gases such as ammonia, chlorine and sulphur dioxide which may show immediate or delayed symptoms. Others such as nitric oxide, phosgene, fluorine and ozone may cause delayed symptoms (48–72 hours after exposure) of pulmonary oedema leading to respiratory distress.

A *sensitiser* is a substance that can trigger an allergic reaction in the respiratory system leading to occupational asthma. It may be of chemical, metal, animal or plant origin and once sensitisation has taken place, further exposure to the substance, however minimal, will produce symptoms. Sensitisation is unpredictable, as only some individuals at risk will be affected (5–25%) and the effect may be latent, occurring after months or years of exposure. Symptoms tend to disappear once exposure has stopped, but will return on re-exposure even after years of avoidance. Symptoms may occur immediately on exposure or be delayed several hours. This is relevant, as workers may not realise their condition is related to work if symptoms occur in the evenings or during the night. However, any reports that the condition improves during days off or holidays would lead to suspicion that the condition was related to work. Different substances sensitise at different concentrations. Research studies are being undertaken to identify what the 'safe' levels are for some of the main sensitisers but no safe levels have been identified to date.

What are they?

5.8   The symptoms of respiratory sensitisation are asthma, rhinitis and conjunctivitis. Asthma is characterised as periodic bouts of wheezing, chest

Table 1: Substances most frequently responsible for occupational asthma

Substance	Work activities
Isocyanates	Vehicle spray painting; foam manufacture
Flour, grain or hay	Harvesting, milling, drying, malting, handling flour, grain or hay (bakers, dock workers, farmers)
Soldering flux (colophony fume)	Welding, soldering, electronic assembly
Laboratory animals (urine and dander)	Handling laboratory animals
Wood dusts (African teak/ iroko, western red cedar)	Sawmilling, woodworking, carpentry
Glues and resins	Any activity curing epoxy resins

tightness and breathlessness caused by constriction of the airways due to the immune system's response to the presence of a certain substance. Rhinitis is a constantly runny or stuffy nose and conjunctivitis is watery and prickly eyes, symptoms similar to hay fever but constant irrespective of the season. Rhinitis and conjunctivitis (and sometimes a dry cough) could lead to asthma if the contact with the substance continues and should not be ignored.

Other substances which can cause sensitisation include:

- antibiotics (ampicillins, penicillins, cephalosporins);

- inorganic substances (chromium, cobalt, nickel, platinum);

- organic substances (glutaraldehyde, azocarbonamide, carmine, chloramine T, certain reactive dyes);

- animal origin (cockroaches, crustaceans, egg proteins, cow or pig skin or urine, storage mites);

- plant or microbial origin (latex, mist form oil-in-water cutting fluids, castor bean dust, green coffee bean dust, guar gum, henna etc; and

- proteolytic enzymes (amylase, cellulase, bromolein, papain, subtilisins, xylanase).

Respiratory diseases resulting from inhalation of biological substances, that may occur in the work setting include extrinsic allergic alveolitis, legionnaires' disease, hypersensitivity pneumonitis, asthma.

Extrinsic allergic alveolitis

5.9 Extrinsic allergic alveolitis is a collection of conditions (farmers lung, bird-fanciers lung, mushroom pickers lung) which share the same symptoms irrespective of the external agent. The symptoms present as a flu-like illness, developing over a four to six hour period, with pains in the limbs, fever, dry cough and shortness of breath (dyspnoea). Significantly there is no wheeze. After two to three days the symptoms subside but the symptoms will return on repeated exposure to the external agent (mouldy hay spores, bird droppings, mushroom compost). Repeated attacks can lead to chronic changes in the lungs and progressive respiratory lung failure.

Hypersensitivity pneumonitis

5.10 Hypersensitivity pneumonitis (HP) is a term used to describe a collection of respiratory symptoms caused by repeated exposure to bioaerosols of microbial or animal origin. The term is sometimes used to include some of the conditions listed as extrinsic allergic alveolitis (see above), but is more accurately concerned with conditions caused by microbiological contamination of metal working fluids (MWFs) and mists from standing water (found in humidifiers).

The symptoms of HP range from an acute flu-like illness with cough, possibly leading to recurrent bouts of what appears to be pneumonia, to a chronic shortness of breath on exertion with a productive cough and weight loss. Symptoms can develop four to twelve hours after exposure. The disease can progress over a few weeks or a few years and will improve or show a complete recovery if exposure is stopped at an early enough stage. Prolonged exposure, however, could lead to permanent lung damage.

The reduce the risk of employees developing HP, control measures must be implemented to avoid the multiplication of microbiological agents in humidifier mists and metal working fluids and employees educated about the risks and how to avoid them. Health surveillance may be required.

Endotoxins

5.11   The term endotoxin refers to a portion of the outer wall of gram-negative bacteria which is associated with respiratory symptoms (cough, chest tightness, shortness of breath, inflammation) and fever, headache, nose and throat irritation. Gram-negative bacteria occur naturally in the environment and endotoxin levels have been detected in air, dust and water. Endotoxin exposure is highest when the water containing the endotoxin is aerolised. This most commonly occurs at wastewater (sewage) treatment sites, within agricultural settings and industrial waste processing settings.

The risk of exposure to endotoxins can be reduced by limiting employee exposure to aerolised contaminated water, adequate ventilation and provision of respiratory protection. Any respiratory symptoms should be investigated to identify the cause and controlled accordingly.

Legionella

5.12   Although the incidence of legionnaires' disease usually affects the general population rather than employees, the employer has a responsibility to protect the public from the operations of the business. Legionnaires' disease, which originates from the legionella bacteria, is widespread in the environment and is found in natural sources of water including lakes, rivers and streams. The bacteria are also found in many re-circulating and hot/cold water systems found in large buildings such as hotels, hospitals, offices and factories. Despite this, infection by the bacteria is unlikely unless a series of events occur which leads to the bacteria multiplying in large numbers and breathable droplets being created. Multiplication of the organism is encouraged where the water temperature ranges between 20–45ºC and there is sludge, scale, rust, algae or organic matter to provide nutrients. Breathable droplets are formed in cooling towers and air conditioning systems where water is used to cool or warm air, or in hot/cold water systems such as showers, spa baths or indoor water features.

The symptoms of legionnaires' disease include high fever, chills, headache and muscle pains. The sufferer may have a dry cough and most experience breathing difficulties, about half may become confused and delirious and one third also develop diarrhoea and vomiting. Legionnaires' disease can be treated with antibiotics, but can be fatal in 12% of reported cases; this figure rises if the population is particularly susceptible (elderly, immuno-suppressed, chronically ill, smokers).

Assessing the risks

5.13 Legionella cannot be prevented from entering water systems, but risk assessment should be used to identify and control high-risk operations. The precautions required to reduce the risk include:

- pipes and cisterns should not allow water to stand undisturbed for long periods;

- cisterns should be covered to prevent dirt and debris entering, and should be inspected periodically;

- water temperatures should *not* be kept between 20–45°C. Hot water should be stored at 60°C and cold water protected from the heat;

- cooling towers need to be well designed, maintained and operated to avoid the risk of legionella building up and being transmitted into the environment;

- cooling systems should be cleaned and disinfected at least every six months; and

- cooling system water should be treated to prevent a build up of scale, corrosion and microbiological growth.

In addition to the legal requirements stated at 5.2 *et seq*, there is an HSE Approved Code of Practice and Guidance for the control of legionella bacteria in water systems ('Legionnaires' disease: The control of legionella bacteria in water systems', January 2001). This should be consulted if any of the water systems noted above are within the workplace.

Skin disorders

What are they?

5.14 A *skin irritant* is a substance that can cause irritation at the sight of exposure if exposure is sufficiently prolonged or the substance is in sufficient concentration. Common skin irritants are some acids and alkalis, soaps, detergents and some solvents. Skin irritant chemicals may be identified on the chemical data sheet by one of the 'risk phrases', for instance R38, R34, R35 or R66 (for the complete listing of risk phrases, see 6.12). Some chemicals can cause deep burns (hydrofluoric acid) or acne (cutting oils and chlorinated napthalenes). Once exposure is removed the inflammation, dryness or cracking the chemical has caused will heal and the condition may not return on subsequent exposures unless the contact is again sufficient and prolonged. Repeated episodes, however, could leave the skin susceptible.

The symptoms of skin sensitisation are inflammation (redness and swelling), defatting (loss of the skin's natural oils) leading to dry, cracked and scaly skin, blistering and sloughing of the skin layers. The symptoms of allergic contact and irritant dermatitis are similar and it may not be possible to determine the exact diagnosis without medical consultation and skin testing.

The following substances are commonly responsible for skin sensitisation:

- epoxy resins;
- germicidal agents such as hexachlorophene;
- mercury and its salts;
- nickel and its salts;
- cobalt and its salts;
- rubber accelerators and antioxidants;
- formaldehyde;
- dyes such as paraphenylenediamine;
- topical anaesthetics such as procaine;
- dichromates.

Occupational groups that have been shown to carry the greatest risk from occupational skin conditions are:

- catering and food processing;
- hairdressing;
- cleaning;
- construction;
- rubber;
- engineering;
- agriculture;
- printing;
- health care; and
- offshore.

Assessing the risks

5.15 Following the principles laid out by the HSE guidance 'Five Steps to Risk Assessment' (HSE, 2002), the employer should:

- Look for the hazards

  Identify whether there are any respiratory or skin irritants or sensitisers in the workplace by considering the nature of the work undertaken and the tasks of those involved (see list of possible occupational groups and agents known to cause health effects). Consult the data sheets for all chemical and biological agents in the workplace to identify all with risk phrases relating to health effects.

  The most notable are:

  o R37: 'Irritating to the respiratory system';

  o R38: 'Irritating to the skin';

  o R42: 'May cause sensitisation by inhalation';

  o R43: 'May cause sensitisation by skin contact';

  o R49: 'May cause cancer by inhalation'; and

  o R66: 'Repeated exposure may cause skin dryness or cracking'.

  (For the complete listing of risk phrases, see 6.12.)

  Consultation with employees and safety representatives may reveal hazards that are not obvious at initial assessment. All stages of the work process must be considered from the point of delivery through to the distribution of a product or the disposal, cleaning, disinfection and sterilisation of any waste or by-product.

- Identify who might be harmed and under what circumstances

  Identify each category of employee (and others affected by the work) who may be at risk given the agents identified under any of the risk phrases listed above. Consider all staff from delivery through to disposal or distribution.

- Evaluate the risk and whether current precautions are adequate

  The most important part of the process is to *assess the likelihood* that any of the agents used in the workplace will cause respiratory or skin problems and *whether existing precautions and control measures are sufficient*. Factors such as how often and how large the contact with the agent must be considered. The number and variety of individuals involved should also be noted. Disease, accident data and 'near miss' records may indicate which areas are at greatest risk and where additional control measures are required.

- Measures to prevent and control the risks should be detailed in the assessment under the *Control of Substances Hazardous to Health Regulations 2002 (SI 2002/2677)*. These might include:

o Substituting an alternative substance that carries no or less risk, to health.

o Changing the work method (fully enclose, automate process) so that exposure is no longer a factor.

o Providing adequate local extraction and ventilation.

o Minimising the chance of spills, leaks or other escape of hazardous agents.

o Providing personal protective equipment required (masks and gloves appropriate to the agent exposed, overalls, aprons, goggles, etc).

o Training and providing information for employees about the hazard involved, the safe working procedures and personal protective equipment required for the task, what symptoms to report and what will happen if they are found to have an occupational condition.

o Providing hand washing facilities to include hand cleaner that is designed to remove the agent without unnecessary abrasion or de-fatting.

o Implementing health surveillance to detect early signs of disease, monitor the effectiveness of control measures and comply with *Regulation 11*.

Once the risk assessment has been completed and adequate control measures and precautions identified, record the findings in writing and ensure that the risk assessment is reviewed and revised when necessary.

5.16

Case study 1– Risk assessment in a bakery

Scenario

A 45-year-old man has worked in the bakery trade for the last 17 years working on the fancy pastries section making danish pastries and chelsea buns. He was not a smoker and had no pre-employment history of asthma. He complained of increasing breathlessness, wheezing and discomfort that had become increasingly obvious over the last two years. He also complained of runny eyes and sneezing which he had always attributed to hay fever. He found that the wheezing worsened during the course of the week, but sometimes the symptoms did not start until late in the evening or at night. There was a definite improvement during annual leave. When the baker consulted his GP he was treated for asthma and referred him to a specialist for investigations into flour dust allergy. The results showed that he was allergic to flour and the disease was reported to the HSE. The company was investigated by the HSE and found to have failed to assess the risks from flour dust.

What the risk assessment should have considered

- The hazards:
  - Flour dust, known to be a respiratory sensitiser and listed as a reportable condition under the *Reporting of Injuries, Diseases and Dangerous Occurrences Regulations 1995 (SI 1995/3163) (RIDDOR)*.
  - Specific HSE document relating to risk assessment and flour (EH72/11) has been published.
  - Long-term exposure limit, $10mg.m^{-3}$, short term exposure limit, $30mg.m^{-3}$.

- Who might be harmed and under what circumstances?
  - Workers on the pastry line who generate flour dust clouds due to pastry making procedures.
  - Cleaners who clear the excess flour from floors and surfaces.
  - Maintenance personnel who work on bakery equipment involved in dry mixes.

- Evaluation of risk (assessment of who is at risk):
  - The flour dust levels during the making of pastries exceeded the long-term time weighted average of $10mg.m^{-3}$.
  - There was no extraction near to the source of the dust generation.
  - No personal protective equipment was issued (dust masks).
  - Flour could not be substituted with another substance.

- Review existing precautions and assess what additional measures required:
  - Provide extraction (local exhaust ventilation) near to the source of the flour dust.
  - Provide and enforce the use of dust masks or respiratory protection.
  - Move the worker who is affected by flour dust to a less dusty area or retire on health grounds if sensitive to even minute concentrations.
  - Commence regular respiratory health surveillance conducted by medical personnel.
  - Inform, train and instruct all employees on the hazard involved, how to protect themselves (train all of the bakers not to generate so much dust during pastry making), what symptoms to report and what will happen if they do suffer with a work-related condition.
  - Keep a written record of the findings and safe working procedures required.

Blood borne viruses

Introduction

5.17   Blood borne viruses (BBVs) are carried in the blood and body fluids of infected humans and may be passed on to others. BBVs can cause anything from mild to very severe disease or, in some cases, individuals may display no symptoms at all, but become carriers. Occupational contact with BBVs is relevant to a range of occupations (see 5.18) and will require an adequate risk assessment to be carried out and appropriate precautions introduced to protect the workforce. The following guidance will provide information on what blood borne viruses are relevant to the work setting, risk assessment, the legal duties of the employer and employee and the action to be taken following a possible contact and infection with a BBV.

What are they?

5.18   The main BBVs of concern in the workplace are hepatitis B virus (HBV), hepatitis C and hepatitis D viruses and Human Immunodeficiency Virus (HIV). Hepatitis B, C and D all cause inflammation of the liver, which may be severe, debilitating, and could lead to chronic ill-health. Infection with the HIV may lead to Acquired Immune Deficiency syndrome (AIDS) which affects the immune system and leads to recurrent, severe and sometimes fatal infections or cancers.

The viruses are found in blood, semen, vaginal secretions and breast milk. Contact with other body fluids such as urine, faeces, saliva, sputum, sweat, tears and vomit are only a minimal risk unless they contain visible blood. BBVs are mainly transmitted by direct exposure to infected blood or body fluids through unprotected penetrative sexual intercourse, innoculation (ie penetration with needles, sharp instruments, broken glass), contact with broken skin (open wounds, eczema,) or splashes into the eyes, nose or mouth.

Work areas and workers at risk:

- health care (nursing and medical staff, pathology technicians, cleaners, chiropodists and anyone in contact with blood or body fluids);
- workers in the Emergency Services (police, ambulance, fire, rescue workers);
- custodial services (police officers, prison officers, cleaners);
- funeral services (embalmers, morticians and crematorium workers);
- laboratories (forensic scientists/technicians, research scientists/ technicians, cleaners) ;
- social services (particularly workers involved with drug abusers, prostitutes);

- local authority services (street cleaners, refuse collectors, public lavatory cleaners, park maintenance, house clearance workers);

- sewage treatment (sewerage and sewage treatment workers, maintenance personnel);

- plumbing and drainage clearance;

- tattooing, ear or body piercing;

- beauty and hairdressing salons (particularly beauticians using needles as part of the treatment); and

- first aiders.

This list is not exhaustive: other jobs that may involve contact with blood or body fluids in such a way that contamination could occur should be risk assessed.

Assessing the risks

5.19   Following the principles laid out by the HSE guidance 'Five Steps to Risk Assessment' (HSE, 2002), the employer should:

- Look for the hazards

  Identify whether there are any BBV hazards in the workplace by considering the nature of the work undertaken (potential contact with blood or body fluids contaminated with blood, semen, vaginal secretions and breast milk) and the tasks of those involved (see list of possible occupations). Consultation with employees and safety representatives may reveal hazards that are not obvious at initial assessment. All stages of the work process must be considered from delivery through to distribution or disposal, cleaning, disinfection and sterilisation.

- Identify who might be harmed and under what circumstances

  Identify each category of employee (and others affected by the work) who may be at risk. All stages of the work process must be considered from the point of delivery through to the distribution of a product or the disposal, cleaning, disinfection and sterilisation of any waste or by-product. There is a legal duty for organisations to inform all contractors of the risks on site and the need for health surveillance. The provision of health surveillance is the responsibility of the contractor. The implications of accidental spillage and contamination by BBVs must also be considered.

- Evaluate the risk and whether current precautions are adequate

  The most important part of the process is to assess the likelihood that BBVs will cause ill-health problems and whether existing precautions and control measures are sufficient. Factors such as how often and how large the contact with blood or body fluids may be must be considered and the number and variety of individuals involved. Accident data and 'near miss' records may indicate which areas are at greatest risk and where additional control measures are required.

• Measures to prevent and control the risks should be detailed in a safe system of work. This should include:

o Prohibition of eating, drinking and applying cosmetics in work area.

o Prevention of puncture wounds (the introduction of alternative equipment designed to avoid the chance of puncture wounds should be considered).

o Prevention of injuries from other sharps such as glass, metal, scalpels, scissors by the introduction of alternative materials, blunt ended scissors, self-shielding implements.

o Protection from splashes into the eyes and mouth by the provision of visor, goggles, safety spectacles or mask or the adaptation of work procedures (eg avoiding hosing or high pressure water jetting).

o Avoidance of contamination of clothing by provision of suitable work-wear (water-resistant if needed) and adequate arrangements for their decontamination or disposal. Arrangements should be made for contaminated clothing to be washed by a reputable cleaning company (not at the employee's home) at a temperature of at least 80ºC, dry cleaned at elevated temperatures or incinerated.

o Provision of rubber boots or plastic overshoes to be worn if floor is likely to be contaminated.

o Procedures to contain and decontaminate contaminated surfaces. HIV has been found a risk of infection in dried and liquid blood for several weeks and HBV is even more resilient. The methods should be identified and include the appropriate chemical disinfection solution (usually hypochlorite, formaldehyde or gluteraldehyde substitutes) or heat (autoclaving, boiling or dry heat) to be employed. More detailed information on decontamination of waste is available in the guidance 'Protection against blood-borne infections in the workplace: HIV and hepatitis' (HSC Advisory Committee on Dangerous Pathogens (ACDP), HSC, 1995).

o Procedures for the disposal of contaminated waste. Information about disposal may be obtained from the local Environment Agency office (general enquiry office tel: 0845 9333111 or Scottish Environment Protection Agency Tel: 01786 457700). More detailed information on disposal of contaminated waste is available in the guidance 'Protection against blood-borne infections in the workplace: HIV and hepatitis' (HSC Advisory Committee on Dangerous Pathogens (ACDP), HSC, 1995).

o Introduction of good hygiene practices such as hand and face washing prior to eating, drinking and smoking or leaving the work area. Covering of all cuts and abrasions and exclusion of those suffering with open, exposed eczema or dermatitis.

Once the risk assessment has been completed and adequate control measures and precautions identified, record the findings in writing and ensure that the risk assessment is reviewed and revised when necessary.

5.20

Case study 2 – Risk assessment of sewage treatment workers

Scenario

Large sewage treatment works employing 100 staff. Jobs range from general administrative duties to stores, sewage operatives, fitters, electricians and control room staff.

What the risk assessment should have considered

- The hazards:
  - o Sewage containing blood, semen or breast milk.
- Who might be harmed and under what circumstances?
  - o Sewage treatment operatives who monitor the flow of the sewage through the site, take samples and clean areas that have been contaminated with sewage containing blood.
  - o Maintenance workers (fitters and electricians). Fitters maintain, mend and unblock pumps, equipment and mechanical parts. Clear blockages that may contain needles, syringes, sharp objects etc. (Electricians maintain and mend electrical equipment not usually contaminated with sewage and probably low risk from BBVs.)
  - o Sewerage workers who work in the sewers, clearing sewers, removing congealed fat, detritus and gravel, mending brick walls, lock gates and access points. Blockages may contain hospital waste (blood, body fluids, clinical sharps, needles) or waste from restaurants. Some is cleared mechanically, but much is done manually.
- Evaluation of risk (assessment of who is at risk):
  - o Health data was used to determine the likelihood of contracting a BBV under the work circumstances. A study was undertaken to identify the number of sewage treatment staff who had gained immunity to hepatitis A and B prior to offering immunisation. The study revealed that only the fitters and sewerage workers (sewermen) were at a greater risk than the general population from contracting Hepatitis A and none of those surveyed were at greater risk than the general population from contracting hepatitis B.

(cont'd)

---

o Company health data and sickness absence data was also used to identify potentially high-risk jobs. It was shown that the only reports of hepatitis A were found in the fitters and sewerage workers.

o Company data was used to identify the number of needle-stick/sharps incidents and their location. Again the number of incidents were higher amongst fitters and sewerage workers.

o Reports of high levels of contamination by blood was used to identify particular high-risk activities. For example, workers in sewers near to hospital outlets reported high levels of fresh blood being flushed down the sewer at certain times.

• Review existing precautions and assess what additional measures required:

o More mechanical means of clearing sewage debris was investigated and new equipment and methods introduced (a 'fat eating bacteria' was used to break down the fats generated by the restaurants).

o Suitable clothing and equipment (water proof overalls, goggles and visors) was required to avoid the risk of contamination from splashes.

o Procedures for the laundry of overalls was to be introduced to stop workers taking work clothing home.

o Immunisation against hepatitis A was offered to all fitters and sewerage workers.

o A video was produced to inform and train workers about the hygiene precautions required to protect their health and leaflets distributed.

o A health record was started to comply with the *Control of Substances Hazardous to Health Regulations 2002 (SI 2002/2677), Reg 11* (health surveillance).

Zoonoses

Introduction

5.21   Occupational zoonoses is the term used for any infections that can be transmitted from animals to humans during a work activity. The current incidence of these diseases is unknown: many are rare (anthrax, brucellosis) and have not occurred occupationally for many years; others (leptospirosis hardjo and lyme disease) remain a problem and the Health & Safety Executive (HSE) consider there is gross under-reporting. Occupational zoonoses may cause anything from mild to severe disease, which in some cases could be fatal if not treated promptly or appropriately. The signs and symptoms of many of the occupational zoonoses can be easily confused with general viral illnesses such as influenza. It is essential, therefore, that all those who are at risk of contracting a zoonotic disease are identified and provided with information about the potential risk so that they may seek and receive prompt and appropriate treatment. A thorough risk assessment is therefore required to identify those at risk, to assess whether existing precautions are adequate to protect employees and whether additional precautions should be introduced.

The following guidance will identify the key occupations that should be considered and the most common occupational zoonoses found in the UK. The guidance will also guide the reader through the risk assessment process for occupational zoonoses. There are hundreds of zoonotic infections, particularly if primates are included, but it is outside the scope of this book to attempt to include them all. Further information about specific diseases may be found in the HSE document 'The Occupational Zoonoses' (HSE, 1993), from trade or professional publications and organisations, trade unions and veterinary advisers.

What are they?

5.22   Occupational zoonoses are infections transmitted from animals to humans during any work activity. Zoonoses can also affect visitors to work premises, especially farms open to the public, with infection by organisms such as escherichia coli 0157 (E coli 0157) and Cryptosporidium parvum being of particular note. Special precautions must be implemented to protect this group.

Listed below are some of the more common occupations where zoonoses may be a hazard. The list is not exhaustive, but is provided as a guide.

The HSC's Advisory Committee on Dangerous Pathogens (ACDP) has concluded that there is no evidence of risk of bovine spongiform encephalopathy (BSE)/variant Creuzfeldt Jacob disease (vCJD) being transmitted to people exposed to BSE through contact with live cattle in normal farming practices or in dealing with their intact carcasses. There have been no cases reported of vCJD or BSE being occupationally transmitted; however, it is recommended that the general occupational hygiene precautions prescribed for zoonoses are adopted where there may be a risk of contact with the agent.

Assessing the risks

5.23   When considering the need for risk assessment the first step is to consider whether there is an association between animals and animal products handled and occupational zoonotic disease or whether there is an

Table 2: Occupations where zoonoses a common risk

Occupation	Infection
Animal farmers and farm workers	Leptospirosis hardjo, Q fever, bovine TB, brucellosis, cryptosporidiosis, ringworm, orf, anthrax, psittacosis, ovine chlamydiosis, hantavirus, streptococcus suis, lyme disease
Animal handlers at quarantine kennels	Rabies
Animal laboratory workers	Leptospirosis icterohaemorrhagiae, leptospirosis hardjo, psittacosis, Q fever, hantavirus, bovine TB, brucellosis, cryptosporidiosis, rabies, Newcastle disease
Animal technicians	Psittacosis, Q fever, Newcastle disease
Bone/bone meal processors	Anthrax
Construction workers	Leptospirosis icterohaemorrhagiae, psittacosis, anthrax
Dog handlers	Hydatid disease
Dog wardens	Rabies
Fish farmers	Leptospirosis icterohaemorrhagiae
Grooms	Ringworm
Knackermen	Anthrax, bovine TB, brucellosis, leptospirosis hardjo, Q fever, ringworm, streptococcus suis
Leisure industry water sports	Leptospirosis icterohaemorrhagiae, hantavirus, lyme disease
Meat workers	Q fever, streptococcus suis, brucellosis, anthrax, orf
Poultry workers	Pssitacosis, newcastle disease
Sewage and water workers	Leptospirosis icterohaemorrhagiae, hantavirus;
Shepherds	Q fever, ovine chlamydiosis, hydatid disease, orf
Slaughterhouse workers	Streptococcus suis, bovine TB, brucellosis, leptospirosis hardjo, Q fever, ringworm, orf, anthrax
Tanneries	Anthrax
Vets, veterinary assistants/nurses	Psittacosis, streptococcus suis, bovine TB, brucellosis, leptospirosis hardjo, Q fever, ringworm, orf, anthrax, ovine chlamydiosis, hydatid disease, cryptosporidiosis, Newcastle disease, rabies

association between the occupation and a zoonotic disease. Information about association can be found in trade and professional publications, from trade unions and by seeking veterinary advice.

The current incidence of the disease in the UK and incidence in the animal reservoir is a relevant factor in the risk assessment. Such information is available from the Public Health Laboratory Service.

The following aspects must also be considered when undertaking the risk assessment:

- Route of transmission and infectivity of organism

  The risk depends upon the work method and route of transmission. For example, if the particular zoonotic organism is caught by aerosol transmission (fine droplets or dust particles in the air that are breathed in) and the work method does not generate aerosols then there may be no risk to those in contact with the organism.

- Vulnerability of individual

  The risks of contracting a zoonotic disease depends on factors such as the infectivity of the organism, infective dose of organism, route of entry, individual's resistance to disease and an individual's own personal hygiene standards. In other words, how easy it is to contract the disease. Particular consideration should be given to screening the health of those exposed to ensure that their resistance to disease is not lowered due to conditions such as leukaemia, HIV, cancer or reduced immunity.

- Severity of disease

  The risk assessment must also consider the seriousness of the disease. If the disease is short-term, self-limiting and amenable to treatment the level of risk and the control measures required will be considerably lower than if the disease is potentially fatal. The severity of the disease may be determined by its Hazard grouping published by the Health and Safety Commission's Advisory Committee on Dangerous Pathogens (ACDP) and entitled 'Categorisation of Biological Agents according to Hazard and Categories of Containment'.

- Prevention and controls

  Prevention is best obtained by eradicating the disease from the animal reservoir, this has been virtually achieved for brucellosis and bovine TB, with anthrax and rabies tightly controlled, however wild animal reservoirs such as leptospirosis in rats and psittacosis in pigeons are virtually impossible to eradicate.

  Where contact with the disease organism cannot be prevented, control may be achieved by reducing the numbers of employees exposed to the biological agent and designing work processes and engineering controls to prevent or minimise the release of the agent into the environment. Plans must be drawn up to deal with accidents involving biological agents and specify the decontamination and disinfection procedures required. Procedures for the safe handling, storage and disposal of contaminated waste must be detailed and enforced. Where contact with the biological agent cannot be avoided or adequately controlled by the above mentioned means, employees should be provided with appropriate protective clothing, access to washing facilities and education about the personal hygiene strategies required to protect them. In some cases, where employees are not already immune, employees may be offered immunisation at the employer's expense. Eating, drinking, smoking and the application of cosmetics must be prohibited in the work area where there is a risk of contamination by biological agents.

Health surveillance

5.24   Every worker in contact with a zoonotic disease should receive information about the potential health hazard of their work. Additionally, health surveillance is required under the *Control of Substances Hazardous to Health Regulations 2002 (SI 2002/2677), Reg 11* if *all* of the following criteria apply:

- there is an identifiable disease;

- there is a reasonable likelihood of occurrence (determined by the risk assessment); *and*

- there are valid detection techniques available.

In many cases of exposure to zoonoses it would not be reasonable to expect an employee to submit to a blood test every day, so health surveillance may only take the form of the maintenance of a health record (this is the minimum requirement). The health record must contain the employee's full name, sex, date of birth, address, National Insurance number, date of commencement of current employment, history of exposure to substances requiring health surveillance in current employment. The employee should also be provided with a medical contact card for presentation to an examining doctor if taken ill. The employee's health should be periodically assessed and records updated, not necessarily by a medical professional, but through the assessment of accident and incident records, sickness absence records, etc to determine whether there are any health concerns relating to exposure.

In addition, employers must keep a list of employees exposed to Group 3 or Group 4 agents, indicating the nature of the work and the zoonotic disease concerned and record any exposures, accidents or incidents. All health records must be kept for a minimum of ten years and under some cases specified in Schedule 3, Part 1, Section 11(3) of the General COSHH ACOP (HSE Books, 1999 – revised edition available from 6 December 2002).

Case study 3 – Risk assessment for construction workers and zoonoses

Scenario

The site of an old tannery is about to be demolished and cleared in preparation for new factory outlets to be built.

What the risk assessment should have considered

- The hazards:
  - o Construction activities near areas where birds roost and congregate (psittacosis)
  - o Construction activities where rats may run or nest (leptospirosis icterohaemorrhagiae)
  - o Demolition of site where anthrax may harbour (abattoirs, tanneries, bone/bonemeal manufacturers, hair and bristle factories)
- Who might be harmed and under what circumstances?
  - o Workers who come into contact with dust or aerosols contaminated with bird faeces or nasal discharge (eg pigeons roosting in the derelict building).
  - o Workers who may be in contact with the urine of rats through cuts, abrasions, lining of the nose, mouth and conjunctiva. This may be through work near potentially infected waters such as rivers, lakes, reservoirs or in sewers or rat infested buildings
  - o Workers who work on infected sites (old tanneries, crypts, old buildings with animal hair plaster binding, infected pasture land).
- Evaluation of risk (assessment of who is at risk):
  - o There is a potential risk from contact with psittacosis, leptospirosis and anthrax due to the circumstances involved. There are birds roosting in the building, there are rats nesting in the area, and the area may have been contaminated with anthrax.
  - o The site should have been investigated for contamination in the initial stages to identify potential problems relating to anthrax (through soil samples and history of the factory), so anthrax could be excluded at an early stage.
  - o The severity of the diseases depends on the route of transmission, with anthrax it is potentially fatal if inhaled and

(cont'd)

leptospirosis potentially fatal if unrecognised and untreated. As the route of transmission for anthrax and psittacosis is by inhalation of dusts, the generation of dust during demolition would increase the risk considerably.

o The vulnerability of the all workers was assessed to determine whether certain individuals should be excluded. For example, anyone suffering from chronic ill-health may be more susceptible to the more severe effects of any of the diseases mentioned above. Health assessment involved the completion of a general health questionnaire and medical advice was sought where any individual stated they had a medical condition.

- Review existing precautions and assess what additional measures required:

  o Control rat and bird infestation

  o Provision of masks (respirators for those at highest risk), goggles and suitable overalls for work in dusty environments

  o Provision of laundry facilities and disposal of anthrax contaminated personal protective equipment;

  o Reduction of dust generated by damping down, ventilation and mechanical extraction

  o Information, training and education of workforce to ensure they understand the signs and symptoms of the diseases concerned, the importance of early reporting and the hygiene precautions required (hand washing before eating drinking and smoking, coverage of all cuts and abrasions, early reporting of disease).

  o Provision of a medical contact card

  o Health surveillance (health record for leptospirosis and pssittacosis, skin checks for anthrax).

Travellers' health

Introduction

5.26   Employers are responsible for the health and safety of their employees whilst at work. This includes the employee who travels abroad on company business. There are a number of major diseases that might be a risk to the employee depending on the location visited and the circumstances under which the employee lives and works. A risk assessment is required for all employees travelling abroad, but particularly those travelling *outside* Northern Europe, North America and Australia/New Zealand. A risk assessment is required therefore, as with the other biological hazards, to identify the risks and determine adequate control measures and precautions. Expert advice is available from reputable travel health clinics or from organisations such as the Department of Health (www.doh.gov.uk/traveladvice), TRAVAX (http://www. fitfortravel. scot.nhs.uk/) and World Health Organisation (www.who.int/ith/).

Risk assessment must be carried out well in advance of any travel to ensure that immunisation schedules can be completed in sufficient time. To confer protection, immunisations should be commenced at least one month in advance, though some immunisations will require a second booster to be fully protective and so three months would be better.

In addition the suitability of the employee should be considered. Are they fit to travel? Do they have any notable medical conditions that might preclude them from travel, prevent them from receiving the immunisations they need, or make it unwise for them to travel to particular areas or engage in certain work activities? These will need to be considered in the risk assessment and control measures (such as medical assessment) introduced.

What are the risks?

5.27   The major diseases cited by the Department of Health are:

- typhoid;
- tetanus;
- polio;
- hepatitis;
- meningitis;
- malaria;
- tuberculosis (TB);
- cholera;
- yellow fever;
- tick-borne encephalitis;
- japanese encephalitis;
- diphtheria;
- bilharziasis; and
- dengue.

Typhoid

5.28   Typhoid fever is a serious illness that could be fatal if untreated. The disease is caught through the consumption of contaminated food and water.

The symptoms take between three–six days to develop leading to fever, headache, abdominal pain, constipation or diarrhoea. Employees who are travelling to areas known to have endemic typhoid, particularly if sanitation is primitive, should be offered immunisation and advised of the general precautions needed to protect them against food borne disease (see 5.37).

Tetanus

5.29   Tetanus is a leading cause of death in many developing countries due to a lack of immunisation and poor hygiene and treatment facilities. The bacteria enters the body through open wounds (often very minor and insignificant) leading to damage to the nervous system and muscles resulting in paralysis and spasm (often known as 'lock-jaw'). In the UK most individuals should have been immunised in childhood, but may need a booster to protect them. Those that have never been immunised may need a course of three injections before travel. The individual should be instructed to seek advice from their GP.

Polio

5.30   Polio is a serious viral disease spread by food or drink contaminated by infected faeces or person to person via the mucous from the nose and throat. It is endemic in countries with low levels of hygiene and low immunisation levels in the general population. Employees travelling to countries outside Northern and Western Europe, North America, Australia and New Zealand are particularly vulnerable and must be immunised. As with tetanus, most UK individuals should have received an initial course in childhood and will need a booster every ten years, those that have never received the initial course will need three oral doses to confer immunity. The individual should be instructed to seek advice about immunisation from their GP and advised of the general precautions needed to protect them against food borne disease (see 5.37).

Hepatitis

5.31   Viral hepatitis is an infection of the liver resulting from infection which can be fatal or leave permanent damage. There are three main types that are significant to the traveller: hepatitis A, B or C.

Hepatitis A is caught by consuming food or water contaminated with infected faeces. The disease is particularly prevalent where sanitation is primitive. The employee should be advised of the general precautions needed to protect them against food borne disease (see below) and immunised against the disease.

Hepatitis B is generally a more serious disease transmitted through blood-to-blood contact (unscreened transfusions, contaminated needles or equipment used in medical treatment, tattooing, ear-piercing) or unprotected sexual intercourse. A risk assessment should be undertaken to determine whether the employee is travelling to high-risk areas, particularly if medical care is basic. If the risk assessment shows the area to be a high-risk, then the employee should be immunised against hepatitis B and provided with a travel kit for medical emergencies.

Hepatitis C is increasing world-wide and is spread in the same way as hepatitis B. As yet there is no vaccination available. The employer must carry out a risk assessment as for hepatitis B and the employee advised to avoid the high-risk activities (unprotected sexual intercourse, blood to blood contact) and provided with a travel kit for medical emergencies.

Malaria

5.32 Malaria is a parasitic disease spread by the bite of infected mosquitoes. The disease is prevalent in parts of Africa, Southern and Central America, Middle East, Far East and the Indian Sub-continent. The employee may be at risk if working, visiting, or travelling through these areas. The risk assessment should identify whether there is a risk and the precautions required. Advice will be required from a medical practitioner about the medications required for the area to be visited and the employee must receive instruction about how to avoid mosquito bites (use of insecticides, covering exposed areas, avoiding high-risk times of day or locations).

Tuberculosis

5.33 Tuberculosis (TB) is increasing world-wide. It is particularly prevalent in Africa, Asia, Central and South America. Those who will be staying in international-style hotels for short periods will not need to be immunised but those who will be living and working closely with the indigenous population and those who are going to stay for more than a month in these areas should have their TB status checked and immunisation given (BCG) if required at least two months prior to travel.

Cholera

5.34 Cholera causes severe diarrhoea leading to dehydration and can be fatal. It is prevalent in areas with poor sanitation, particularly in South America, the Middle East, Africa and Asia and is spread by contaminated food. There is no effective immunisation available, so employees working in high-risk areas must be instructed in the general precautions required to avoid food borne disease (see 5.37).

Yellow fever

5.35 Yellow fever is transmitted via the bite of a mosquito. The disease is found in parts of Africa and South America. Immunisation is available and lasts ten years. Some countries demand a certificate of immunisation particularly if travelling form one potential source country to another.

Other diseases

5.36 Meningitis, tick-borne encephalitis, japanese encephalitis, diphtheria, bilharziasis and dengue are less common, but advice should be sought about precautions from the Department of Health leaflet 'Health advice for travellers' if the risk assessment identifies them as a potential risk for the countries to be visited or worked in.

Food borne disease

5.37 The general precautions needed to protect against food borne disease:

- if there are any doubts about the safety of the water supply, boil, sterilise or use bottled water (from containers with intact seals) for drinking, washing food and brushing teeth;
- avoid ice in drinks or to keep food cold unless known to be made from safe water sources (ie bottled, sterilised or boiled);
- hot tea, coffee, carbonated drinks, packaged or bottled fruit juices, beer and wine are generally considered safe;
- avoid cooked food that has been left to keep warm unless it is piping hot and cooked thoroughly;
- avoid uncooked food unless it can be peeled or shelled by the consumer;
- beware uncooked shellfish such as oysters as it can be suspect in some countries;
- only buy ice cream from reputable sources;
- avoid unpasturised milk;

Other general precautions:

- sufficient supplies of prescribed medications should be taken with a covering letter from the GP to avoid difficulties in some countries;
- avoid sunburn;
- avoid sunstroke and heat exhaustion;
- avoid insect, snake and animal bites;

- avoid swimming in fresh water lakes, unfiltered or unattended swimming pools;

- use vehicles (cars, motorbikes or pedal cycles) that are well maintained and from a reputable source;

- avoid making important decisions if suffering from jet-lag.

Travel health is often omitted by organisations when undertaking risk assessment. It is, however, as important as any other health and safety issue and must be considered when planning an employee's work schedule.

Food health

5.38   Any organisation that is in the business of production, processing, storage, distribution or sale of food (whether to employees or the general public) must be aware of the obligations imposed on them by the *Food Safety Act 1990* and supporting regulations. Risk assessment is part of the process of ensuring that the food produced for sale is safe to eat. It is not within the scope of this book to cover food safety as this is covered by many existing documents and manuals.

6   Chemical Hazards

Introduction

6.1   Many thousands of chemical substances are used in the workplace: the Twelfth Edition of the Merck Index has entries for 2,000 'common' organic chemicals and laboratory reagents (Budavari, S, 'The Merck Index', Merck and Co Inc, 1996). Some chemical substances may damage the skin by direct contact at room temperature, eg sulphuric acid or sodium hydroxide; some may be harmful by ingestion, eg lead compounds; some may be harmful by inhalation, eg chlorine or hydrogen cyanide; and some can penetrate the intact skin and enter the bloodstream, eg benzene or carbon disulphide. The consequences of exposure to chemical substances can include skin or respiratory sensitisation, cancer, damage to the kidneys/liver/lungs/unborn child, genetic damage, reduced fertility, irritation, dizziness or drowsiness. In addition, substances in the workplace can enter the environment via finished products, eg adhesives in carpets or solvents in paints, or by eventual disposal. That is, hazardous substances in the workplace have the potential for causing harm in the workplace, in the home and in the environment.

To ensure that the adverse health effects arising from substances in the workplace are either prevented or controlled, the *Control of Substances Hazardous to Health Regulations 2002 (SI 2002/2677) (COSHH)* require that an employer shall not carry on any work which may expose his employees to hazardous substances unless a suitable and sufficient risk assessment has been carried out. The purpose the risk assessment is to enable a valid decision to be made about measures necessary to control hazardous substances arising from any work. Guidance on carrying out a risk assessment is given in CHAPTER 10. Useful help in undertaking a *COSHH* assessment can also be found at http://www.coshh-essentials.org. uk/Home.asp.

The essential precursor to such a risk assessment is to determine the hazards associated with any substances prior to their introduction to the workplace. It has been suggested, therefore (see Zapp, JA and Doull, J, 'Industrial Toxicology: Retrospect and Prospect', in 'Patty's Industrial Hygiene and Toxicology', John Wiley & Sons, 1993), that the potential manufacturer or user should ask himself three questions about any substance:

- Can it be manufactured safely?
- Can it be used safely for its intended purpose?
- Can it be disposed of safely into the environment during manufacture and after its intended use?

If the answer to any of the above questions is 'No', it would be imprudent to manufacture or use the substance. For some substances, particularly those which can cause cancer, there is a long delay between exposure and the development of adverse health effects, eg there is generally a delay of at least 20 years between exposure to beta-napthylamine and development of bladder cancer. It is therefore critical that the *lack of evidence of harm* is not taken as *evidence of lack of harm*. Unless there is clear evidence of lack of harm it is prudent to assume that harm may occur. That is, if the answer to any of the above questions is 'I cannot say Yes', it would be imprudent to take the chance that the substance will not cause harm. Consequently, unless the answer to all three questions is a definite 'Yes', it would be imprudent to manufacture or use the substance.

In practice, completely new substances are produced by only a very small number of companies, most of whom are fully aware of the need for thorough testing and evaluation of new substances. The vast majority of employers are therefore likely to manufacture or use chemical substances for which hazard information is available. However, although such information is available, it may not be easily accessible, and it may not be comprehensible to a small employer who lacks the resources to interpret and apply the information to his own products or workplace.

The critical requirement for most manufacturers and users of chemical substances is, therefore, to be able to find, understand and use the relevant information regarding any hazards associated with the substance of interest. Both national and European legislation has been introduced to ensure that adequate information on the safety and heath hazards associated with substances are available for users of many substances and that no-one will introduce new substances without obtaining the necessary hazard information and passing it onto users.

Legal requirements

6.2   The provision of hazard information in the UK is covered by the *Health and Safety at Work etc Act 1974* (as amended) and the *Chemicals (Hazard Information and Packaging for Supply) Regulations 2002 (SI 2002/1689).*

Health and Safety at Work etc Act 1974

6.3   The *Health and Safety at Work etc Act 1974, s 6* (as amended) specifies:

'**General duties of manufacturers etc as regards articles and substances for use at work**

6(1)   It shall be the duty of any person who designs, manufactures, imports or supplies any article for use at work–

(a) to ensure, so far as is reasonably practicable, that the article is so designed and constructed as to be safe and without risks to health when properly used;

(b) to carry out or arrange for the carrying out of such testing and examination as may be necessary for the performance of the duty imposed on him by the preceding paragraph;

(c) to take such steps as are necessary to secure that there will be available in connection with the use of the article at work adequate information about the use for which it is designed and has been tested, and about any conditions necessary to ensure that, when put to that use, it will be safe and without risks to health.'

From *section 6* it is clear that the necessary testing and evaluation must be carried out and that information on how to use the product safely must be provided to the user.

Chemicals (Hazard Information and Packaging for Supply) Regulations 2002

6.4   The *Chemicals (Hazard Information and Packaging for Supply) Regulations 2002 (SI 2002/1689) (CHIP Regulations)* are intended to implement the EU *Dangerous Substances Directive (67/548/EEC)* (as amended) to cover 'substances dangerous for supply' and apply to the majority of chemical substances manufactured, used or imported into the EU. Substances regarded as dangerous for supply are listed in the Approved Supply List ('Approved Supply List: Information approved for the classification and labelling of substances and preparations dangerous for supply', HSC, 2002)

Outlines of the critical regulations are discussed below.

Regulation 2 – Interpretation

6.5   Substances are often provided as mixtures or solutions of two or more substances. Such mixtures or solutions are defined as 'preparations'. All duties applicable to substances are also applicable to preparations.

Regulation 3 – Applicability

6.6   The *CHIP Regulations* apply to any dangerous substance or preparation unless otherwise defined, eg they do not apply to specified medicines, drugs, cosmetics, waste, food, animal feed, radioactive substances or medical devices.

Regulation 4 – Classification of dangerous substances and dangerous preparations

6.7   No person shall supply a dangerous substance unless it has been classified in accordance with this regulation. Such classification shall be as listed in the Approved Supply List.

New substances shall be classified in accordance with the *Notification of New Substances Regulations 1993 (SI 1993/3050).* A substance not listed in the Approved Supply List shall be classified in accordance with the *CHIP Regulations, Sch 2.* The person applying such classification shall make himself aware of all relevant information.

If a substance is classified as carcinogenic, mutagenic or toxic for reproduction, the person undertaking the classification will supply relevant information to the Health & Safety Executive.

Regulation 5 – Safety data sheets

6.8   When dangerous substances are supplied for occupational use, a safety data sheet (SDS) shall be supplied which gives the information specified in the Approved Code of Practice ('Safety data sheets for substances and preparations dangerous for supply', HSC, 1996). The SDS should contain the following information, as specified in the *Chip Regulations, Sch 4*:

- identification of the substance/preparation and supplying company;
- composition/information on ingredients;
- hazards identification;
- first-aid measures;
- fire-fighting measures;
- accidental release measures;
- handling and storage;
- exposure controls/personal protection;
- physical and chemical properties;
- stability and reactivity;
- toxicological information;
- ecological information;
- disposal considerations;
- transport information;
- regulatory information;
- other information.

The SDS shall be provided free of charge and shall be provided not later than the date when the substance was first supplied to the user. When an SDS has been revised, the supplier shall provide a copy of the revised SDS to every person who has received the substance or preparation within the preceding twelve months and who has requested a copy of the SDS.

Regulation 8 – Labelling

6.9 Unless otherwise specified, no person shall supply a dangerous substance unless labelled with:

- full name, address and telephone number of the supplier;

Table 1: Categories of danger and packaging symbols

Physio-chemical properties		*Symbol*	
Explosive		E	
Oxidising		O	
Extremely flammable		F+	
Highly flammable		F	
Flammable		none	
Health effects	*Symbol*	*Health effects*	*Symbol*
Very toxic	T+	Mutagens:	
Toxic	T	Category 1 – confirmed	T
Harmful	Xn	Category 2 – likely	T
Corrosive	C	Category 3 – possible	Xn
Irritant	Xi		
Sensitising by inhalation	Xn	Toxic for reproduction:	
Sensitising by skin contact	Xi	Category 1 – confirmed	T
		Category 2 – likely	T
Carcinogens:		Category 3 – possible	Xn
Category 1 – confirmed	T		
Category 2 – likely	T		
Category 3 – possible	Xn		

- the name of the substance as shown in the Approved Supply List, if listed, or an internationally recognised name if not listed; and

- any indication of danger, ie the risk phrases (see 6.12), set out in full.

For dangerous preparations, the trade name of the preparation will be given in addition to the above information

Schedule 2

6.10 Dangerous substances and dangerous preparations should be classified under the headings shown in TABLE 1.

Schedule 3 – lower limits of concentration

6.11 For preparations to which the *CHIP Regulations, Sch 3* applies, every preparation containing more than the specified amount of a substance shall be given the same classification as that substance: see TABLE 2.

Risk phrases

6.12 The Approved Supply List classifies substances into general hazard categories and assigns one or more *risk phrases* which identify the particular

Table 2: Lower limits of substance concentration

Category of danger	*Limiting concentration*	
	Gaseous preparations %vol/vol	Other preparations %weight/weight
Very toxic Toxic Carcinogenic Category 1 or 2 Mutagenic Category 1 or 2 Toxic for reproduction Category 1 or 2	≥ 0.02	≥ 0.11
Harmful Corrosive Irritant Sensitising Carcinogenic Category 3 Mutagenic Category 3 Toxic for reproduction Category 3	≥ 0.2	≥ 1
Dangerous for the Environment Dangerous for the Environment N Dangerous for the Environment Ozone	– – ≥ 0.1	≥ 1 ≥ 0.1 ≥ 0.1

Table 3: Indication of particular risks

Risk phrases (R)		Risk phrases (R)	
1	Explosive when dry	35	Causes severe burns
2	Risk of explosion by shock, friction, fire or other sources of ignition	36	Irritating to the eyes
3	Extreme risk of explosion by shock, friction, fire or other sources of ignition	37	Irritating to the respiratory system
4	Forms very sensitive explosive metallic compounds	38	Irritating to the skin
5	Heating may cause an explosion	39	Danger of very serious irreversible effects
6	Explosive with or without contact with air	40	Possible risk of irreversible effects
7	May cause fire	41	Risk of serious damage to eyes
8	Contact with combustible material may cause fire	42	May cause sensitisation by inhalation
9	Explosive when mixed with combustible material	43	May cause sensitisation by skin contact
10	Flammable	44	Risk of explosion if heated under confinement
11	Highly flammable	45	May cause cancer
12	Extremely flammable	46	May cause heritable genetic damage
14	Reacts violently with water	48	Danger of serious damage to health by prolonged exposure
15	Contact with water liberates extremely flammable gases	49	May cause cancer by inhalation
16	Explosive when mixed with oxidising substances	50	Very toxic to aquatic organisms
17	Spontaneously flammable in air	51	Toxic to aquatic organisms
18	In use may form flammable/explosive vapour-air mixture	52	Harmful to aquatic organisms
19	May form explosive peroxides	53	May cause long term adverse effects in the aquatic environment
20	Harmful by inhalation	54	Toxic to flora
21	Harmful in contact with skin	55	Toxic to fauna
22	Harmful if swallowed	56	Toxic to soil organisms
23	Toxic by inhalation	57	Toxic to bees
24	Toxic in contact with skin	58	May cause long term adverse effects in the environment
25	Toxic if swallowed	59	Dangerous for the ozone layer
26	Very toxic by inhalation	60	May impair fertility
27	Very toxic in contact with skin	61	May cause harm to the unborn child
28	Very toxic if swallowed	62	Possible risk of impaired fertility
29	Contact with water liberates toxic gas	63	Possible risk of harm to the unborn child
30	Can become highly flammable in use	64	May cause harm to breastfed babies
31	Contact with acids liberates toxic gas	65	Harmful: may cause lung damage if swallowed
32	Contact with acids liberates very toxic gas	66	Repeated exposure may cause skin dryness or cracking
33	Danger of cumulative effects	67	Vapours may cause drowsiness or dizziness
34	Causes burns		

hazard(s) associated with each substance: see TABLE 3. For example, xylene, a solvent widely used in paints, is classified as 'harmful' and is assigned the following risk phrases: R10: 'Flammable'; R20/21: 'Harmful by inhalation or contact with the skin'; and R38: 'Irritating to the skin'.

For dangerous substances not listed in the Approved Supply List, the supplier is responsible for assigning the general hazard classification and the relevant risk phrases.

Dangerous substances must be supplied in containers clearly marked with the symbols assigned to the general hazard classification, the risk phrase numbers assigned and the full text of each risk phrase. From such information, the user should be able to identify the hazards associated with the substances manufactured or used in the workplace.

If a preparation contains more than a specified proportion of a particularly hazardous substance or mixture of substances, the same risk classification applied to such substance or substances applies to the entire preparation.

Comment

6.13   The major limitation of the *CHIP Regulations* is that where the supplier assigns his own risk phrases, there is no explicit duty of competency unless the substance or preparation is classified as Category 1 or 2 carcinogenic, mutagenic or toxic to reproduction. That is, the regulations do not demand competency for the decision *not* to assign a substance as Category 1 or 2 carcinogenic, mutagenic or toxic to reproduction.

Chemical substances in the 'real world'

6.14   Notwithstanding the requirements of legislation, there are frequent difficulties in the real world in obtaining the necessary information on chemical substances from product suppliers: some suppliers deliberately withhold such information as being 'commercially sensitive'; some suppliers fail to provide adequate safety data sheets (SDS); some products contain proprietary products which are not listed in the Approved Supply List and the hazard classifications in the Approved Supply List can be less stringent than assigned by other authorities.

Even where an apparently adequate SDS is supplied, it can be difficult to independently check that information provided is accurate, primarily because many substances have more than one name. Nomenclature is therefore important.

Commercial confidentiality

6.15 Many companies provide only the minimum possible information on the basis that more detailed information may be of use to a competitor. It is this author's experience that a suggestion that the SDS does not meet the requirements of the *Chemicals (Hazard Information and Packaging for Supply) Regulations 2002 (SI 2002/1689) (CHIP Regulations)* and/or that unless a thorough independent hazard assessment can be made, the product will not be bought, tends to help a more thorough safety data sheet to be provided.

Chemical nomenclature

6.16 Many substances have more than one name. For example, methyl ethyl ketone, widely used in paints and printing materials, is also called 2-butanone, butan-2-one, butanone 2, butanone, MEK, ethyl methyl ketone and EMK. It is listed in the Approved Supply List only as butanone.

Many substances have been registered with organisations such as the Chemical Abstract Service (CAS) or the European Inventory of Commercial Chemical Substances (EINCS) and assigned a CAS or EINCS registry number respectively. These registry numbers permit efficient searching on computerised databases or publications such as the Merck Index (Budavari, S, 'The Merck Index', Merck and Co Inc, 1996) or Sax's Dangerous Properties (Lewis, RJ, 'Sax's Dangerous Properties of Industrial Materials', 1996). For example, butanone has been assigned the CAS registry number 78-93-3 and the EINCS registry number 606-002-00-3. The Merck Index and Sax can both be searched by CAS number.

However, it is not currently possible to search the Approved Supply List by synonym or CAS or EINCS number. It can be difficult, therefore, to identify the substance of interest in the Approved Supply List.

The safety home page of the Physical and Theoretical Chemistry Laboratory at Oxford University offers a web page which permits identification of common chemical names from CAS numbers. Access to the Oxford University website is free of charge at http://physchem.ox.ac.uk/MSDS/. Use of the Oxford University web page may enable some substances to be identified in the Approved Supply List.

Inadequate safety data sheets

6.17 Inadequate safety data sheets (SDS) are very common. Over the past five years this author has been involved in a number of studies in the paint spray and printing industries and has never been presented with an adequate SDS without contacting the supplier and requesting further information, even though some of the suppliers have been major multi-national companies.

For example, the SDS for one coloured paint noted that it contained 1–2.5% by weight of chromium (VI) compounds. No hazard classification under the *Chemicals (Hazard Information and Packaging for Supply) Regulations 2002 (SI 2002/1689) (CHIP Regulations)* or risk phrases were given in the SDS for these compounds. The occupational exposure limit (OEL) was given as a maximum exposure limit (MEL) of 0.05 mg/m^3. The SDS was dated 1998. Although chromium VI compounds were not listed in the earlier Approved Supply Lists, the Supplement to the third edition of the Approved Supply List ('Supplement to the third edition of the Approved Supply List', HSC, 1997)) identified a number of such compounds as Category 2 Carcinogens which were assigned risk phrases R45: 'May cause cancer', or R49: 'May cause cancer by inhalation'. The failure to assign a general classification of carcinogen or risk phrase R45 or R49 to chromium VI compounds is therefore surprising. In 2000, the revised publication on OELs ('Occupational Exposure Limits', HSE, 2000) noted the assignment of risk phrase R49: 'May cause cancer by inhalation', to such compounds.

As specified in the *CHIP Regulations*, the SDS should have been updated immediately new information was available and a revised SDS should have been supplied to the user. Unless the user had been made aware of the hazards associated with chromium VI compounds, significant exposures to a confirmed carcinogen could have occurred. Such exposures may be occurring with other users of the same product who may not have been supplied with an SDS identifying the current risk phrases for these compounds.

Proprietary or difficult to identify products

6.18   Many commercially-available products contain proprietary products or difficult to find substances which are not listed in the Approved Supply List, for which no hazard data may be provided by the supplier and for which no relevant data can be found in the scientific literature.

For example, one component of a two-pack paint contained bis(2-dimethylaminoethyl) (methyl) amine. No CAS or EINCS number was given. In the safety data sheet (SDS) this substance was classified as Toxic and assigned the risk phrases: R 24: 'Toxic in contact with the skin'; R34: 'Causes burns'; R22: 'Harmful if swallowed'. This substance was not found in the Approved Supply List or Sax's Dangerous Properties (Lewis, RJ, 'Sax's Dangerous Properties of Industrial Materials', 1996). It was therefore not possible to independently check the correctness of the risk phrases assigned to this substance in the supplier's SDS.

EU hazard classifications may be less stringent than other authorities

6.19   The lead chromate paint noted at 6.17 also illustrates the differences between the Approved Supply List which regards lead chromate as a suspected carcinogen whereas the National Institute for Occupational Safety and Health (NIOSH) in the USA considers all chromium (VI) compounds as potential carcinogens. NIOSH has assigned a recommended exposure limit (REL) of 0.001 mg.m^{-3}, as chromium VI, to such compounds, NIOSH (1997). In the UK a maximum exposure limit (MEL) of 0.02 mg.m^{-3}, as chromium VI, is assigned to such compounds.

The UK MEL is therefore substantially less protective than the NIOSH REL. Note that to comply with both the REL and MEL it is necessary to minimise exposures.

It should be noted that under the European *Carcinogens Directive* (90/394/EEC) any exposure to Category 1 or 2 carcinogens must be reduced to as low as technically possible. It is therefore critically important in terms of controlling exposures to airborne substances to determine whether carcinogens are present in the product.

The safety home page of the Physical and Theoretical Chemistry Laboratory at Oxford University lists about 450 known and suspected carcinogens. The Oxford University list of known and suspected carcinogens contains substantially more substances than given in the Approved Supply List.

The large number of known and suspected carcinogens listed on the Oxford University website suggests that the Approved Supply List may be unduly conservative in its hazard classifications and that the severity of hazard associated with a significant number of substances may increase in the future. In the meantime persons may be inadequately protected.

It should be noted that in the Approved Supply List risk phrase R 40: 'Possible risk of irreversible effects' is assigned to all suspected (Category 3) carcinogens. Given the conservatism of the EU hazard classification procedures, it is strongly considered that any substances assigned risk phrase R40 should be regarded as R45 or R49 in the case of Category 3 carcinogens.

Assessing the risks

6.20   Before any substance or preparation is manufactured or used in the workplace, a thorough independent hazard assessment should be made as an essential part of the risk assessment. The concepts of 'hazard' and 'risk' are described in CHAPTER 10. To carry out such an assessment, it is necessary to be able to identify all substances which may be present.

The starting point in the hazard assessment is to demand that the supplier provides an up-to-date safety data sheet (SDS) which:

• identifies all substances present, or likely to be present in the preparation; and

• identifies the hazard(s) associated with each constituent.

All constituents should be identified in a form which permits an independent literature search to be carried out to identify any reported hazards. Any hazards should be identified in the form of the general hazard classification and risk phrases defined in the *Chemicals (Hazard Information and Packaging for Supply) Regulations 2002 (SI 2002/1689) (CHIP Regulations)* or in the form of a thorough report from the supplier's database, preferably corroborated by a thorough literature search of the independently published literature.

If it is not possible to obtain a valid SDS, the supplier should asked in writing for an SDS which complies with the requirements of the *CHIP Regulations* and warned that the Health & Safety Executive will be informed if a valid SDS is not immediately forthcoming.

Once received, the validity of the SDS should be checked to see what proportion of the product has been identified, eg for the paint described in 6.17, the substances identified in the SDS accounted for not more than 12% of the product. What health or safety hazards were associated with the other 88% of the product?

It must be appreciated that any employer who uses any substance or preparation without an adequate SDS is *indisputably liable* in both criminal and civil law for any harm which results. Consequently, if the supplier cannot or will not provide an adequate SDS, or an explicit statement that no adverse health or safety hazards are associated with his product, it would be imprudent to use the product.

Once all the substances present have been identified, the hazard classifications and risk phrases given in the SDS should be checked against the Approved Supply List for accuracy. Care should be taken if any substances are assigned risk phrase R40: 'Possible risk of irreversible effects', as such risk phrase is assigned to Category 3 carcinogens. In such situation it would be prudent to consult the list of known and suspected carcinogens on the Oxford University website noted at 6.16.

If the substances were noted in that list, it would be prudent to carry out a search of MEDLINE on the web. A number of search engines offer free searches on MEDLINE and permit abstracts of cited references to be downloaded. MEDLINE can be accessed free of charge, for example at http://www.nlm.nih.gov/medlineplus/. A charge is generally made for a printout of the full paper. Only if the MEDLINE search is clear, should the substance or product be used without assuming that such substance or product is a carcinogen. For example, the lead chromate content of the paint discussed at 6.17 is classified in the Approved Supply List as a Category 3 carcinogen. However, the Oxford University list of known and suspected carcinogens recommends that this substances should not be used if an alternative safer product is available, and that if used, it should be handled as a carcinogen. A MEDLINE search strongly indicated that lead chromate should be regarded as at least a Category 2 carcinogen to which risk phrase R49: 'Many cause cancer by inhalation' would apply.

Once the risk phrases have been checked and found accurate, the occupational exposure limits listed in the SDS should be checked against the current edition of the Health & Safety Executive publication EH 40 (Health & Safety Executive, 'Occupational Exposure Limits', EH40 (2002)) to ensure that the current occupational exposure limits are used in the risk assessment.

As a final check, particularly if Category 1 or 2 carcinogens, mutagens or substances toxic to reproduction have been identified in the product, the necessity of using such substances should be carefully evaluated and the reason for use of such substances clearly defined and justified.

7　Physical Hazards

Introduction – what are physical hazards?

7.1　Physical hazards are those hazards that arise from physical aspects of the environment. These include, sound, vibration, temperature, light, static electricity, ionising and non-ionising radiation and the physical structure of the surroundings. As with other hazards of a chemical or biological nature, the risk to a person's health and safety will depend on how these hazards present themselves and how they might cause harm. This chapter discusses the nature of physical hazards and the health risks arising from them.

For information about sound and noise, see 7.2; for vibration, see 7.8 *et seq*; for temperature, see 7.15 *et seq*; for light, see 7.25 *et seq*; for ergonomic aspects, see 7.31 *et seq*; for the workplace, see 7.59 *et seq*; for static electricity and non-ionising radiation, see 7.66 *et seq*; and for ionising radiation, see 7.78 *et seq*.

Sound and noise

7.2　It is important to distinguish between 'sound' and 'noise'.

Sound is a physical phenomenon in which waves of pressure pass through the air and are received by the ear and then interpreted by the brain. Although sound has a physical property it is only because it is sensed by the ear that we interpret it as sound. The same physical phenomena occurring above (ultra sound) and below (infra sound) the frequency response of the ear cannot be heard. The physical property of the sound wave is measured in terms of the air pressure (the acoustic pressure) and the frequency (ie the number of times the pressure wave repeats in a given time). Pressure is measured in Newtons per square metre (Nm^{-2}) or Pascals: one Pascal is one Nm^{-2}. The ear is extremely sensitive and can detect minute changes in air pressure, whereas the highest pressures encountered can be millions of times greater. In order to compress this wide range of sound energies into a useful scale, the logarithmic decibel scale is used. A three-decibel (3 dB) increase represents a doubling of the sound intensity. Another complication is that since the ear is frequency dependent we are usually interested only in the sound intensity at the frequencies which causes a response in the ear, ie the audible range. Consequently, the decibel (A) scale (dB(A)) is often used as a measure of the sound intensity in the audible range. Frequency is measured in hertz (Hz) where 1 Hz is one cycle per second.

Noise is often defined as unwanted sound. Noise is therefore either a physiological or psychological response which expresses an individual's adverse response to sound energy. Some sounds may be perceived as pleasant and desired (such as listening to a chosen CD), but the same music coming from a neighbour's house may cause annoyance and be regarded as noise. The sounds of a colleague talking loudly on the telephone or a hum from the air conditioning unit may all be perceived as unwanted and, therefore, a source of annoyance, anger, frustration and stress. These are the psychological effects of noise. The physiological effects relate to damage to the hearing mechanism which can occur after excessive or prolonged exposure to high levels of sound: this is called *noise-induced hearing loss*.

Heath effects of noise

Psychological effects of noise

7.3   Noise is a subjective phenomenon and people will vary widely in their tolerance of other people's sounds. The perception of noise, however, also depends on circumstance and what the individual is doing at the time he or she is exposed to noise. If you are having lunch in a crowded restaurant the background conversation will usually not be too disturbing, but the same level of background conversation in an open-plan office, when you are trying to concentrate, would be unacceptable. There are also individual differences in tolerance: some people will not be too upset by background noise, whereas others will be disturbed by the least amount of distraction.

Whether noise is annoying or distracting depends on the nature of the sound. Loud sounds are more distracting and cause more annoyance if they are intermittent and unexpected. There is an ability to habituate to some extent to low level continuous sounds (like the background sounds from the air conditioning system), but it is not possible to adjust to infrequent or intermittent sounds (like low flying aircraft or telephones ringing). Loud sound (such as a pneumatic drill outside the window) is also difficult to adjust to and can cause annoyance.

The most frequent sources of noise in modern office workplaces which people find most disturbing are other peoples' conversations, office machinery (such as photocopiers) and telephones ringing. Other research has found that the more people who share a workplace the more complaints there are of noise. Open-plan workplaces are therefore a frequent source of noise distraction.

Noise can also affect performance. The effects of noise on performance depend on whether or not the person is able to habituate to the sounds. Intermittent and unpredictable sounds, and sudden increases in sound intensity, cause the largest reduction in task performance. The more complex the task, and the more mental processing, vigilance and attention required, the more likely it is that background noise will adversely affect performance. Only the simplest tasks are unaffected by noise.

In most workplaces the ability to communicate is essential and noise can interfere with this. Effects on communication can cause errors and may be a safety risk; but in terms of health effects, poor communication will be annoying, frustrating and stressful. This stress may be felt both by the person who is speaking who cannot be heard, and by the listener who cannot understand what is being said. To be heard effectively, speech must be about 10 dB(A) louder than background sound. It is therefore important to keep background levels to below 50 dB(A) so that speech doesn't have to exceed 60 dB(A), for above this level strain on the vocal cords is likely. The BS/EN/ISO Standard 9241 Part 6, which applies to the environment around computer workstations, recommends a limit of 55 dB(A) for high concentration tasks, and 60 dB(A) for other tasks, but this recommendation is set in order to reduce the likelihood of *performance* effects. If there is need for effective voice communication, whether on the telephone or openly, a limit of 50 dB(A) is recommended.

Prolonged disturbance by noise in the workplace (as also in the home) will lead to stress. Stress occurs when a person feels he or she cannot cope with the situation he or she is in and is made worse when the individual feels that he or she has no control over the factors which are causing the stress. Obviously this applies to many things, but in the case of noise the person will feel unable to cope with the annoying, disturbing or irritating effects of being unable to concentrate and, additionally, will feel helpless in controlling the source of the noise. People suffering from noise stress will complain of inability to sleep (even if it is quiet at night), fatigue, headaches, irritability, intolerance of other people and an inability to concentrate.

Noise-induced hearing loss

7.4   Noise-induced hearing loss, or occupational deafness, is caused by damage to the cochlea of the ear. Hearing loss can be temporary or permanent.

Temporary hearing loss occurs when the ear is subjected to high levels of sound for a relatively short period of time. For a short while afterwards the ability to hear is diminished, but will recover. The degree of hearing loss and the time it takes to recover fully depend on the level and duration of sound exposure. Normally, temporary hearing loss recovers within 24 hours.

Permanent hearing loss is usually the result of accumulated damage over a long period of time. Hearing ability becomes increasingly poor over several years until a significant disability exists. Occasionally permanent damage to the ear can be caused by a sudden loud sound such as an explosion.

Permanent hearing loss can nearly always be prevented and failing to take the necessary precautions to minimise the risk of noise-induced deafness can expose the employer to liability and considerable damages for personal injury.

Legal requirements

7.5 There is no specific legislation which applies to the risk of psychological effects of noise. There are general duties, however, under the *Health and Safety at Work etc Act 1974, s 2*; and a specific duty under the *Management of Health and Safety at Work Regulations 1999 (SI 1999/3242)* which require a risk assessment to be made of noise in the workplace. The *Noise at Work Regulations 1989 (SI 1989/1790)* provide a statutory duty to assess the risk of hearing damage and to implement controls to limit the risk.

Assessing the risks

7.6 If you believe that any part of the workplace might subject employees to excessive levels of noise, then the *Noise at Work Regulations 1989 (SI 1989/1790)* require that a noise assessment is carried out by a competent person. A rule of thumb is that if people have to shout or have difficulty hearing ordinary conversation at two metres away, then there is likely to be a problem.

It is very important that the person undertaking the assessment understands the requirement of the Regulations, has the appropriate training and means of measuring sound levels (ie properly-calibrated equipment) and knows how to interpret the results. These are the essential requirements for competence. Under the Regulations noise exposure is measured as $L_{ep,d}$. This is a measure of the average exposure to noise over an eight-hour working day and there is a prescribed method for calculating this from the sound measurements that are taken. Again, the competent person must know how to make this calculation.

The *first action level* under the Regulations is defined as 85 dB(A) $L_{ep,d}$. If the average daily exposure is found to be below 85 dB(A) then there is still a legal obligation to reduce the risk of hearing damage to the lowest level reasonably practicable. If the average daily level is found to be above 85 dB(A) then there is not only a requirement to reduce the risk of hearing damage to the lowest level reasonably practicable, but this must include providing appropriate hearing protection to those likely to be exposed. There is, however, *no* legal requirement on the part of the employee to wear the provided hearing protection at the first action level.

Average daily exposure of 90 dB(A) and above is the *second action level* under the Regulations. At this level there is a requirement to reduce noise exposure by means other than hearing protection (ie by employing engineering solutions) and to demarcate hearing protection zones. At the second action level employees *do have* a legal obligation to wear the hearing protection provided when they are in an ear protection zone.

There is also a *peak action level*, set at 200 Pascals (Pa) (equivalent to 140 dB(A)), which represents the peak sound pressure when there is impulsive noise, such as from cartridge operated tools or rivet guns. If the peak level reaches or exceeds 200 Pa the same legal requirements exist as for the second action level, even though the $L_{ep,d}$ may not exceed 90 dB(A).

Health surveillance

7.7   Health surveillance is not a legal requirement under the *Noise at Work Regulations 1989 (SI 1989/1790) (Noise Regulations)*, but it is a requirement under the *Management of Health and Safety at Work Regulations 1999 (SI 1999/3242)*. Under the 1999 Regulations (and their Approved Code of Practice), health surveillance is required where all the following criteria apply:

- there is an identifiable disease or adverse health condition related to the work concerned;

- valid techniques are available to detect indications of the disease or condition;

- there is a reasonable likelihood that the disease or condition may occur under the particular conditions of work; and

- surveillance is likely to further protect the health and safety of the employees to be covered.

In this case, the valid technique for health surveillance is *audiometry*. Staff who are regularly exposed to noise at work, whether they wear hearing protection or not, should be required to have regular hearing checks by audiometry. This is also a specialised test which must be undertaken using appropriate and calibrated equipment and by someone who is competent to perform the test and interpret the results. The test can be conducted using portable equipment but the results are often misleading due to the masking effect of external sounds in the vicinity of the test area. Such screening must be undertaken in the very quietest of locations and any suspect or positive test must be followed up by a full test using a sound proof booth. Ideally, audiometry should always be undertaken using a sound proof booth so unless the facility is available in the workplace this will mean sending staff to a local occupational health clinic or hospital audiology department. Anyone exposed to noise at work who complains of tinnitus should have their hearing checked because this is often the sign of early hearing damage.

Records must be kept of all assessments under the *Noise Regulations* and any individual audiometry results. The legal requirement is to keep records only until the next assessment is carried out, but it is good practice to keep comprehensive historical records so that any future litigation can be properly defended. It is also good practice, if you are recruiting into a job that will expose a worker to noise, to have a baseline audiometric test done on starting work. This will put on record whether there is any existing hearing impairment at the time the person entered your employment.

Figure 1: Assessing the risk from noise

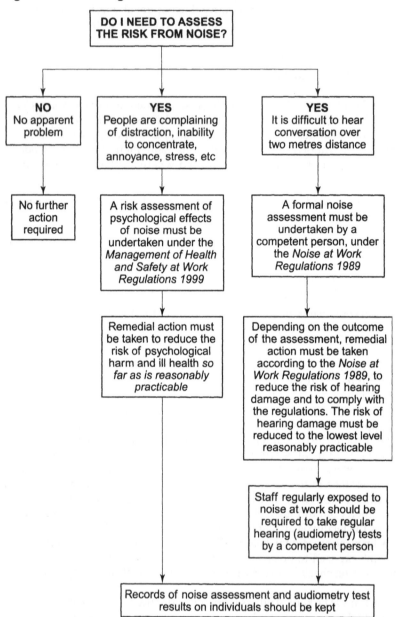

Vibration

7.8   It is surprising how many industries and processes subject employees to vibration and, therefore, put staff at risk of vibration injury. Anyone using a hand-held tool such as a drill, riveter, grinder, mower, floor cleaner or polisher (and these are but a few examples) will be exposed to the hazard of vibration. The most common health effects of vibration are those which arise from vibration of the hand and arm by use of such hand-held tools, called *hand-arm vibration*. However, in some circumstances, *whole body vibration* can occur when the entire body is subjected to vibration (eg when sitting or standing on machinery) and this has different effects on the body.

Vibration is an oscillatory motion in an object. When a person is in contact with the oscillating object, this motion is transmitted to the body. The oscillatory motion can occur in any axis in relation to the body. It can be a fore and aft motion (called the x-axis), a sideways (lateral motion, called the y-axis) and an up and down motion (the vertical or z-axis). When an object vibrates it moves in one direction with a given velocity and acceleration and when it reaches the end of movement in that direction it moves back again with a given velocity and acceleration. The number of times in a given time that it repeats this movement is called the frequency. Frequency is measured in the unit of hertz (Hz) where 1 Hz is one cycle per second. Velocity is measured in metres per second (m.s^{-1}) and acceleration (the rate of change in velocity) is measured in units of metres per second per second (m.s^{-2}). Characterising a vibration can be very complex, therefore. To simplify measurement of vibration, and to provide a measure that correlates well with health effects, the acceleration alone is normally used. This can be measured using an accelerometer.

Health effects of vibration

7.9 Whilst the health effects of vibration include both hand-arm vibration and whole body vibration (discussed below), they may present as generalised symptoms of fatigue, sleeplessness, headache and digestive disorders. It should be borne in mind, therefore, that these are common symptoms of someone under stress and may not be due directly to vibration.

Hand-arm vibration

7.10 Hand-arm vibration can lead to damage of the nerves, muscles, joints and blood vessels of the hand and arm. The most common ill-health effect is *vibration white finger* (VWF). VWF is probably caused by cumulative damage to the nerves which control the blood vessels supplying blood to the fingers or to the blood vessels themselves. The condition often starts in the finger tips of one or more fingers. Exposure to the cold, either working in cold air or the hand in contact with cold objects, will precipitate constriction of the blood vessels causing the affected finger tips to blanch. Blanching is also often associated with numbness and tingling. The condition then progresses to involve more fingers and more phalanges (the sections of the fingers between the joints). There are a number of ways of describing the severity of VWF, but one of the common methods is that devised by the Stockholm Workshop (see TABLE 1).

Table 1: The Stockholm Workshop Scale for describing the severity of vibration white finger

Stage	Grade	Description
Cold-induced blanching		
0		No attacks
1	Mild	Occasional attacks affecting only the tips of one or more fingers
2	Moderate	Occasional attacks affecting the distal (finger tip) and middle phalanges of one or more fingers
3	Severe	Frequent attacks affecting all phalanges of most fingers
4	Very severe	As in Stage 3 with trophic skin changes in the finger tips
Sensorineural effects		
0_{sn}	—	Exposed to vibration but no symptoms
1_{sn}	—	Intermittent numbness with out or without tingling
2_{sn}	—	Intermittent or persistent numbness, reduced sensory perception
3_{sn}	—	Intermittent or persistent numbness, reduced tactile discrimination and/ or manipulative dexterity

The cold-induced blanching (Raynaud's Phenomenon) is often tested by immersing the hands in cold water. The staging in the Stockholm Workshop Scale is made for both hands separately.

VWF is a very debilitating disease. It prevents the person feeling accurately with the fingers which means they cannot properly hold or pick things up. As a consequence, their ability to perform a whole range of tasks which normally requires manual dexterity is severely affected, limiting their ability to work and to undertake social activities. The loss of sensitivity in the fingers can also be a significant safety factor.

As well as VWF, other effects of vibration are recognised. These are neurological (caused by nerve damage), muscular (effects on muscles) and articular (effects on joints). *Neurological effects* include numbness (without blanching and therefore distinct from VWF), tingling, elevated sensory threshold for touch, pain, and temperature and reduced nerve conduction velocity. *Muscular effects* include weakness, reduced muscle mass (wasting of muscle in the arm) and reduced grip strength. Reduced grip strength can have serious safety implications when using a power tools or other hand-held tools. Some evidence exists that vibration causes *damage to the joints* of the fingers, wrist and elbow and this seems to be most commonly associated with using percussion tools that send low frequency shock waves along the length of the arm. These injuries can lead to a variety of arthritic-type conditions although the scientific evidence linking these specifically to hand-arm vibration is scanty.

Whole body vibration

7.11   Whole body vibration is caused by standing or sitting on industrial machinery or vehicles such as lorries, tractors, fork-lift trucks or motorcycles. Low frequency motion may induce vertigo or nausea (similar to travel sickness) but people who are prone to these effects will usually avoid working in situations which provoke their sickness. Aside from whole body vibration actually making someone feel ill, it will often cause severe discomfort. This subjective discomfort will vary with individual perceptions of the vibration and personal reactions to it. The threshold at which people will begin to feel discomfort is 0.01 m.s^{-2} and the subjective sensation of discomfort will increase linearly with increases in vibration magnitude.

Whole body vibration has also been linked with damage to the spinal column, including displacement and damage to the intervertebral discs and degeneration of the spinal vertebrae. Whilst it is quite likely that vibration of the spinal column will increase the risk of spinal damage, other causes cannot be ruled out. Posture and heavy lifting associated with the job may also play a part. It is good practice to include whole body vibration when assessing the risk of back injury in a job which also involves lifting and carrying and working in poor postures.

Legal requirements

7.12   There is currently no *specific* legislation which requires a risk assessment for vibration. However, the *Management of Health and Safety at Work Regulations 1999 (1999/3242), Reg 3*, requires an assessment to be made of the risks to which employees are exposed whilst they are at work. Where employees are exposed to vibration there is a clear legal requirement, therefore, to assess the risks to health but, unfortunately, without a framework of specific regulations governing how that assessment should be carried out. This situation is set to change in the next few years, however, with the adoption of the EU *Physical Agents (Vibration) Directive 2002 (2002/44/EC)*. It will have to be adopted in the UK by mid-2005, although there are derogations for certain industries up to 2014. It would be prudent to work towards adopting the requirements of the EU Directive as soon as is practicable; although in many circumstances this will be challenging.

For hand-arm vibration the exposure action level averaged over an eight-hour day will be 2.5 m.s^{-2} and the exposure limit will be 5.0 m.s^{-2} (Note that these limits are more stringent than that currently recommended: see TABLE 2). The values for whole body vibration will be set at 0.5 m.s^{-2} over an eight-hour day with a limit of 1.15 m.s^{-2}.

Assessing the risks

7.13   A risk assessment for vibration must start with identifying those employees who use hand-held power or pneumatic tools, use percussion tools (such as hammer and chisel) or who use mechanical equipment (such as floor polishers, mowers, etc) or any other equipment that is likely to transmit vibration to the hand and arm. In addition, employees who use ride-on machines, means of transport or other equipment which is likely to cause whole body vibration must also be identified. Under current legislation there is a need to assess the risk to health but there are no enforceable exposure limits. There is, therefore, no legal obligation to measure vibration dose. As mentioned at 7.12, this will change in mid-2005 when UK legislation to enforce the EU *Physical Agents (Vibration) Directive 2002 (2002/44/EC)* is introduced. The daily average and limit values specified above will then need to be met.

At the present time guidance on exposure dose is contained in HS(G)88 (HSE), which in turn is taken from the British Standards Institute's guidance BS 6842. It is recommended that the exposure dose over an eight-hour working day is limited to an average of 2.8m.s^{-2}. If the length of the working day is shorter, then higher averages are allowable (see TABLE 2). If it is decided to have measurements of vibration dose made then they will have to made by a competent person and should conform to the standards set down by the British Standards Institute (BS 6841 for whole body exposure and BS 6842 for hand-arm vibration).

The risk assessment will need to assume that the risk is high for people who regularly use vibrating hand tools and equipment as a necessary part of the job. Other risk factors include working in the cold and smoking. If it is decided that measurements should be taken, then currently exposure dose should at least be within the limits recommended by the HSE in HS(G)88.

Table 2: Average hand-arm vibration levels over a working day that would give an average of 2.8m.s^{-2} over an eight-hour day

Length of working day(hours)	16	8	4	2	1	½
rms (root mean square) average vibration level (m.s^{-2}) over working day to give an eight-hour dose of 2.8 m.s^{-2}	2	2.8	4	5.6	8	11.2

Figure 2: Assessing the risk from vibration

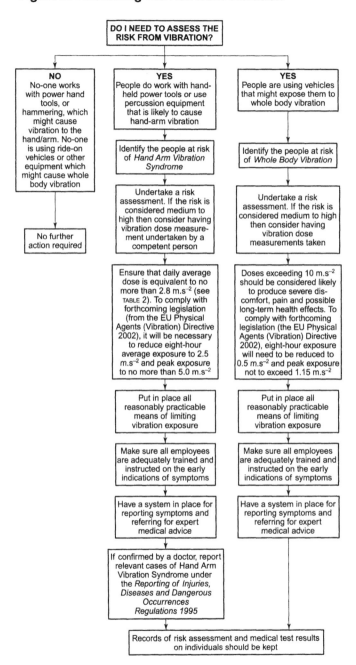

Whilst again there is, as yet, no statutory requirement to adhere to these limits, the Court of Appeal has endorsed them and has used them as a basis for determining liability in civil claims for damages.

Risk management will need to consider a range of options to reduce exposure to vibration. These include reducing the time of exposure, perhaps by job rotation or building in frequent rest breaks, providing personal protection (eg gloves to protect against cold and vibration, although the effectiveness of gloves in reducing transmission of vibration is very limited), and making sure equipment is properly maintained and lubricated. It may be necessary to replace old tools with new tools which have been better designed to limit vibration.

Health surveillance

7.14   Anyone working with vibrating equipment must be kept under health surveillance. There is a legal requirement for this under the *Management of Health and Safety at Work Regulations 1999 (SI 1999/3242)* and their Approved Code of Practice. The form that health surveillance takes is at the discretion of the employer, but it must be sufficient to detect early signs of vibration illness and further protect the health of the employee. In an industry which has a large number of employees at high risk of vibration illness it would be normal practice to employ an occupational health nurse backed up by referral to an occupational health physician to undertake regular screening. In smaller companies, however, a nurse may be contracted to undertake a screening programme on an occasional basis. In the very smallest companies, or where the risk of vibration illness is considered low, then self-monitoring would be an acceptable means of health surveillance. If self-monitoring is employed, staff must be familiar with the symptoms and must be aware of how, and to whom, they should report any concerns. The company must, in turn, have access to medical advice in order to refer anyone who complains of early symptoms.

The main symptoms of hand-arm vibration are:

- tingling and numbness in the fingers;
- loss of sensation in the fingers and reduced manual dexterity;
- coldness and/or blanching of the fingers (starting in the finger tips) after exposure to vibration or exposure to the cold; or
- aching fingers and limbs.

In addition, anyone exposed to whole body vibration should report:

- back ache/back pains;
- leg ache/pains;

- frequent digestive upsets;

- balance problems or dizziness;

- visual disorders;

- headaches; or

- sleeplessness.

Hand arm vibration syndrome (HAVS) is a reportable disease under the *Reporting of Injuries, Diseases and Dangerous Occurrences Regulations 1995 (SI 1995/3163)*. Strictly this is only reportable when it occurs as a result of working with certain types of equipment. These are listed in Sch 3 of the 'Guide to the Regulations' (HSE, L73). (For further discussion of these Regulations, see CHAPTER 2.)

Less informative advice is available for whole body vibration, although British Standard 6841 suggests that whole body exposure above 15m.s$^{-1.75}$ (equal to about 10 m.s^{-2}) is likely to be associated with severe discomfort, pain and injury. This is a value which might be considered to be excessive and efforts should be made to reduce average exposure to values considerably below this.

Forthcoming legislation, based on the EU *Physical Agents (Vibration) Directive 2002 (2002/44/EC)* (see 7.12), will require eight-hour average exposure to be limited to 0.5 m.s^{-2} and peak values not to exceed 1.15 m.s^{-2}.

Temperature

7.15 From an occupational health point of view, the temperature of our surroundings is of great importance. It affects us in two main ways:

- very high or very low temperatures can alter the body temperature, and cause *severe physiological effects* which can be life-threatening; and

- moderately high or low temperature can cause *discomfort*.

Working in hot environments

7.16 The normal body (core) temperature is 37°C and needs to be controlled within fairly small limits around this value. A rise in body temperature above 37°C is termed *hyperthermia* and is not well tolerated. A rise to only 41°C is serious and a temperature of 43°C is nearly always fatal. The body has a number of very effective mechanisms for maintaining its temperature at the normal value. These include flushing the skin with blood (*vasodilation*) and sweating to lose heat. Working in very hot environments can overload the normal body control mechanisms and lead to anything from a moderate to severe rise in the body temperature.

Factors associated with a risk of hyperthermia are:

- High workload

  High workload increases the amount of heat generated by the body. Someone engaged in heavy work will typically generate 450 watts of heat. This heat has to be dissipated in order to keep the body temperature constant. If the work is being carried out in a hot environment then it may be impossible for the body to lose this heat and the body temperature will rise.

- Too much body insulation (clothing) or impervious clothing

  Too much insulation reduces the ability of the body to lose heat. It may be necessary sometimes to wear protective clothing in a hot environment and this may have an adverse effect on the ability of the body to lose heat. Equally, clothing made of materials which are impervious will quickly become saturated with moisture vapour inside and prevent the body losing heat by sweating.

- High dry bulb temperatures

  The *dry bulb temperature* is the measure of the air temperature using an ordinary thermometer.

- High radiant heat loads

  Radiant heat is the heat absorbed by the body from hot surfaces in the environment around the person. This can be a very significant source of heat gain in many industries: for instance, working with molten metal or glass, or in kitchens. Radiant heat can also be significant when working outdoors where the heat source is the sun.

- High humidity

  High humidity can seriously affect the body's ability to lose heat because it inhibits the effectiveness of sweating. Sweating is an effective way of losing heat by a mechanism called the latent heat of vaporisation. This means that when the sweat evaporates it removes heat from the skin surface and this in turn cools the blood flowing through the skin. Evaporation will not occur if the air around the skin has a higher level of moisture than the skin itself. In high humidity therefore the body produces sweat but it does not evaporate, making the person feel wet and uncomfortable and increasing the risk of the body temperature rising.

- Low air velocity

  Air velocity affects the rate at which sweat evaporates from the skin but this depends on a number of factors. If the air has high humidity then even high air velocities will not increase the rate of heat evaporation. In fact, if the air has a high humidity and is also at high temperature, a high rate of air movement over the body may actually add heat to the body by a process known as convection. If the body is substantially covered by clothing or with impervious clothing, then increased air velocity will not influence the rate of sweat evaporation. To be maximally effective the air should be cooler than the body surface, should be at low humidity and the body surface should be largely exposed: in those circumstances increased air velocity will hasten the evaporation of sweat and increase the rate of heat loss.

Heat stress disorders

7.17   Responses to a hot environment vary depending on the amount of heat strain imposed on the body. A number of possible heat stress disorders can occur. In a hot environment, in which the body is attempting to lose heat, the blood vessels in the skin will be dilated and blood pressure may fall.

A common response to this condition is *heat syncope* (fainting). This is not usually a serious condition (although injury may result when the victim falls).

Sweat contains water and salts and if a substantial amount of sweat is lost the body can become dehydrated and can suffer from salt imbalance. This disturbance of the body's fluid and salt balance leads to *heat exhaustion* a more serious condition than heat syncope. Classic symptoms of heat exhaustion are hyperventilation (over-breathing), dizziness, nausea, numbness in the fingers and toes and around the mouth. Typically the body temperature in someone with heat exhaustion is between 37–39°C. If untreated this progresses to confusion, collapse and possibly fits. If a person has been sweating profusely another condition can occur, prickly heat (*miliaria*). This is caused by the sweat gland ducts swelling and blocking, creating reddened and painful itchy weals.

The most serious form of heat illness is *heat stroke*. This usually occurs when a person has been undertaking hard physical exercise in a hot humid environment and the body temperature has risen quickly to above 39°C. There is a sudden failure in the thermoregulatory mechanism and sweating stops. The victim is hot and dry to the touch and becomes semi-conscious or comatose. Without sweating the body temperature rises quickly and there is a high risk of death.

Legal requirements

7.18   Anyone working in a hot environment must be assessed for the risk of developing a heat stress disorder: this is a legal requirement under the *Management of Health and Safety at Work Regulations 1999 (SI 1999/3242)*. The complexity of the risk assessment will depend on the nature of the likely exposure to heat. The Regulations require that the risk assessment is 'suitable and sufficient', which means that someone expected to perform hard physical work in a hot humid environment exposed to radiant heat will require a more thorough assessment of all the factors involved than someone who is sedentary in only a moderately hot environment.

Assessing the risks

7.19   There are many ways in which a person's expected response to a hot environment can be assessed. Many of these are highly technical and normally only used where people are required to work in extreme environments. Most of them use measures of environmental heat load and work rate to calculate tolerance times or work-rest regimes. For all but the simplest hot environments it would be necessary to engage the help of an experienced occupational hygienist to undertake the required measurements and apply the most appropriate heat stress index. The most widely used index, and among the simplest, is the *wet bulb globe temperature* (WBGT). This requires two measurements: the wet bulb temperature (WB) and the globe temperature (GT):

- the WB is the temperature of the air taken with a thermometer covered by a wet wick; when compared to the dry bulb temperature this is the measure of humidity; and

- the GT is the measure of radiant heat provided by a thermometer covered by a black bulb.

The WBGT is then calculated from:

WBGT = 0.7 WB + 0.3 GT (for indoor environments)

or

WBGT = 0.7 WB + 0.2 GT + 0.1 DB (for outdoor environments),

(where DB is the dry bulb temperature).

Table 3: Summary of WBGT reference values from ISO 7243

Metabolic rate class	Total Metabolic rate (W)	Reference value (WBGT °C) (person not acclimatised)
0 (resting)	<117	32
1	117–234	29
2	234–360	26
3	360–468	22 (no sensible air movement)
		23 (with sensible air movement)
4	>468	18 (no sensible air movement)
		20 (with sensible air movement)

These values are a summary only. Different values (slightly lower) can be applied if the person is acclimatised to the heat. The total metabolic rate applies for a person with an average skin surface area of 1.8m² but for accuracy should be adjusted for different body sizes. Full details of the references are contained in ISO 7243.

Table 4: Work-rest regimes recommended by the American Conference of Industrial Hygienists

Work-rest regime		Workload		
		Light	*Moderate*	*Heavy*
Work (minutes each hour)	*Rest (minutes each hour)*	*WBGT (°C)*		
Continuous work		30.0	26.7	25.0
45	15	30.6	28.0	25.9
30	30	31.4	29.4	27.9
15	45	32.2	31.1	30.0

American Conference of Industrial Hygienists. Threshold Limit Values for 1994–95 (ACGIH, Cincinnati, 1994)

The WBGT value is useful because it can be compared with reference values to estimate the maximum WBGT value that a normally fit and normally clothed individual could work without suffering heat stress disorders. Reference values are contained in an international standard ISO 7243 (see TABLE 3).

The WBGT can also usefully be used to determine work-rest regimes. The American Conference of Industrial Hygienists (ACGIH 1994), recommends different work-rest regimes according to the WBGT and the workload, as shown in TABLE 4.

Working in cold environments

7.20   Many people work in a cold environment. In Northern Europe and Scandinavia most outdoor workers will be exposed to the cold, and in winter this can sometimes be severe. Many indoor workers, in cold stores and open warehouses for example, will work in extremely cold conditions. As with heat, the body has several mechanisms for maintaining the body temperature despite the temperature of the surroundings. In the case of cold, the mechanisms are constriction of the blood vessels in the skin to restrict heat loss and an increase in heat production. Increases in heat production are graded according to the cold threat. With mild exposure, shivering will start in small groups of muscles but will spread to whole body shivering if the cold exposure increases. If the cold exposure is prolonged or intensifies, the body will start to produce hormones, such as adrenaline, noradrenaline and thyroxin, to increase the metabolic rate.

Any fall in the temperature below the normal core body temperature of 37°C is termed *hypothermia*, and if it drops to around 32°C a state of severe hypothermia exists resulting in mental confusion and loss of consciousness. Such a low temperature is not, however, incompatible with life: people have survived deep body temperatures of as low as 17°C. Nevertheless, any state of hypothermia is serious and potentially life threatening. In addition to the risk of the body temperature falling, cold presents a risk of injury to the extremities (frostbite).

Factors associated with a risk of hypothermia are:

- Low workload (low metabolic rate);

- Loo little body insulation (clothing or impervious clothing);

- Low dry bulb temperatures;

- High levels of conductive heat loss to the extremities (causing cold injury); and

- High air velocity (wind chill).

Legal requirements

7.21   The legal obligation to undertake a risk assessment for people working in cold environments falls within the *Management of Health and Safety at Work Regulations 1999 (SI 1999/3242)*.

Assessing the risks

7.22   Assessing the risk of cold stress is not nearly as well developed as assessing heat stress. The method normally used is to estimate the wind chill index (WCI) from measurements of the dry bulb temperature and the air velocity. The WCI is actually a measurement of the rate at which heat is lost from the body (in watts per square metre of body surface, ie Wm^{-2}). Although this is a useful measure of the likely adverse effects of cold exposure, it fails to take into account one important factor, namely the amount of clothing and the insulative value of the clothing worn.

The WCI is calculated as follows:

$$WCI \ (kcal.m^{-2}.h^{-1}) = (33 - t_a) \ (10v^{0.5} - v + 10.45)$$

(where t_a is the ambient (dry bulb) temperature and v is the air velocity in metres per second ($m.s^{-1}$))

This formula calculates the kilocalories per square metre of body surface per hour; this is then divided by 1.16 to derive the WCI in watts per square metre (W.m^{-2}). The WCI can then be related to an equivalent *chilling temperature*, which is perhaps the most useful application of the WCI for most purposes. The chilling temperature is the temperature equivalent if the air had been calm. So, for example if the ambient temperature is –1°C and the air velocity is 16m.s^{-1} the wind chill is equivalent to being in a still-air temperature of –21°C (see TABLE 5).

Table 5: Wind chill equivalent temperatures

Air velocity m.s^{-1}	Dry bulb air temperature (°C)							
0 (Still Air)	–1	–7	–12	–18	–23	–29	–34	–40
2	–3	–9	–15	–21	–26	–32	–38	–44
4	–9	–16	–23	–30	–36	–43	–50	–57
6	–14	–21	–29	–36	–43	–50	–58	–65
8	–16	–24	–32	–40	–47	–55	–63	–71
10	–18	–26	–34	–42	–51	–59	–67	–76
12	–19	–28	–36	–44	–53	–61	–70	–79
16	–21	–30	–38	–46	–55	–64	–73	–82

Siple, PA, and Passell, CP, 'Dry atmospheric cooling in sub-freezing temperatures', Proc Am Phil Soc 89: 177–199, 1945 (adapted from Oakley, EHN, Heat and Cold, Chapter 15 in 'Hunter's Diseases of Occupation', 9th Edition (Arnold, London, 2000)

Thermal comfort

7.23 The aspect of the thermal environment that affects more people than any other is that of thermal comfort. Comfort describes the complete satisfaction with one's surroundings. *Thermal comfort* relates to satisfaction with the thermal environment, in other words it is a feeling of being neither too hot nor too cold. Thermal comfort is therefore a subjective phenomenon. A group of people sharing the same environment are likely to differ considerably in their perception of satisfaction with it, and will therefore express varying perceptions of comfort. When the deep body temperature is normal, we base our feelings of thermal comfort on skin temperature and on the feeling of dampness of the skin. We also base the feeling of comfort on lack of perception of any differences in skin temperature between different parts of the body. In particular, most people will be uncomfortable if they sense that their feet are cooler than the upper parts of their body. The temperature of our surroundings is detected by a network of temperature sensors in the skin. These sensors feed back information to the brain and provide us with a conscious awareness of whether the skin is hot, neutral or cold. It is the differences in interpretation of what the skin sensors are telling us about the temperature of our skin which leads to differences in preferences in environmental temperature. Some people will prefer to be in a warm environment and others will prefer a cooler environment.

In addition to general activity levels (work rate), the factors which affect thermal comfort are:

- The amount (and insulative value) of clothing

  The *amount of clothing* and the *level of activity* will influence thermal comfort by altering the amount of heat generated by the body and the rate at which it can be lost. Any imbalance in this will adversely affect comfort.

- The dry bulb temperature

  The *dry bulb temperature* is closely related to thermal comfort. The range of acceptable temperatures varies according to the work being performed and the work environment. A person engaged in sedentary work indoors for example, will demand a higher temperature for comfort than someone performing hard physical work.

- Radiant heat/radiant cold

  Radiant heat refers to the warming of the skin by heat radiated from objects which are hotter than the skin surface. Typical sources indoors would be a radiator or a cooker in a kitchen. Outdoors, working in the sun or close to a fire would be obvious examples.

  Radiant cold refers to the heat lost from the skin surface by being radiated to an object nearby, such as a window, which is colder than the skin. Even if the dry bulb temperature is at a reasonable value, being exposed to a radiant heat source or being close to a radiant cold source can cause considerable discomfort.

- Relative humidity

  Recommendations for comfort temperatures are discussed later. At any given temperature, the *relative humidity* (RH) is a measure of the proportion of moisture in the air, compared to the maximum amount of moisture the air can carry. It is expressed as a percentage, so 50% RH means the air is 50% saturated with water. We are not very sensitive to relative humidity so a wide range of RH values is usually acceptable. However if the humidity falls too low (ie the air is dry) then the resultant drying of the eyes, nose, throat and skin can be very uncomfortable. A high relative humidity (especially if the temperature is also high) can prevent sweat evaporating from the skin leaving it feeling moist, which is also perceived as uncomfortable. Recommended values for humidity are discussed later.

- Air velocity

  Air velocity (air movement) can either help comfort or add to the discomfort. If the air temperature is too warm, a sensible air movement (such as breeze outdoors or a fan indoors) will help cool the skin and contribute positively to comfort. However a strongly directional air movement (on the back of the neck or around the feet for example) or a movement of air which is very cold (see wind chill at 7.22) will be sensed as very uncomfortable.

- Time of day

  One further factor may be added to this list and that is time of day. Thermal comfort has a *circadian rhythm*. The conditions which are most comfortable during the day will often be sensed as too cold at night, with obvious implications for night workers. Temperatures usually need to be about 2°C higher at night to maintain the same level of thermal comfort.

Legal requirements

7.24 There is no specific legislation covering hot and cold environments, but there are a number of legal obligations under general legislation. Apart from the obligations under the *Health and Safety at Work etc Act 1974, s 2(1)* and *(2)* to provide a safe and healthy working environment, there are duties under the *Workplace (Health, Safety and Welfare) Regulations 1992 (Workplace Regulations) (SI 1992/3004)* and the *Health and Safety (Display Screen Equipment) Regulations 1992 (DSE Regulations) (SI 1992/2792)*. These apply to indoor environments and in the case of the *DSE Regulations* specifically to environments in which DSE users are working.

The *Workplace Regulations, Reg 7* requires that the temperature in all workplaces *is reasonable* during working hours. The Approved Code of Practice to these Regulations sets out the minimum temperature of 16°C at all times people are at work, except where work involves considerable physical effort, in which case it reduces to 13°C. These are minimum temperatures and no maximum is provided except that any higher temperature must be *reasonable*. The lower temperature is not always feasible to maintain, for example in cold storage areas, in which case adequate protective clothing and rest breaks out of the cold area must be provided in order to ensure the reasonable comfort of the employees.

Display Screen Equipment users are covered by the *DSE Regulations*. *Schedule 3(e)* states:

> '... equipment belonging to any workstation shall not produce excess heat which could cause discomfort to operators or users'.

An interpretation that should be taken to mean that the environment of DSE workstations is not uncomfortable to users (regardless of where the heat comes from) would be in line with the BS EN ISO Standard 9241(6). This standard on the work environment of DSE workstations recommends a temperature of 19–23°C. *Schedule 3(g)* of the *DSE Regulations* sets the requirement that:

'... an adequate level of humidity should be established and maintained'.

What is 'adequate' can again be taken from the recommendation in BS EN ISO Standard 9241(6) that humidity should be maintained at between 40–60% RH.

Although more of a safety issue, the *Provision and Use of Work Equipment Regulations 1998 (SI 1998/2306), Reg 13* requires that any equipment which is at very high or very low temperatures must have protection to prevent burn, scald or sear. Any risk to health from more extreme hot and cold environments must be assessed under the *Management of Health and Safety at Work Regulations 1999 (SI 1999/3242)*.

Assessing the risks

7.25   Although the factors which contribute to thermal comfort can be measured they cannot usefully predict a person's thermal comfort. Since comfort is a subjective response it can only be measured by subjective means. The usual way of measuring comfort is to apply a thermal comfort rating scale such as that drawn up by the American Society of Heating and Refrigeration and Air Conditioning Engineers (the ASHRAE scale). This is shown in TABLE 6.

Table 6: The ASHRAE Thermal Comfort Scale

Numerical scale	Descriptor
1	Hot
2	Warm
3	Slightly Warm
4	Neutral
5	Slightly Cool
6	Cool
7	Cold

This is used by asking subjects to circle the number which most closely fits the way they feel at the time. The object is get the thermal conditions sufficiently right so that the majority of people will vote at the neutral point. However, the proportion of people who vote neutral is often no more than 70% even when all the comfort factors are optimal. Small changes in the ambient temperature will affect this rating significantly. A temperature of just 3°C lower or higher than the one found to be optimal for a group of people will reduce the comfort rating from 70% to about 30%. Because

Table 7: Thermal comfort questionnaire

Please answer the following questions concerned with *your thermal comfort*.

1. Indicate on the scale below how you feel *now*:
    ❑ Hot
    ❑ Warm
    ❑ Slightly Warm
    ❑ Neutral
    ❑ Slightly Cool
    ❑ Cool
    ❑ Cold

2. Please indicate how you would like to be *now*:
    ❑ Warmer   ❑ No Change   ❑ Cooler

3. Please indicate how you *generally* feel at work:
    ❑ Hot
    ❑ Warm
    ❑ Slightly Warm
    ❑ Neutral
    ❑ Slightly Cool
    ❑ Cool
    ❑ Cold

4. Please indicate how you would *generally* like to be at work:
    ❑ Warmer   ❑ No Change   ❑ Cooler

5. Are you generally satisfied with your thermal environment at work?
    ❑ Yes   ❑ No

6. Please give any additional information or comments which you think are relevant to the assessment of your thermal environment at work (eg draughts, dryness, clothing, suggested improvements, etc).

Thank you.

BOHS Technical Guide No 8, 'The Thermal Environment', 1990. Reproduced by permission of the British Occupational Hygiene Society.

Figure 3: Assessing the risk of hot and cold environments

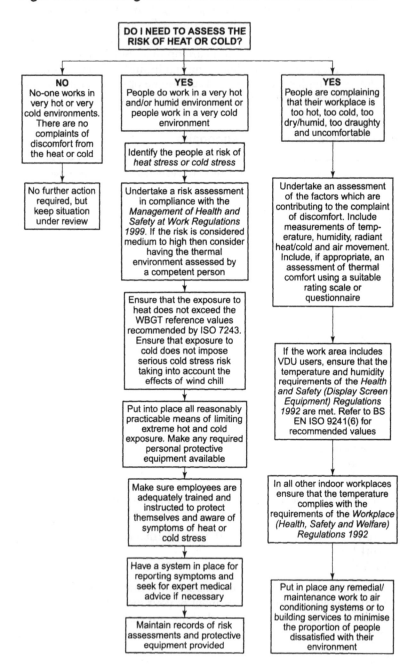

thermal comfort is very subjective, it will often not be possible to satisfy everyone's preferences: this is especially true in indoor environments and where large numbers of people have to share a common air-conditioned space. Even when the thermal comfort conditions suit the majority, there will be a significant minority who will complain of discomfort.

One of the disadvantages of the one-off Thermal Comfort Scale (see TABLE 6) is that it measures a person's feeling of comfort at the moment in time it is taken. It is sometimes better to gain a longer-term overall view of the average feeling of satisfaction with the thermal environment and this can be done by a questionnaire similar to that published by the British Occupational Hygiene Society (1990) (see TABLE 7).

Light

7.26 The lighting environment should be designed to achieve four main goals:

- safety;

- provision of a pleasing and comfortable environment;

- performance of the task; and

- general health and the avoidance of eyestrain.

A safe and pleasant environment

7.27 It is beyond the scope of this book to discuss in detail the very complex areas of lighting design and colour. However, the provision of artificial lighting or a mix of natural and artificial lighting and the colour of surroundings which together provides a pleasing and comfortable environment can have very positive effects on wellbeing.

Lighting can also have a major impact on safety. Adequately lit stairwells, and walkways, properly lit outdoor areas such as car parks, and in machine shops are just a few examples of where sufficient levels of light are essential for safety. Safety may also be an issue where there are explosive or inflammable atmospheres where light fittings will need to be intrinsically safe, and in the provision of emergency lighting for escape routes in the event of a power failure.

These issues are dealt with in a series of lighting codes and other literature published by the Chartered Institution of Building Services Engineers (CIBSE).

Performance of the task

7.28   Well-designed and adequate levels of light are essential to any task that requires vision. Whilst there are many technical ways in which light can be measured the illuminance is the most commonly used. *Illuminance* is the amount of light falling onto a surface divided by the area of the surface onto which it is falling. The units are lumens per square metre or, more usually now, the SI unit of the lux. The CIBSE provide guidance on the levels of illuminance required for different tasks and in different industries in their lighting guides (eg 'Code for Lighting' (CD ROM (2002) available from the Chartered Institution of Building Services Engineers, 222 Balham High Road, Balham, London SW12 9BS). For example, in a frozen food processing area 200 lux is an acceptable illuminance, hand decorating in a bakery requires 500 lux and fine machine and finishing in woodwork shop requires 750 lux. Very fine detailed work in manufacturing and printing inspection may require 1,500 lux. General office tasks require 500 lux and computer workstations between 300–500 lux. The HSE also produces guidance on lighting at work (HSE, 1998).

Colour – In addition to illuminance the other important aspect of lighting is colour. The colour of artificial light depends on the source. Different types of lamp will produce different colour of light which will alter the way the eye sees the colour of the surroundings. Sometimes colour rendition is designed for aesthetic purposes to match a particular light and design ambience that is being created. Halogen-phosphate fluorescent tubes are available as cool white, white and warm white. Each of these emphasise yellows but have different effects on the green and blue part of the spectrum providing a range of colour rendition from bluish 'cold' to yellow-red 'warm' light. Where colour matching or accurate rendering of colours is required for particular tasks (such as inspection or drawing) then artificial daylight or full-spectrum lighting is required.

Glare – Task performance may also be adversely affected by glare. Glare is the situation where there is excessive contrast in the visual field. Two forms of glare are recognised: disability glare and discomfort glare. *Disability glare* occurs when a bright source of light in the field of vision prevents the eye from seeing anything else. An example would be a computer VDU located in front of a window with sun shining through it. The high intensity of the sunlight in the operator's eyes compared with the intensity of light around the computer screen (high contrast) prevents the eye seeing details of the screen image. *Discomfort glare* does not usually affect task performance but the presence of high contrasts in the field of vision will cause discomfort. Over a period of time this discomfort may result in eyestrain and headache. Discomfort glare usually results from poorly-designed interior lighting.

Age – Lighting can affect task performance in other ways. If the lighting conditions cause visual fatigue (see 7.29) then that, in turn, will cause a reduction in performance. Age will also affect visual performance. Above about the age of 40 there is a marked decline in the efficiency with which light is transmitted through the eye. As a result, the illuminance required for visual tasks (such as reading print) will need to be increased. Many people, particularly as they get older, may like to use task lights (individual desk lamps) so that they can have personal control over the illuminance of the task independent of the levels of light provided by the background lighting. Task lighting can very successfully provide individual control over lighting conditions, but the possibility that one person's desk lamp causes glare to another person has to be considered.

General health and eyestrain

7.29   Light can have profound effects on the general health of people. Natural sunlight has stimulating and arousing effects on the body, which are often lost when people spend long periods exposed to artificial and low intensity light sources. On a bright sunny day outdoors, the illuminance levels are about 10,000–12,000 lux compared to the usual levels of 300–500 lux indoors. This low intensity of light, together with differences in the colour of artificial light, is not stimulating and in fact produces hormonal changes that increase the feeling of fatigue and sleepiness. This may be part of the cause of *sick building syndrome* (see 7.60). The beneficial effect of sunlight is evident from the 15% or so of the population who suffer from *seasonal affective disorder* (SAD or winter depression). Sufferers can be severely depressed by the lack of sunlight in the winter months, but for many people this can be alleviated by daily exposure to a bright source of light (phototherapy). Much research has been done to investigate the possibility of reproducing the beneficial effects of sunlight indoors. The only solution so far is the introduction of full-spectrum lighting which produces light similar to the spectral quality (colour) of sunlight. Whilst there is some evidence of the beneficial effect of this, it does not overcome the problem of illuminance levels. The eye needs to receive at least 3,000 lux to produce the full stimulating effects on the brain and, as mentioned earlier, this level of light indoors would produce high and unacceptable levels of glare. The incorporation of natural light during the daytime in buildings is advantageous but practically very difficult, especially in deep-plan buildings.

General health is also affected by poor lighting design and the poor positioning of equipment in relation to light sources. Eyestrain is a condition that arises when the small muscles within and around the eye become fatigued. This results in a heavy, tired feeling in the eyes and pain which can spread to become a headache. Factors which contribute to visual fatigue and eyestrain include the following:

* visual task involves seeing minute detail;

* high concentration required for task;

* excessively low contrast between task and background;

* reflections and glare from surfaces associated with the task;

- background discomfort and disability glare;

- task involves tracking movement;

- inadequate illuminance of the task; and

- flicker from light sources.

In addition to these environmental causes, poor eyesight, eye disease (such as glaucoma) or inappropriate spectacles will also contribute to eyestrain.

The frequency of fluorescent lights is also thought to play a part in determining adverse heath effects. Fluorescent lights flicker at a rate which is twice the power supply frequency (ie 100 hertz (Hz) where 1 Hz is one cycle per second). At this rate, the brain fuses the individual flickers and interprets it as continuous light. However, it appears that the brain still reacts to this low frequency flicker and there is evidence that it can cause headache and possibly fatigue. A solution introduced in recent years is high frequency lighting in which the fluorescent tube is driven much faster, at many thousands Hz. This can have beneficial effects in significantly reducing the severity and frequency of complaint of headache. There are commercially available light sources that combine the benefits of high frequency and full-spectrum lighting.

Legal requirements

7.30   The provision of 'suitable and sufficient' lighting is required by the *Workplace (Health, Safety and Welfare) Regulations 1992 (Workplace Regulations) (SI 1992/3004), Reg 8*. The Approved Code of Practice to these Regulations also states that dazzling lights and annoying glare should be avoided. *Regulation 8* requires that, so far as is reasonably practicable, lighting should be by natural light. The *Provision and Use of Work Equipment Regulations 1998 (PUWER) (SI 1998/2306), Reg 21* requires that:

> '...every employer shall ensure suitable and sufficient lighting which takes account of the operations to be carried out, is provided at any place where a person uses work equipment'.

The *Health and Safety (Display Screen Equipment) Regulations 1992 (SI 1992/2792), Sch 3* applies where DSE users are at work. This requires that any room lighting or task lighting provided shall ensure satisfactory lighting conditions and appropriate contrast between the screen and the background. Disturbing glare and reflections on the screen must be prevented and windows must be fitted with a suitable means of adjustable covering (usually blinds).

What is 'suitable and sufficient' is partly defined by the lighting design in relation to the task (suitability) and the level of illuminance (sufficiency of light). Guidance on this is available from BS EN ISO 9241(6), which

Figure 4: Assessing the risk from light

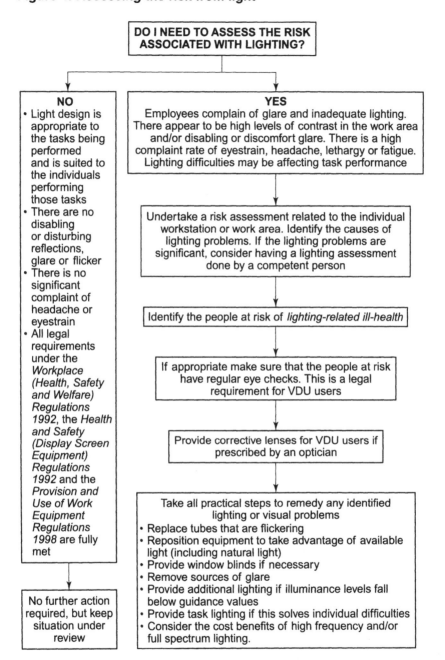

DO I NEED TO ASSESS THE RISK ASSOCIATED WITH LIGHTING?

NO
- Light design is appropriate to the tasks being performed and is suited to the individuals performing those tasks
- There are no disabling or disturbing reflections, glare or flicker
- There is no significant complaint of headache or eyestrain
- All legal requirements under the *Workplace (Health, Safety and Welfare) Regulations 1992*, the *Health and Safety (Display Screen Equipment) Regulations 1992* and the *Provision and Use of Work Equipment Regulations 1998* are fully met

No further action required, but keep situation under review

YES
Employees complain of glare and inadequate lighting. There appear to be high levels of contrast in the work area and/or disabling or discomfort glare. There is a high complaint rate of eyestrain, headache, lethargy or fatigue. Lighting difficulties may be affecting task performance

Undertake a risk assessment related to the individual workstation or work area. Identify the causes of lighting problems. If the lighting problems are significant, consider having a lighting assessment done by a competent person

Identify the people at risk of *lighting-related ill-health*

If appropriate make sure that the people at risk have regular eye checks. This is a legal requirement for VDU users

Provide corrective lenses for VDU users if prescribed by an optician

Take all practical steps to remedy any identified lighting or visual problems
- Replace tubes that are flickering
- Reposition equipment to take advantage of available light (including natural light)
- Provide window blinds if necessary
- Remove sources of glare
- Provide additional lighting if illuminance levels fall below guidance values
- Provide task lighting if this solves individual difficulties
- Consider the cost benefits of high frequency and/or full spectrum lighting.

169

recommends illuminance levels of 300–500 lux for computer workstation environments; and CIBSE lighting guides, which recommend 300–500 lux for computer workstations and 500 lux for general office work. For work areas other than offices and DSE workstations which fall under the *Workplace Regulations 1992* and *PUWER*, lighting design must be appropriate to the requirements of the task and the individuals performing the task. Guidance on illuminance levels for different types of work is contained in the CIBSE lighting guides.

Ergonomic aspects

7.31 Ergonomics is concerned with the fit between people and the things they use. Ergonomics applies scientific information about human abilities, attributes and limitations to help ensure that tools and equipment, tasks, workstation, environments and the work organisation are designed to suit people. As well as reducing the potential for ill-health, applying ergonomics principles should also result in safer work systems, greater efficiency and improved performance.

Health effects related to ergonomic risks

Musculoskeletal disorders

Overview

7.32 The term *musculoskeletal disorders* (MSDs) refers to disorders affecting the muscles, tendons, ligaments, nerves, joints or other soft tissues of the body. They most commonly affect the back, neck and upper limb and are the most common work-related condition affecting the general population in Britain.

MSDs give rise to symptoms such as pain, numbness, tingling, and usually also result in some functional changes (eg reduced ability to use the part of the body affected and restrictions to movement or strength).

It is increasingly recognised that both physical factors (eg poorly-designed equipment, furniture, tasks and environments) and psychosocial factors (eg management support, control over work, etc) contribute to the development of MSDs.

Back disorders

7.33 Back pain is generally cumulative in nature, rather than caused by a single injury, although a minor incident may be seen as the final straw that triggers discomfort. Back discomfort can arise from manual handling activities; awkward postures such as twisting, leaning, bending, stretching and prolonged static postures; poor seat design (including car seats); and exposure to whole body vibration.

Upper limb disorders

7.34 *Upper limb disorders* (ULDs) are injuries to the soft tissue of the upper limbs (fingers, hands, wrists, arms, shoulders and neck). The term covers specific conditions such as tenosynovitis and carpal tunnel syndrome as well as non-specific disorders which have been know as RSI (repetitive strain injury). The term 'ULDs' or 'WRULDs' (work-related upper limb disorders) is preferable to the term 'RSI' as it is less specific about the causation of these problems. These disorders are usually cumulative in nature, arising from a series of micro-traumas.

The main physical risk factors in the development of ULDs are application of force, repetitive movements, and awkward or static postures. It is usually the interaction of at least two of these risk factors that leads to disorders. Exposure to hand-arm vibration is also a risk factor.

Lower limb discomfort

7.35 *Lower limb disorders* are less common, and often less debilitating, than other MSDs. Lower limb discomfort can be caused by prolonged standing, particularly on concrete floors; heavy or inappropriate (particularly hard soled) footwear; operation of foot controls; and a lack of adequate foot support if sitting.

Stress

7.36 Stress arises as a result of a mismatch between the demands of the job or situation and the abilities of the individual. Stress can lead to health effects such as headaches, indigestion, disturbed sleep, smoking or drug taking, loss of concentration, irritability and loss of self-esteem. Work-related stress may be caused by lack of appropriate training, high workload, lack of control over work, poor communication, inadequate feedback, or repetitive or boring work, ie if tasks, jobs and systems are not designed with full consideration of the users.

Other health outcomes

7.37 Other health outcomes which may arise due to inappropriate design of the task or environment include:

- visual strain due to inappropriate lighting or high visual demands of the task;

- hearing loss due to exposure to excessive noise; and

- heat or cold strain due to exposure to extreme thermal environments.

Ergonomic risk factors

Posture

7.38   To work comfortably and reduce the risk of musculoskeletal injury, the body should be able to adopt 'neutral' postures. A neutral posture is one in which the joints are at about the midpoint of their comfortable range of movement and where the muscles are relaxed (eg arms hanging by the side of the body). Awkward postures (ie when the posture deviates from the neutral) place a strain on the muscles and soft tissue and can lead to discomfort. Awkward postures such as bending, twisting and stretching, reaching the arms behind the shoulders, and reaching above shoulder height or below knee height should be avoided as far as possible: this can be achieved through careful selection, positioning and adjustment of the equipment and furniture used.

Static postures (ie postures in which there is no movement for a period of time) can also lead to discomfort. Introducing movement and changes in posture through the design of the task can help alleviate discomfort.

Force

7.39   Application of frequent or excessive force (eg gripping, pushing, etc) will place a strain on the muscles involved and may lead to injury.

Repetition

7.40   Frequent, repetitive movements require the same muscles to contract and relax over and over again. If the movements are very rapid or continue for a long period of time the muscle can become fatigued and this can lead to discomfort.

Task design

7.41   The task that the person is required to do will influence their activities eg the postures adopted, amount of force applied, repetition and duration of exposure to these risk factors.

Rest breaks and changes in activity (eg job rotation) help alleviate both mental and physical fatigue. Infrequent breaks can lead to increased discomfort and reduced performance. Prolonged periods looking at a display or screen without a break can also lead to visual discomfort. Short, frequent breaks are better than long, less frequent breaks. During breaks workers should undertake different activities to those they perform in their usual task (eg avoid reading small print if work involves looking at a screen). Where operators rotate between jobs these should be sufficiently different (in terms of postures, movements required, and forces applied) so as to vary in the demands placed on them.

Pacing of work (by a machine or process) will dictate the speed of movements and amount of recovery. Machine pacing may be too fast or too slow, either of which can lead to problems (lack of recovery time for muscles and soft tissue; or frustration, stress, etc). As far as possible, work should be self-paced rather than machine-paced. Both excessively busy periods and quiet periods can lead to stress and discomfort and should be avoided.

Equipment design

7.42   Equipment design can have an impact on posture and movements made; poor design can contribute to musculoskeletal disorders. Equipment should be designed and selected for those who will use it, taking account of the task to be completed and the conditions under which it is used.

Hand tools should be designed to allow neutral arm, wrist and finger postures in operation. Angling either the workpiece or the tool handle can help reduce the amount of wrist deviation required; however, the potential need to vary the orientation of the tool on the workpiece may limit the benefit of this.

Risk factors include:

- handles that create any pressure on the soft tissue of the hand, ie handles should be sufficiently long, not having finger contouring or excessive ridges;

- excessively smooth handle surfaces (as this requires greater grip strength to hold securely);

- handles or controls that require excessive stretching to reach or activate (eg two handled tools such as pliers);

- excessively heavy tools;

- uneven distribution of weight of the tool.

These risk factors also apply to other items that have to be held in the hands (eg excessive stretching of the fingers should not be required to hold work items).

Workstation design

7.43   The workstation should be: an appropriate size for all the equipment required to be laid out conveniently; of a height that will allow a good posture; and any necessary equipment/tools/components should be arranged to allow good posture and acceptable movements.

Work surface

7.44   The work surface height (whether designed for sitting or standing tasks) should be such as to avoid users stooping or reaching to its surface. Depending on the task, the working height should generally be level with the user's elbow height (slightly higher for precision tasks such as writing; slightly lower for non-precision tasks).

The front edge of workstations should be bevelled to prevent point pressure on the forearms if the arms are rested on them.

There should be sufficient legroom underneath the work surface to allow the user to be able to sit comfortably and sufficiently close to the workstation.

Sitting versus standing

7.45   Sitting can help to reduce discomfort in the lower limbs and back, as long as the chair provides adequate support and the feet are also supported. Tasks that require generally static postures (with limited or no trunk movement) should be undertaken while sitting. However, prolonged sitting and inappropriate seating can lead to discomfort. Seating should provide adequate support to the back and legs without creating excess pressure. Some users will find a backrest with more pronounced lumbar support is comfortable, while others will prefer a flatter backrest. Adjustability in seat height, backrest height and angle are recommended; adjustment in seat depth can also be beneficial. Armrests should not compromise posture eg by coming into contact with the workstation or forcing the user to stretch to the work. Some individuals may require a footrest to allow them to sit at a comfortable height; this should be large enough to support both feet evenly, without creating point pressure on the underside of the foot.

Standing is beneficial if the task requires a range of body movement, or handling of heavy items. However, prolonged standing, particularly with little walking or on a concrete floor, can result in workers experiencing lower limb and lower back discomfort.

Whether sitting or standing, workers should be able to vary their posture and should be able to take short, frequent breaks away from the workstation.

Workstation layout

7.46   To allow a good working posture, the equipment and items used to complete the tasks should be within convenient reach of the user ie without the need to stretch. To facilitate their use, equipment and tools can be arranged by sequence of use or frequency of use (with those used most frequently positioned closest to the user). Controls that are operated by the hand should be located between elbow and shoulder height.

Items to be viewed should be positioned directly in front of the user and slightly below eye height to allow comfortable neck and eye posture. The required viewing distance depends on the person's visual ability, the size of the item being viewed and the lighting levels. A viewing distance of between 500–750mm should be suitable for most items, but a shorter viewing distance may be required for fine work.

Physical work environment

Noise

7.47 Exposure to high levels of noise can lead to hearing damage. Annoying noises (eg those that are unexpected, infrequent, high frequency and those over which the listener has no control) can contribute to stress.

See further 7.2 *et seq.*

Vibration

7.48 Exposure to vibration (both whole body and hand-arm) is associated with musculoskeletal disorders and other health problems.

Whole body vibration usually occurs via the feet or seat when the person is working in a vibrating environment (eg transport systems). Low frequencies of vibration (such as those from motor vehicles) can lead to chest pains, difficulties in breathing, back pain and impaired vision.

Hand-arm vibration can be experienced when using hand held power tools. It is a known risk factor in the development of hand arm vibration syndrome (HAVS) which affects the blood supply and nerves to the hand. Transmission of vibration increases as the gripping force increases and where tight gloves are worn.

See further 7.8 *et seq.*

Thermal environment

7.49 Body temperature is affected by the ambient conditions (air temperature, humidity, radiant heat and air velocity), the activity being undertaken (and therefore the heat produced by the body) and the clothing worn. Body temperature needs to be maintained within a relatively narrow range for health; deviations from this can lead to reduced performance, fatigue, discomfort and ill-health. In extreme circumstances this can be fatal.

Low temperatures reduce manual dexterity and where this is required the hands should be kept warm (eg through appropriate gloves). If the hands are sweaty operators will tend to grip a tool or work item more tightly to hold it secure in the hand and this can lead to discomfort.

Manual handling injuries are more likely in extreme thermal environments.

See further 7.15 *et seq.*

Lighting

7.50   Inappropriate lighting can lead to visual fatigue (symptoms include red or sore eyes, blurred vision, headaches) and can also force users to adopt poor postures in order to view items more easily. Risk factors include:

- excessively high levels of illuminance, or insufficient light levels;
- bright lights or glare in the field of view;
- uneven light distribution; and
- unclear text or displays, eg due to inappropriate contrast, colours, size, etc.

See further 7.25 *et seq.*

Clothing and personal protective equipment

7.51   Clothing and personal protective equipment (PPE) can have an impact on the user's interaction with the tools/equipment. For example, wearing gloves usually results in operators gripping a tool handle more tightly. Some clothing can restrict movement and posture.

PPE acts as a barrier between the wearer and the environment; thus it can prevent heat being lost from the body or sweat being evaporated, so that some forms of PPE (particularly non water vapour permeable garments) can increase the risk of heat strain.

See further CHAPTER 9.

Psychosocial risk factors

7.52   There is strong evidence of the role of work-related psychosocial factors (ie those affecting the worker's psychological response to work and workplace conditions) in the development of musculoskeletal disorders.

Relevant factors include the design, organisation and management of work, the context of the work (overall social environment) and the content of the work (the specific impact of job factors). Specifically, repetitive, monotonous tasks, excessive or undemanding workloads, lack of control over the task or organisation of the workplace, working in isolation, poor communication and lack of involvement in decision making have been implicated.

Individual differences

7.53 Some people may be more likely to develop an MSD than others. These include new employees who may need time to develop the necessary skills/rate of work; those returning from holiday or sickness absence; older/younger workers; new/expectant mothers; and those with particular health conditions. Account should also be taken of differences in body size which may require awkward postures/reaches.

Specific tasks

Manual handling

7.54 Manual handling activities (lifting, moving, carrying, etc) pose a risk of musculoskeletal injury, particularly to the back. The risk of injury is effected by:

- the nature and characteristics of the load (eg weight; size; ease of holding; distribution of weight; stability or predictability of the load; and intrinsically harmful characteristics such as sharp edges, hot or cold surfaces);

- the environment in which the handling is conducted (eg any constraints on posture; floor surfaces; stairs or variations in levels; cold, hot or humid conditions; strong air movements; poor lighting conditions);

- the task (vertical and horizontal handling distances; postures required, such as stretching, bending, stooping; strenuous pushing or pulling; repetitive handling; handling at a specified work rate; frequency of handling, etc);

- the capabilities of the individual (task requires unusual capabilities; may pose a hazard to those with a health problem or who are pregnant; special information or training may be required); and

- clothing which may hinder movement and posture.

Display screen equipment work

7.55 Work at display screen equipment (DSEs) (also known as visual display units (VDUs)) has been associated with a range of health problems. Musculoskeletal disorders (particularly upper limb and back disorders) are associated with this work due to poor postures that may be adopted (potentially due to inappropriate furniture or layout of equipment), long periods spent at the keyboard, highly repetitive keying activities and/or mouse work, and application of force. Work at DSE does not cause eye damage but may make workers with pre-existing vision defects more aware of them. Temporary visual discomfort (sore or red eyes, headaches, etc) can result from work at DSE due to static postures and high concentration associated with this work, poor position of the screen, poor legibility of the screen or source documents, poor lighting, or a flickering image on the screen. Fatigue and stress can arise from the type of jobs which involve DSE use (eg repetitive tasks) or frustration with the software.

Work at DSE has not been known to induce epileptic seizures. Complaints of facial dermatitis associated with DSE use is relatively rare. The levels of electromagnetic radiation generated by DSE are such as not to pose a significant risk to health. Scientific evidence does not show a link between work with DSE and miscarriages or birth defects.

Legal requirements

7.56   Under the *Management of Health and Safety at Work Regulations 1999 (SI 1999/3242)*, risk factors should be assessed, and appropriate action taken to reduce the risk of injury. While there is no specific legislation which encompasses all aspects of ergonomics, several pieces of legislation have ergonomics requirements in them, including the *Manual Handling Operations Regulations 1992 (SI 1992/2793)*, the *Health and Safety (Display Screen Equipment) Regulations 1992 (SI 1992/2792)*, the *Personal Protective Equipment at Work Regulations 1992 (SI 1992/2966)* and the *Provision and Use of Work Equipment Regulations 1998 (SI 1998/2306)*.

Assessing the risks

Understanding if there is a problem

7.57   Existing company data (eg productivity, accident and ill-health data, and information from safety meetings) can often be used to identify any particular ergonomics issues, and the extent of the problem. Data can be analysed by work area or type of injury in order to help prioritise areas for risk reduction measures.

Surveys or discussions can be undertaken to obtain users' views on equipment, tasks or workplaces. Discomfort surveys, which ask workers about the extent and severity of any discomfort they experience, can be used to identify in which parts of the body operators are experiencing discomfort and also to identify any trends in relation to the work tasks or work areas. They can also be used as a baseline against which the benefit of any interventions can be evaluated. This sort of survey can be used in conjunction with risk assessments to help interpret risks and set priorities.

Figure 5: Assessing the risk of musculoskeletal injury

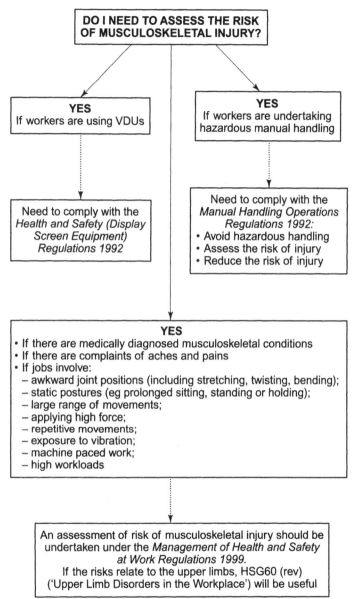

Risk assessments

7.58 Ergonomic risk assessments can identify the risk of injury, accident or reduced performance due to ergonomic deficiencies in the work or tasks. Checklists can be used to ensure all elements within the task are covered, ie person, task, workstation, work environment and work system. One example of a simple ergonomics checklist is provided in 'Ergonomics for Beginners' (Dul and Weerdmeester, Taylor and Francis, 2001).

A risk assessment checklist concerning the risks of manual handling is provided in the *Manual Handling Operations Regulations 1992 (SI 1992/2793)*. A list of factors to consider in the assessment of the risk of injury through DSE work is included in the *Health and Safety (Display Screen Equipment) Regulations 1992 (SI 1992/2792)*. The revised HSE guidance, 'Upper Limb Disorders in the Workplace' (HSG60 (rev)), also contains a thorough risk assessment checklist for upper limb disorder risks.

Many people can contribute to the design of the workplace or task. These may include planners, procurers, human resources as well as those who undertake the task itself. Involvement of the relevant people in any proposed changes is important to ensure that it is acceptable. In particular, involvement of those who undertake the task in risk assessment, redesign and evaluation is key to ensuring that the task is thoroughly understood, and that any redesign, new equipment or changes are acceptable to the users. This can be achieved, for example, through questionnaires, discussions, and trials of new equipment.

Assessment of risk should identify appropriate measures that could be taken to reduce the risk of ill-health. With musculoskeletal disorders the greatest risk reduction benefits will be achieved by tackling both physical and psychosocial risk factors in the workplace.

The workplace environment

7.59   There are many aspects of the physical environment at work which impact on a person's health. Many of these, such as noise, vibration, lighting and ergonomic design, are considered in more detail earlier in this chapter (see 7.2 *et seq*, 7.8 *et seq*, 7.25 *et seq* and 7.31 *et seq* respectively). This section deals with those aspects of the work environment which relate to buildings and the effects building design and services may have on employee health. Some of these factors relate to safety issues and will not be dealt with in detail here but that is not to underestimate their importance. Other factors associated with buildings are related to chemical hazards (such as air pollutants) and biological hazards (such as legionnaire's disease), which are dealt with in more detail in CHAPTER 6 and CHAPTER 5. Sometimes these factors operate within buildings to produce a high level of complaint of ill-health which has come to be known as sick building syndrome (SBS). SBS however, has a complex causation and involves not only physical components of the building but also psychological and psychosocial elements: again, these issues are dealt with in more detail in CHAPTER 8.

Sick building syndrome

7.60 *Sick building syndrome* (SBS) describes an unusual level of ill-health complaints which occur in a single building (or sometimes in one part of a building), and for which no single cause can be easily attributed. What characterises a 'sick building' is the large proportion of the building's occupants who appear to have similar ill-health complaints, usually exceeding 50% of the workforce. In many cases, the causes are related to the building and its services (such as the ventilation and air conditioning system) and to indoor air pollution. Sometimes, however, the symptoms are not caused by building-related factors but by work organisation, work pressures and managerial issues that lead to work stress.

Where SBS is suspected it must be taken seriously. The problem will not go away on its own, and without suitable intervention it can have serious repercussions for the organisation. Sick buildings get a reputation, which can affect recruitment and retention. It badly affects staff attitudes to their work and results in poor morale. Sickness absence, poor performance and efficiency have been estimated to cost at least 1% of payroll costs.

What is it?

7.61 There is no agreed definition of SBS. It is a convenient term used to describe a range of symptoms which are, or at least appear to be, associated with working in a particular building. Because the symptoms are commonly encountered in the population it is important to be sure that:

- the number of people complaining of the symptoms exceeds the proportion normally expected from such a group of people; and

- that people complaining have a definite association between the building (or being at work) and the onset or worsening of their symptoms.

Suggestions for how to determine the prevalence of symptoms and their association with work are given below at 7.63 *et seq.*

The common symptoms of SBS (in order of frequency) are:

- headache;

- lethargy;

- eye irritation and soreness and dryness;

- nasal irritation, nasal blockage (rhinitis), and dryness;

- throat irritation and soreness.

Not all of these symptoms need to be present together in the building nor together in the same individuals. However, it is usual for two or three of the symptoms to be present at significantly increased prevalence within the building.

Other symptoms, such as chest tightness, wheeze and menstrual disorder, have from time to time been reported, but these seem to be uncommon and may not be part of the Sick Building Syndrome. It is important to distinguish SBS from other building and work-related conditions such as humidifier fever, building-related asthma, legionnaire's disease and effects of exposure to specific toxic substances. It is also important to recognise that stress can cause many of the symptoms of SBS and that work-related stress and job factors must be considered as a potential cause. Other specific complaints found in office environments such as upper limb disorders must be dealt with on their own merits and not be considered as part of SBS.

Any worker can be affected by SBS. There is some evidence that women suffer more than men, but this may be because a higher proportion of women work in office environments where SBS is most commonly found. SBS can be found in almost any type of building but it is *most frequently* encountered in buildings:

- which are relatively modern (post-1980);

- which are large and open-plan in design allowing little individual control over the environment;

- which are air conditioned;

- which have large areas of glazed exterior;

- which are office environments employing people in routine clerical work; and

- which are operated in the public sector.

Legal requirements

7.62 There is no specific legislation dealing with SBS. However, employers have a general duty under the *Health and Safety at Work etc Act 1974, s 2(1),* to 'ensure so far as is reasonably practicable, the health, safety and welfare of all his employees'. This specifically includes maintaining a place of work which is safe and without risks to health. The legal requirement is strengthened further under the *Management of Health and Safety at Work Regulations 1999 (Management Regulations) (SI 1999/3242). Regulation 3* requires a 'suitable and sufficient' assessment of the risks to the health and safety of employees to which they are exposed whilst at work. *Regulation 7* requires that this risk assessment, (and any other health and safety measures), are carried out by competent persons. Under *Regulation 3(6),* where the employer has five or more employees, the significant findings of the assessment must be recorded.

Many aspects of SBS are likely to have legal duties under the *Workplace*

(Health, Safety and Welfare) Regulations 1992 (SI 1992/3004). Regulation 5 deals with the maintenance and cleaning of the workplace and equipment (including ventilation systems). *Regulation 6* deals with the adequacy of ventilation, *Regulation 7* with temperature and *Regulation 8* with lighting. *SI 1992/3004, Regulation 9* requires all workplaces, furniture, furnishings, fittings and surfaces to be kept clean, and *Regulation 10* deals with room dimensions and minimum space.

In order to comply with the law therefore you must:

- list the hazards that might lead to SBS;

- assess the risk of SBS occurring;

- take any reasonable remedial steps to reduce the risk;

- keep the risk assessment under review;

- ensure that specific workplace requirements under the *Workplace (Health, Safety and Welfare) Regulations 1992* are met; and

- record the findings (legal requirement where there are five or more employees).

To reduce the risk of civil litigation you should in addition:

- investigate any collective or individual complaints of ill-health thought to be related to the work or the workplace;

- take all reasonably practicable steps to reduce or remove identified causes of discomfort or illness; and

- ensure that staff receive competent occupational health advice on their ill-health complaint.

It is a sensible precaution to keep records of any investigations, remedial actions and referrals for medical advice.

Assessing the risks

7.63   The risk assessment can be used in this case to serve one of two purposes:

- to determine the risk of SBS arising and so prevent it so far as is possible; and

- to determine likely causes and prioritise actions after a case is suspected.

It is a sensible precaution to assess the risks of SBS arising before any evidence of a problem emerges, especially if your building has many, or all, of the features above which increase the risk of it becoming associated with SBS. If anecdotally there appear to be a large number of complaints of SBS-like symptoms then a systematic and thorough assessment of the potential causes (hazards) is necessary in order to try find solutions.

The *Management of Health and Safety at Work Regulations 1999 (1999/3242)* require persons undertaking risk assessments to be 'competent'. That is they should have sufficient training and experience or knowledge to undertake the assessment properly. Before assigning an employee to undertake an assessment of SBS, managers should ensure that the person has sufficient understanding of what is to be done and what is to be looked for, so that the assessment is carried out properly. The assessor should also recognise his or her limitations and the Company be prepared to call upon external expertise if that is required to complete the assessment. This may be necessary, for example, if it is decided that measurements of microbiological or chemical contaminants are necessary or measurements of lighting or noise need to be undertaken.

For more detailed information on carrying out a risk assessment, see CHAPTER 10.

Hazards

7.64   The following are possible hazards associated with SBS. Each will need to be positively eliminated as a possible cause or if not then it must be further investigated. The list is not exhaustive and other hazards may be present in particular environments.

- Physical environment:

    o noise;

    o temperature;

    o humidity;

    o lighting;

    o electromagnetic radiation;

    o static electricity;

    o workstation design and layout.

- Chemical environment:

    o fumes;

o odours;

o solvents;

o tobacco smoke;

o air pollution from outside drawn into the ventilation system;

o dusts and fibres;

o gases (such as ozone from laser printers and photocopiers and formaldehyde from composite fibre and chip boards).

- Biological environment:

  o moulds and mould spores;

  o insects and mites;

  o bacteria and viruses (although there is little evidence that SBS is caused by infectious micro-organisms, the rapid spread of infectious illness – such as coughs and colds – is often reported in sick buildings, and may be caused by people working in close proximity).

- Building maintenance:

  o poor maintenance and function of the ventilation system (inadequate air exchange and fresh air supply);

  o poor maintenance and function of the air conditioning system. Inadequate control of temperature, humidity and air movement to meet thermal comfort needs;

  o poor maintenance of lighting system (lights flicker, faulty lights not replaced, etc);

  o poor standard of general repair and maintenance;

  o poor standards of cleanliness (dust accumulating on high surfaces, areas difficult to access not being vacuumed, etc).

- Job-related factors:

  o poor job design (eg routine work with little job variation);

  o perceived lack of stimulation/job satisfaction;

  o little or no control over workload or pacing;

  o excessive workload/time pressures;

  o poor working environment/crowding, distractions, inability to concentrate, etc;

  o poor staff/management relationships.

Figure 6: Assessing the risk of sick building syndrome

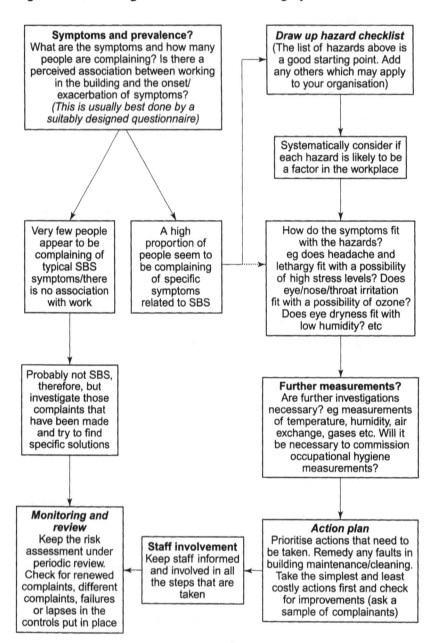

7.65

Case study – Reducing the risk of sick building syndrome

Building X had 300 employees. It was a new construction of modern design with open-plan working on all but the top floor. It was built speculatively and the current occupants designed the interior to meet their own requirements. The tenant was a software development company producing software for a highly specialised market. It had its own customer support service and telephone help line and a telephone sales team. Soon after staff moved into the building, complaints started to surface about headache, eyestrain and lethargy. They were initially anecdotal having been brought up at health and safety meetings, but with no detailed evidence as to the extent of the complaint or its precise nature.

The Company decided to have a detailed study made. A questionnaire was designed which asked anonymously for information on what complaints each member of staff had, when they started in relation to moving into the building, and how often symptoms now occur. The questionnaire also asked when during the day symptoms started and if symptoms occurred on days off. The results showed that 75% of the 300 employees had complaints of headache and eyestrain more than twice a week and almost as many (60%) complained of lethargy. Only a few (less than 5%) complained of eye, nose or throat irritation or dryness. Most employees reported that their symptoms came on during the day and were worse by mid-afternoon. A significant number were leaving work early complaining of being unwell. As this was not recorded there was no apparent increase in sickness absence. Most staff felt the problem had been there in the old building but had got much worse since the move.

The risk assessment did not reveal any obvious problem with the temperature and few people complained about being too hot or too cold or had complained of dry eyes. It was unlikely, therefore, to be low humidity or poor performance of the air conditioning system. Examination of the ventilation system however revealed that the filters were not being regularly maintained: there was a possibility, therefore, of a reduced fresh air exchange rate. Inspection of the building and talking to staff revealed that many complained of glare and reflection on their computer screens. This was consistent with the high complaint of headache. An occupational hygienist with experience of office lighting was commissioned to undertake a study of the lighting in the offices and make recommendations. A reduction in overall intensity of lighting, some alterations in desk positioning, together with better blinds on the south facing side of the building were recommended. A recommendation was also made to make sure that everyone knew how to adjust their computer screen to avoid glare and reflection. The ventilation engineers were asked to make sure that the filters were on a regular maintenance schedule. These relatively simple measures made a significant difference to the complaints of headache and lethargy. A repeat questionnaire after six months revealed that the level of complaint was down to under 15% – a figure which was consistent with expected rates for headache and post-lunch lethargy.

Static electricity and non-ionising radiation

Static electricity

7.66 *Static electricity* is the build up of electrical charge on surfaces. The crackle when you place your hand near to a television screen is caused by static discharge from the screen surface. The party trick of rubbing a balloon and making it stick on the wall is caused by the generation of a static charge on the balloon surface. Many materials including most man-made fibres, plastics and wool, can carry large static charges when they are rubbed. Television and computer screens (cathode-ray types) carry static charge because of the high electrical charges on the inside of the screen.

Static charge is normally encountered in indoor environments but static can be a problem in outdoor environment, especially on days when the humidity is very low. Static can also create problems in vehicles.

Health effects of static electricity

7.67 Static electricity has been associated with three health problems

- visual display unit (VDU) erythema;

- cable bugs; and

- micro shocks.

Visual display unit erythema

7.68 This condition causes a skin reddening or even a full dermatitis, caused by air-borne particulates being concentrated on the face and hands when sitting for long periods of time in front of a computer screen. The computer screen may have 30,000 or more volts of static charge on it's surface. The operator sitting about half a metre away is sitting in a very strong electrostatic field, which can repel particles from the air at high velocity towards the operator's exposed skin, usually the face and hands where they then impact. VDU erythema is a relatively rare condition, but when it does arise is very distressing. The characteristics of the condition are that the skin reddening occurs on the bony prominences of the face and along the knuckle line of the backs of the hands. Cases should be referred to a doctor for treatment but the solution lies in removing the static at source. This is achieved by replacing the sufferer's screen with a low-static screen (or better a TFT or LCD screen). If it is not possible to replace the screen, a conductive mesh can be installed over the screen. It is important that this is a type that is electrically conductive (usually made of carbon fibre) and is earthed when it is installed. These measures will almost certainly alleviate the problem.

Cable bugs

7.69   Cable bugs is a condition in which people complain of what appears to be insect bites. These usually occur around the ankles and lower leg, but occasionally around the wrists. Whilst insect bites might actually be the cause, it is often found that static electricity is the culprit. The build-up of static on the body discharges to a metallic object such as the chair or desk leg or the metal desk frame. These discharge points cause a small itchy blemish on the skin which, if scratched, enlarges to a red weal looking very much like an insect bite. The cure to this problem is to eliminate the source of static, by increasing the humidity (see later) or by using anti-static preparations on the chair fabric and carpets.

Micro shocks

7.70   Micro shocks occur when there is a build up of static electricity on the body surface which is then discharged when the person touches a metallic or earthed object such as a door handle or filing cabinet. The same phenomenon occurs when getting out of a car and touching the metal body. This does not cause a health problem as such, but some people find the repeated experience of micro shocks distressing. Some individuals seem to be particularly prone to micro shocks. The reason for this is not certain but is probably due to differences in skin moisture – people with dry skin seem to be more likely to suffer micro shocks. The environmental conditions which increase the risk of micro shocks are a dry atmosphere, the presence of electrical equipment such as computer screens, and people being in contact with fabrics and materials which generate large static charges. The solution is to reduce the amount of static charge by using anti-static preparations and/or increasing the humidity if the air is dry. The use of air ionisers can also be helpful in reducing static electricity.

Humidity

7.71   In addition, humidity plays an important part in determining the levels of static charge on surfaces, except the computer screen which is continuously being charged whilst it is operating. Moist air is more conductive to electricity and so surface charges leak away to air. However, in dry air, with the humidity below 30% RH the surfaces are more likely to accumulate charge. Relative humidity below 20% is almost certain to create static problems especially in carpeted office-type environments.

Non-ionising radiation

7.72   *Non-ionising radiation* is emitted from sources of electrical energy which are time varying. (Static electricity, considered at 7.66, has no time variation and therefore does not create an electromagnetic field). Time variation means that the voltage or power of the source is fluctuating in a periodic manner. This gives rise to a radiated field that moves away from the source with the speed of light and is said to be an electromagnetic field. The field has a number of important characteristics that determine how it is transmitted through space and how it may in turn affect a person who is exposed to the field. These characteristics are:

- The magnetic field component (the H field).

- The electric field component (the E field).

- The magnitude of the field (the intensity of the electrical or magnetic radiation).

- The frequency of the radiation.

- The wavelength of the radiation.

The strength of the magnetic field (H) is measured by the current at a particular point, in units of amps per metre ($A.m^{-1}$). The magnetic flux density (B) (in effect the strength of the magnet) is often used in assessing human effects of electromagnetic radiation. This is measured in the unit of Tesla (T). The strength of the electric field component is measured in unit of volts per metre ($V.m^{-1}$). Sometimes, especially with high frequency radiation, the power density of the field is measured. This is the amount of incident radiation falling on a specified area (usually of the body). The unit of power density is Watts per square metre ($W.m^{-2}$). The frequency is the number of times the wave repeats itself in a given time. This is measured in the unit Hertz (Hz) where 1 Hz is one cycle per second. The wavelength is the distance between corresponding points on the wave (say the peak of one wave to the peak of the next wave), and is related to the frequency – as the frequency increases the wavelength decreases. Wavelength is measured in metres. Frequency can be expressed in the following way:

kHz (kilohertz – 1 kHz is 10^3 or 1,000 (1 thousand) cycles per second)

MHz (megahertz – 1 MHz is 10^6 or 1,000,000 (1 million) cycles per second

GHz (giga hertz – 1 GhZ is 10^9 or 1,000,000,000 (1 billion) cycles per second).

Starting at just above zero frequency, non-ionising radiation exists for frequencies rising up to 3×10^{15} Hz (a wavelength of 100 nano metres). Frequencies greater than 3×10^{15} Hz have sufficient energy to cause ionisation in body tissue and are therefore called 'ionising radiations' (see 7.76 *et seq*). The range of frequencies up to and including those in the ionising region is called the electromagnetic spectrum. This is illustrated in FIGURE 7.

Below the infrared region, the spectrum is almost equally divided arbitrarily into frequency bands which are used mainly for communication purposes. Collectively this often called the radio frequency spectrum (or RF radiation). At the lower end of the spectrum (usually defined as up to 300 Hz) is the extra low frequency (ELF) region. This is important because in here lies the

Figure 7: The electromagnetic spectrum

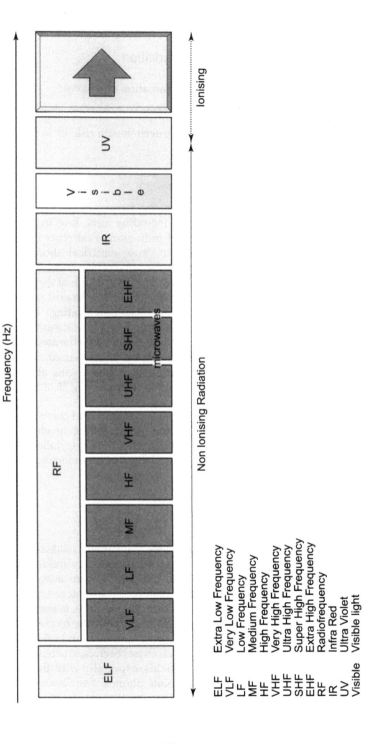

ELF   Extra Low Frequency
VLF   Very Low Frequency
LF   Low Frequency
MF   Medium Frequency
HF   High Frequency
VHF   Very High Frequency
UHF   Ultra High Frequency
SHF   Super High Frequency
EHF   Extra High Frequency
RF   Radiofrequency
IR   Infra Red
UV   Ultra Violet
Visible Visible light

power frequency fields from electrical mains power distribution and usage. In Europe this is 50 Hz and in North America 60 Hz.

Health effects of non-ionising radiation

7.73   The hazards of non-ionising radiation are twofold:

- acute (short term) effect arising from body heating, shock and burn; or
- chronic (the possibility of a long-term health risk, including cancer).

Acute effects

7.74   The *acute* effects depend on the frequency. At low frequencies (typically power frequencies, but including very low frequency radio transmissions) the hazard is one of induction of currents into the body. These currents can be sufficient to cause electrical shock when they discharge from the body and burn at the point of discharge. The likelihood of induced current and shock depends on the strength of the electrical and magnetic field. At frequencies above 100kHz the hazard is one of body heating and tissue damage caused by localised heating. This can have serious effects if the heating occurs in sensitive organs such as the eye (where the risk is of cataract formation). At these frequencies the amount of energy absorbed by the body (or specific areas of the body) is used as a measure to determine risk. The unit of measurement is the specific absorption rate (SAR) measured as watts per kilogram of tissue ($W.kg^{-1}$).

The *chronic* effects (see 7.75) are more contentious but there is evidence of an increased cancer risk with prolonged exposure to electromagnetic radiation. The certainty of the evidence for this, however, falls short of being able to set guidelines on exposure. Guidelines are therefore set to reduce the risk of the acute effects.

Chronic effects

7.75   The cancer risk of exposure to electromagnetic fields is inconclusive. Studies of residential exposure to power frequency fields suggest that average exposures of above 0.4µT (microtesla) are associated with a doubling of the risk of leukaemia in children. The evidence is inconclusive, however and the evidence for a cancer risk in adults is even less certain. Some studies have shown that occupational exposure to power frequency fields is associated with leukaemia, brain tumours and other cancers but again the evidence is uncertain. Research has been conducted on health risk from exposure to radiofrequency fields, especially with the more recent concern about the risk of using mobile phones. The Stewart Committee, which investigated the evidence for health risk from mobile phone technology, concluded that:

'... it is not possible at present to say that exposure to RF radiation, even at levels below national guidelines, is totally without potential health effects, and that gaps in knowledge are sufficient to justify a precautionary approach'. ('Mobile Phones and Health', the Independent Expert Committee on Mobile Phones (the Stewart Report), National Radiological Protection Board, May 2000).

Prolonged mobile phone use has also been associated with headaches, nausea, memory loss, changes in blood pressure and other health effects which have not been replicated scientifically.

Whilst the jury is still out on chronic health risks, adopting a precautionary approach may be the sensible policy. The European Commission considers that the precautionary principle is:

'... relevant in the event of a potential risk, even if the risk cannot be fully demonstrated or quantified or its effects determined because of the insufficiency or inconclusive nature of the scientific data'.

A more complete debate on applying the precautionary principle is to be found in the European Commission Communication (Commission of the European Communities, Communication from the Commission on the Precautionary Principle, Brussels (COM (2000) 1 02.02.2000).

Legal requirements

7.76   There is no specific legislation which applies to exposure to non-ionising electromagnetic radiation. However general duties apply under the *Health and Safety at Work etc Act 1974, s 2,* and a risk assesment is required under the *Management of Health and Safety at Work Regulations 1999 (SI 1999/3242), Reg 3.* Although not a legal requirement, assessment of risk should be undertaken by reference to reputable exposure guidelines such as those issued by the National Radiological Protection Board or International Commission on Non-Ionising Radiation Protection (see 7.77).

Guidelines on exposure

7.77   In the UK, guidelines on exposure to electromagnetic radiation are set by the National Radiological Protection Board (NRPB): see its 'Board Statement on Restrictions on Human Exposure to Static and Time Varying Electromagnetic Fields and Radiation' (NRPB, Vol 4 No 5, 1993); and its website at www.nrpb.org

Internationally, guidance exists from the International Commission on Non-Ionising Radiation Protection (ICNIRP, 1998). In 1999, the NRPB published a statement on the standing of the ICNIRP Guidelines in the UK ('Board

Statement: Advice on the 1998 ICNIRP Guidelines for Limiting Exposure to Time-varying Electric, Magnetic and Electromagnetic Fields (up to 300GHz)' (NRPB, Vol 10 No 2, 1999). These guidelines work in similar ways although the limit values are sometimes different between the two sets of guidelines.

The NRPB guidelines set *basic restrictions*. At frequencies below 100kHz these are set to limit induced currents in the body. Above 100kHz the basic restriction is on the SAR which is set at $0.4\ \text{Wkg}^{-1}$ over the whole body

Figure 8: Assessing the risk from electromagnetic radiation

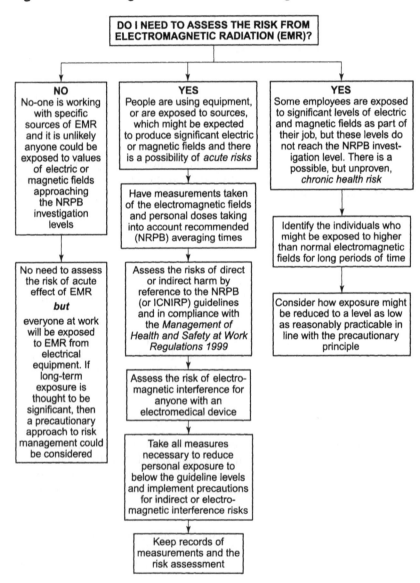

averaged over any 15-minute period. Different values and averaging times are given for the head, the foetus and the limbs. Between 10GHz–300GHz a power density of 100 W.m^{-2} is given, with the averaging time dependent on the frequency.

Basic restrictions are complicated to apply and specialised measurements have to be taken to ensure that they are complied with. NRPB, therefore, also provide *investigation levels* which are simpler measures of electric and magnetic field strengths and power density which, if not exceeded, *should* allow compliance with the basic restriction. Investigation levels are provided in its NRPB Board Statement (NRPB 1993) and the reader is advised to consult this if a risk assessment on employees working with electromagnetic radiation is required.

Acute effects can be *direct*, that is they act by direct interaction with the body; or they can be *indirect*, that is they can cause harm by interacting with external metal objects with which the body may come into contact. Acute effects may also occur as a result of electromagnetic interference with medical devices such as cardiac pacemakers or cochlea implants. The risk of these events must be included in the risk assessment.

Ionising radiation

7.78   If a person has been exposed to penetrating radiation from an external source, he or she will have radiation damage but will not remain radioactive and is not a hazard to others. An example of this is taking an ordinary chest X-ray. Once the source of the radiation is removed then they get no more dose.

If a person has radioactive material on or in their body, then he or she is contaminated. An example of this is contamination by plutonium. As the source of the radiation is actually in them, they continue to receive the radiation even if they leave the area where they were contaminated.

Radiation dose is measured by the amount of that energy that is absorbed by the body:

*   the gray is the unit of dose absorbed by a body; and

*   the sievert is similar to the gray, but takes into account differences in the biological effect of various radiations.

The following principles apply:

*   Distance

    The further one is from the source of the radiation, the less radiation dose one will get. In fact, if you double the distance from a source you reduce the dose by a quarter.

- Time

  The less time one is close to the source, the less radiation dose one will get.

- Shielding

  Most materials will provide some degree of protection, but the denser the better, which is why lead is often used for shielding.

Clearly those working with radiation must have adequate personal protection.

Legal requirements

7.79   Before contemplating work with ionising radiation an employer must study the *Ionising Radiations Regulations 1999 (SI 1999/3232)* and their associated Approved Code of Practice. As mentioned earlier, the key is risk assessment. The Regulations are highly proscriptive and cover, amongst others, authorisation, risk assessment, restriction of exposure, personal protective equipment, dose assessment and classification of employees.

The *Radioactive Substances Act 1993* regulates the use and disposal of radioactive material; and the *Radioactive Material (Road Transport) Regulations 2002 (SI 2002/1093)* regulate the package and transport of radioactive materials. Medical exposures are governed by the *Ionising Radiation (Medical Exposure) Regulations 2000 (SI 2000/1059)* and the *Medicines (Administration of Radioactive Substances) (Amendment) Regulations 1995 (SI 1995/2147)*. A health and safety manager should seek advice from an radiation protection adviser if in any doubt (see 7.81).

Risk assessments

7.80   The *Ionising Radiations Regulations 1999 (SI 1999/3232)* require an employer to designate as *classified* any employee who is likely to exceed a radiation dose in excess of 6 milli-sieverts per year or a dose more than $^3/_{10}$ of any dose limit. Dose assessments of classified workers must be done by an approved dosimetry service.

Radiation protection advisers

7.81   *Radiation protection advisers* (RPAs) are key to working with ionising radiation: it is they who can give practical advice on putting the *Ionising Radiations Regulations 1999 (SI 1999/3232)* into practice. *Regulation 2* gives details of the competence required of an RPA. The National Radiological Protection Board (NRPB) (see 7.77) provides RPA services and enquiries should be made to a local centre.

Regulation 13 specifically requires an employer to consult an RPA on how to observe the regulations, specifically risk assessment; designation of radiation areas; design of work practices and controls; calibration of monitoring equipment and periodic testing of controls. *Regulation 13* describes how to choose an RPA. The RPA is key to work with ionising radiation.

Health surveillance

7.82 Classified workers must also have regular health surveillance by a doctor who has been appointed by the Health & Safety Executive (HSE) or by an employment medical adviser employed by the HSE. The local HSE Office will have a list of such doctors.

Such surveillance includes an assessment before starting, an annual health review and special surveillance following over-exposure. The annual review need not be face-to-face, but the doctor must include a review of sickness absence and radiation dose. The decision of the appointed doctor must be recorded in a health record, which is separate from the medical file.

A classified worker has the right to appeal to the HSE against the decision of the appointed doctor.

In relation to pregnant women and breastfeeding mothers, the key is risk assessment to reduce dose, involving the RPA for advice. When an employer is notified of pregnancy, he must restrict further radiation exposure so that the dose to the foetus is unlikely to be more than 1 milli-sievert. The risk assessment must also take into account that some radioactive substance are concentrated in breast milk.

A health and safety manager needs to be particularly vigilant if he or she is responsible for industrial radiography, where problems in working practices can lead to high doses. Hospital radiologists are a high-risk group, as monitoring their exposure whilst undertaking clinical work can be difficult.

Emergencies

Employer responsibility

7.83 The *Ionising Radiations Regulations 1999 (SI 1999/3232)* place an obligation on the employer to prepare a contingency plan if the risk assessment shows that an accident is foreseeable. The *Radiation (Emergency Preparedness and Public Information) Regulations 2001 (SI 2001/2975)* require emergency planning and if the public is liable to be affected, it must be informed.

Over-exposures

7.84 If a worker has a suspected over-exposure to radiation, the HSE and appointed doctor or employment medical adviser must be informed. In practice, the employee should be seen as quickly as possible by the RPA and doctor and given as much information and support as possible. Usually psychological factors drown out physical concerns.

Unforeseen incidents

7.85 *National Arrangements for Incidents involving Radioactivity (NAIR)* – NAIR is a set of national arrangements that provide a 'long-stop' to other emergency plans. NAIR has been designed to provide advice and assistance to the police in incidents involving radioactivity where members of the public may require protection. The arrangements have been devised around assistance to the police since they will normally be among the first informed of any incident in a public space. In an incident, the police check whether there are plans to deal with the event. If no suitable plans exist, or if plans fail, NAIR assistance should be sought. NAIR assistance may be obtained by means of a 24-hour national notification telephone number (0800 834 153). This connects to the United Kingdom Atomic Energy Authority Constabulary, Force Communications Centre, who will take details of the incident and contact the nearest respondent.

Emergency training

7.86 Trident Medical Services, and the University of Surrey run courses for appointed doctors and how to cope with medical aspects of radiation emergencies, both for the National Health Service and independent sector. They can be contacted on 01483 686690.

8 Occupational Mental Health

Introduction

8.1   The World Health Organisation (WHO) defines health as 'a state of mental, physical and social well-being' ('Health aspects of wellbeing in working places: report on a WHO working group', WHO, 1980). Health is necessary for functional effectiveness in personal, domestic, occupational and community life. It ensures the ability to cope with inevitable stressors in all these domains. Promotion of occupational mental health requires consideration at the following levels: individual; organisational; and environmental.

Since the 1950s stress-related illnesses, anxiety and depression have increased by some 40–50% and are now said to cost more than industrial strife, without counting loss of productivity due to alcohol and drug abuse. In 1995–96 work-related stress cost employers £353–381 million and society £3.7–3.8 billion.

It should be emphasised that effective treatment of stress, anxiety and depression brings as favourable work, domestic and social outcomes as does the treatment of a range of 'acceptable' physical illnesses. However, such relatively minor psychiatric illnesses can seriously impair work performance, cause sickness absence, and costly labour turnover and do need to be addressed. These illnesses are very common, probably accounting for about a third of all GP attenders, although the presenting symptoms may be physical. This prevalence is reflected throughout the workforce, increasing vulnerability to inevitable workplace stressors, which vary according to the size of the organisation, and to the nature of the operation. Unrecognised, more serious, impairment may develop with adverse effects on the work performance of the individual, co-workers, and that of the organisation as a whole. Thus, even a small reduction in the incidence of minor psychiatric illness would be beneficial to productivity and to the economy.

Mental health in the workplace

8.2   The role of work can have positive and negative effects. Correlation between work and positive mental health has long been recognised. Achievement and job satisfaction contribute to self-esteem. There is a need for continuous constructive feedback, both positive and negative, in order to develop trust. Positive feedback from the line-manager, client, or self – the ability to give oneself 'well dones' – is thought to release endorphins, the natural 'feel-good' body chemicals. The capability of realistic positive self-appraisal facilitates self-esteem and confidence, so valuable in combating predictable and unpredictable work-related stressors.

The trauma of enforced retirement, or redundancy, results from cessation of such positive feedback with loss of mental stimulation, and of involvement with co-workers. People who are not prepared for these events due to lack of hobbies, sport, or cultural interests, often succumb, lacking the ability to structure time fulfillingly. Hence there is a sense of loss which can predispose to depression. Reference to obituaries of high-profile people confirm death often follows shortly after retirement. The impact of redundancy obviously depends on the package, whether work has been fulfilling, and the prospect of re-employment for those needing it for economic, or psychological reasons. Again, uncertainty in this context can predispose the individual to anxiety.

A healthy workforce with high morale maximises productivity. *Physical toxicity* can be due to industrial substances such as asbestos, lead and solvents. The latter two can cause organic brain disease with impaired cognitive function. *Emotional toxicity* results from interpersonal tensions between superiors or subordinates. Working from home, now feasible due to new technology, avoids the necessity of commuting, and eliminates the stress of interpersonal tension, but has the adverse effect of isolation. Communication has been revolutionised by the use of e-mail with its advantages and pitfalls. It has changed working practices, and organisational structure.

Stress can cause significant mood changes such as anxiety and depression which are experienced by some 10–25% of people at some time in life (Lucas, G, 'Mental Health at Work', *Employment Gazette*, December 1989). The onset may be precipitated by a major traumatic life-event such as bereavement, divorce, a serious road traffic accident, or the diagnosis of severe physical illness. Depression affects the strong and resolute and is associated with neuro-chemical changes. Its persistence for more than two weeks has clinical significance.

The Health & Safety Executive (HSE) defines stress as 'the reaction to excessive pressure or other type of demand, and worry regarding the inability to cope' ('Survey of work related illness', HSE, 1995). Effects include increased pulse rate and blood pressure, allergies, musculoskeletal pain, headache, migraine, lowered immunity, behavioural changes, impaired sleep, inability to delegate, impaired cognitive function, irritability, verbal and even physical aggression. There is often increased consumption of caffeine/alcohol/nicotine/minor analgesics, and drug abuse, such as of amphetamines or cocaine.

Prevalence of mental health problems

8.3   Only musculoskeletal disorders exceed minor psychiatric morbidity as a cause of sickness absence. Their inter-relationship is recognised. Social workers, teachers, the emergency services, probation officers, police officers, and healthcare professionals are particularly vulnerable. In fact, any occupation is stressful where there is interfacing with a demanding and potentially aggressive section of the community. According to the Health & Safety Executive (HSE), the highest rates of stress, anxiety and depression occur in nurses and teachers ('Scale of occupational stress – A further analysis of the impact of demographic factors and type of job', Contract Research Report 311, HSE, 2000). The risks are high because these professionals are both physically and psychologically vulnerable: they are exposed to demanding and potentially violent children and adults.

At some time during adult life, some 15–30% of the population manifest depression and anxiety including phobic and obsessional disorders. By comparison, the affective psychoses (mood disorders) and schizophrenia respectively, occur in 1% of the adult population.

Epidemiological studies confirm that depression and anxiety which are common in the general population are also common in the workforce. Obviously, those so affected are more vulnerable to inevitable workplace stressors (Jenkins, R, 'Prevalence of Mental Illness in the Workplace', in 'Prevention of Mental Ill Health at Work', HMSO, 1992).

The symptoms of sick building syndrome (SBS) may be misinterpreted as being due to neurosis. There are specific diseases such as humidifier fever, legionnaires' disease, and those due to exposure to toxic agents in the work environment. The prevalence of SBS is difficult to assess since the symptoms are those of common ailments, present in the general population: typical reported symptoms include headaches, nasal problems, eye irritation, dry skin and tiredness. No single specific causative factor has been identified for SBS but there are ergonomic factors which could be implicated (see further CHAPTER 7).

Surveys of work-related illnesses were conducted by the HSE in 1990 and 1995. Another survey by the European Union Statistics Office in 1998–99 (EUROSTAT Ill Health Module Labour Force Survey) had a more restricted coverage than the HSE commissioned studies and, therefore, is not strictly comparable. From the 1995 studies it was estimated that 279,000 individuals in the UK suffered from work-related stress, depression or anxiety. A further 254,000 ascribed a physical condition to 'stress at work'; of these, 102,000 described their condition as hypertension, cardiac disease, or stroke, and 52,000 as gastrointestinal disease. Thus, 500,000 believed that they had experienced work-related stress sufficient to make them ill. Another stress and health at work survey ('Scale of occupational stress: The Bristol health at work study', Contract Research Report 265, HSE, 2000) indicated that almost 20% of the workforce rated their work on a five-point scale into 'very' or 'extremely' stressful categories. Thus five million British workers believe that they are exposed to work stress. The tenfold difference between figures in 1995 and those given in the later survey arises from the measurement of different things: the 1995 survey calculations are based on individuals reporting, unprompted, that work stress was making them ill by causing significant physical or psychological impact on their health; whereas, the later survey represents individuals' assessments generally of the stress levels at work, when questioned.

Risk as a cause of increased anxiety

8.4   Risk taking, whether physical or financial, can be stimulating to some, but unacceptable to others, due to the intolerable anxiety generated. To the chief executive officer of an international blue-chip company or to the proprietor of a corner shop, it is always a potentially serious hazard. The events of 11 September 2001 and, more recently, those in Bali, have increased the need for risk assessment throughout the global village. Since the bombings at Lockerbie, the Baltic Exchange, the Guildford pub and the Arndale Centre in Manchester, escalating risk has already become a feature of daily life in the UK.

Prior to such events, attention was appropriately focused on specific job or process-related risk. Now, the constant re-evaluation of general security that was previously assumed, is causing an enormous change in the attitude of employees. The accepted trade-off between time and remuneration is complicated by the possibility of international terrorism. There is persisting world-wide awareness, with relatively minor incidents receiving major media coverage. This applies particularly to those working in the airline industry and transportation generally, but also to other areas such as the handling of potentially contaminated mail. Workers are questioning whether the adverse effects of being away from partners and children are adequately balanced by the benefits of working in such 'at risk' occupations and organisations. The anxiety-prone employee's perception may sometimes be exaggerated, but even the otherwise phlegmatic can now experience greater occupational stress.

Age and sex-related distribution

8.5   Similar numbers of males and females reported work-related stress. This was most common for the ages 45–retirement. Very few cases failed to remit following early or ill-health retirement. New data from a further survey of work-related illness will soon be available, and preliminary results will be published on the Health & Safety Executive (HSE) website. Additionally, there will be a further year's data regarding a surveillance scheme where a consultant psychiatrist reports cases of work-related mental ill-health. Occupational health and safety information is available on the HSE website at http://www.hse.gov.uk/

Legal requirements

8.6   Every organisation now faces the challenge of the changing nature of working practices. Employee mental health is at risk due to stress and safety issues, and management must constantly be mindful of potential litigation from within, and from outside, due to the prevailing 'blame' culture. The case of *Walker v Northumberland County Council [1995] IRLR 35* illustrates the potential risk to employers. Diana Kloss summarises this landmark case as follows:

> 'John Walker was an area social services officer employed by Northumberland County Council. He was responsible for four teams of field workers in an area where suspected child abuse was prevalent. The volume of work increased considerably, without extra staff being appointed. In 1986 Mr Walker suffered a nervous breakdown. He was off work for three months. He had no previous history of mental disorder. He returned to work with the promise that more support would be provided, but this failed to materialise. In September 1987 he suffered a second breakdown and was awarded damages against his employer for psychiatric injury caused by negligence. The employer knew that the work was stressful, that Walker was vulnerable, and yet failed to take reasonable care to provide additional staff. The defendants stated that, as a local authority, they had insufficient financial resources, but this was not considered a valid defence on the facts. It was, however, regarded as vital that the employer knew of Walker's susceptibility to stress after his first breakdown. It was also important that he had a stable family life and had never before succumbed to stress. If he had had serious problems in his home life, it would have cast doubt on his allegations that his illness was caused by his work.' (Kloss, D, 'Occupational Health Law', p 183, Blackwell Science, 1998.)

Application of the Management of Health and Safety at Work Regulations 1999

8.7   The *Management of Health and Safety at Work Regulations 1999 (SI 1999/3242)* require employers to assess the risks arising from work and to reduce or eliminate significant hazards of whatever nature, whether physical, mental, chemical, biological or situational. This includes preventing exposure to unacceptable demands which are, or could be, detrimental to mental health. There have been examples confirming the responsibility implied in the Regulations, that employers can be held liable for work-related mental impairment. Hence, to comply, the employer must confirm provision for employee mental health within occupational safety and health policy. Explicit reference is made to the identification and elimination of mental health hazards including mental distress, communication problems, bullying, sexual harassment, and excessive workload, all of which could contribute to mental ill-health. Inappropriate unconstructive and unpredictably adverse appraisals are counter-productive. Therefore, the question is not whether employers can afford to address mental ill-health issues, it is that, given the economic, legal and humane reasons, can they afford not to?

The promotion of mental health and the prevention of mental illness should be enshrined within any organisation's occupational health and safety policy: this should aim to reduce sickness absence, labour turnover, workplace disputes, and personal grievance claims. It should also aim to increase motivation, job satisfaction and productivity, while fulfilling legal responsibilities regarding bullying, sexual harassment, and racial discrimination.

This policy should require the organisation to audit needs and hazards, and to prioritise in its planning. Ongoing health education promotes awareness of mental and physical aspects including diet, weight, exercise and relaxation. In-house, or out-sourced, stress management programmes are customised for the structure, working practices and the nature of the organisation.

Disability Discrimination Act 1995

8.8 The *Disability Discrimination Act 1995* identifies the employer's responsibility for mental wellbeing, and culpability for failure to deal with organisational causes which contribute to an employee's mental health impairment. It confirms that mental wellbeing is a crucial aspect of working life. A person is held to have a disability if he or she has:

'... a physical or mental impairment which has a substantial and long-term effect on his or her ability to carry out normal day-to-day activities'.

This encompasses a mental impairment resulting from, or consisting of, a clinically well-recognised mental illness. Employers are required to make reasonable adjustments to accommodate the needs of disabled individuals, and to take reasonable steps to prevent such people from being placed at a substantial disadvantage in determining to whom employment is offered, in determining any term, condition or arrangement, promotion, transfer, training or any other benefit that is offered or afforded, and in relation to any physical features of the premises occupied by the employee.

A psychiatrist is required to give evidence as to whether the diagnosis of the alleged disability can be confirmed, and if so, the degree of severity. A consultant should not expound on a subject unless the opinion given can withstand rigorous scrutiny. It is inadvisable to stray from established areas of expertise. For instance, dyslexia may be claimed as the cause of impaired performance, and it is often very difficult to differentiate from a low IQ. Therefore, assessment by a clinical or educational psychologist, or a speech therapist is essential.

The organisation

8.9 Effective management incorporates administration, marketing, human resources (HR), health and safety, and union or workers' representatives.

The workforce constitutes the organisation's most valuable asset. Stress and interpersonal tension can lead to impaired performance, sickness absence, labour turnover, and even ill-health retirement. Hence the importance of optimising the emotional and ergonomic aspects of the working environment.

Any workforce inevitably divides into:

- workhorses
- stars
- dead wood
- problem children

The aim is to maximise the efficiency of workhorses, eliminate dead wood and transform problem children into stars.

Corporate social responsibility

8.10 An organisation has a range of community responsibilities to those who are both directly or indirectly affected by the nature of its operation. Business should be conducted with people in mind. This obviously conflicts with Milton Friedman's famous quote that the social responsibility of business is to increase its profits. In fact, this is best achieved by considering people first.

Corporate social responsibility has been defined as the continuing commitment by business to behave ethically, and to contribute to economic development whilst improving the quality of life of the workforce and their families, as well as of the local community and society at large (WBCSD, 'Stakeholder Dialogue on Corporate Social Responsibility', Sept 6–8, 1998).

Organisations are now more accountable regarding health and safety, and it is mandatory for any business to evaluate the so-called 'triple bottom line' of social, economic, and environmental factors. Corporate social responsibility requires an organisation to understand what society expects of it, and to express its purposes; in effect to improve and audit performance, to sustain development, and to achieve targets. It is involved in mainstream management, engages with stakeholders, and deals with issues which matter to individuals. Stakeholders are people remote from the commercial value chain.

One study determined the prevalence of workplace bullying in an NHS community trust, and identified the association between bullying and health impairment (Quine, L, 'Workplace Bullying in NHS Community Trusts: Staff Questionnaire Survey', BMJ, 318:228-232, 1999). It concluded that physical or emotional bullying is a significant problem. Systems must be in place for adequate staff support, and to counteract interpersonal conflict. The workplace is an ideal setting within which to encourage awareness of health as it is a definable community in which changes in behaviour and performance can be monitored. Thus the need for psychiatric referral can be identified by a sensitive line manager in conjunction with an occupational health professional, and GP, given the employee's formal permission. Formal job appraisal and interim feedback facilitates this process. Hopefully, when indicated, clinical management is thus more acceptable to the employee, already reassured that their problem is recognised and that appropriate treatment is being supported. Obviously, this eases re-entry to the workplace, when sickness absence has been necessary.

However, if the employee's first approach is to a GP, the perceived adverse consequences of accepting treatment commonly deter its uptake because of concern about confidentiality in relation to the organisation and to his or her own job security. Employees frequently elect to deprive themselves of available corporate medical insurance cover, risking a long delay in accessing NHS facilities, or inappropriately attempt to self-finance private treatments. An unfortunate scenario of denial develops including the using up of precious annual leave instead of sick leave. Inevitably, stigma-related anxiety compounds the situation and compromises the outcome of any treatment programme. An employee's understandable priority is to maintain a strong image within the organisation, and so to avoid perceived weakness, which might jeopardise job security. Inevitably, this is counter-productive.

Occupational health resources

8.11 Occupational health professionals include nurses, psychologists, counsellors and physicians. However, only a relatively low proportion of organisations have an occupational health department, or even any access to a part-time occupational health nurse or physician, or to a GP with occupational health experience (see further CHAPTER 11) ('Occupational health provision at work', Contract Research Report 57, HSE, 1993). Therefore, small or medium-sized enterprises require to have emergency access to local community psychiatric facilities, whether NHS or private, to ensure immediate availability of appropriate assessment and treatment, be it for alcohol or substance abuse, stress, anxiety, depression or potential suicide.

The duration of any sickness absence is critical: it can be counter-productive without some form of urgent treatment and a rehabilitation programme to achieve soonest re-entry into the workplace. The GP faces a dilemma, and is often cajoled into setting up a range of 'high tech' medical investigations which are more acceptable to the patient than their being confronted with a psychiatric diagnosis, however minor.

The key to the successful management of an occupational mental health problem is its early identification and effective intervention. Features to note are change in behaviour, such as spontaneous weeping, irritability, poor timekeeping, performance, and increasing sickness absence. 'Presenteeism' describes the situation where an employee is at work but virtually non-functional, and the mnemonic 'HALT' is helpful in identifying such vulnerability, as follows:

- Hungry.
- Angry.

- Lonely.

- Tired.

It is much easier if identification and sensitive intervention is achieved within the workplace. The patient is then confidentially referred to the occupational health department or occupational health nurse if either is available. The GP is kept informed routinely, subject to the employee's agreement. Preferably, identification is by the individual him or herself, by the line manager, or by the occupational health physician or nurse. A sensitive and immediate response is mandatory with appropriate help, be it 'tea and sympathy', counselling or cognitive behavioural therapy. Urgent psychiatric referral may be necessary. Otherwise, the employee can become frustrated and isolated, with potentially unfortunate consequences, such as suicide.

Clinical management

8.12   Employee assistance programmes and counselling are extremely valuable provided that underlying anxiety and depression are diagnosed, and treated effectively with cognitive behavioural therapy, and, when indicated, antidepressant or anxiolytic medication.

Counselling or psychotherapy (cognitive behavioural therapy or psychodynamic) resolves problems and improves interpersonal skills, achieving appropriate self-assertion without aggression. Also, it enables time-structuring and management, with the insertion of 'cushions of time' between commitments.

It should be clarified in the company's health policy that *psychotherapy* and *psychotropic medication* are complementary and not mutually exclusive: that is, talk for problems, medication for symptoms. However, there are certain jobs such as flying, and in certain other forms of transportation and other hazardous occupations, where psychotropic medication is specifically contra-indicated, and it is the responsibility of doctors to warn patients of its possible adverse effects on their work. In any form of driving, whether private or in public service, the individual has a legal responsibility whilst taking any form of prescribed medication (*Road Traffic Act 1988, Pt I*).

Ongoing rehabilitation and management to avoid or minimise sickness absence to prevent ill-health retirement, and to facilitate sensitive re-entry into the workplace, avoids the huge cost to industry of labour turnover, and loss of productivity. Premature ill-health retirement can consign a relatively young person to 'the scrap heap' and is very costly to the organisation. It is pointless, frustrating and counter-productive to have a health policy which includes mental health, if there is no readily accessible treatment facility.

Following prolonged sickness absence, effective rehabilitation and re-entry entails support from management and co-workers. Provided the rehabilitee agrees, a meeting including the key mental health professional, line manager or Human Resources representative, and partner is invaluable. This helps the employer to better understand work-related issues which may have contributed to the illness, and reduces the initial embarrassment of re-entry by 'breaking the ice' off site. Many managers welcome such an opportunity and themselves feel supported in facilitating re-entry, and in ongoing identification and modification of subsequent stressors. Thus health, performance, and productivity can be monitored to the mutual advantage of the rehabilitee and of the organisation.

A severe psychotic illness may respond well to treatment, and successful resumption of previous work can be achieved. However, a small proportion will have had a more severe psychotic illness necessitating long-term sickness absence and continuing medication. Nevertheless, they may well be capable of resuming some form of employment, given appropriate work rehabilitation.

Identifying common mental ill-health triggers and symptoms

8.13

- Psychosocial:
  - interpersonal relationship problems, partner abuse, or separation;
  - family illness, difficult adolescent behaviour, elderly parents, or bereavement;
  - acute emotional crisis such as unexpected pregnancy, spontaneous abortion or termination.
- Work-related:
  - stress, anxiety and depression, possibly resulting from heavy workload, adverse appraisal, failure to achieve advancement, or over-promotion.
- Health-related:
  - onset of chronic non-life-threatening conditions such as diabetes, respiratory tract infections, arthritides and musculoskeletal disorders. There may be an associated inability to consider underlying psychological factors, and multiple short-term sickness absences may ensue;
  - repeated presentation with somatic complaints (ie physical) with the request for a blood pressure check; other investigations often ensue.

Strategies in the training of occupational health professionals

8.14 It is recognised that Human Resources departments, and health and safety staff are people-orientated professionals and their approach should be appropriately customised to maximise communication. They advise the organisation regarding time-tabling to avoid overload. They enable collaboration with managers to rationalise workers perception of risk, and encourage re-entry following sickness absence. They manage emotional and psychosexual problems, and alcohol, drug and substance abuse, including dependence on minor analgesics. They handle stress, anxiety and depression and psychiatric emergencies including violence and attempted suicide. They understand the whole-person concept of mental and physical disorders, cognitive impairment due to general and psychotropic medication, and the importance of sleep hygiene in reducing reliance on hypnotics. Thus a comfortable balance is facilitated between home, work and community life.

Destigmatisation and discrimination in the workplace

8.15   The whole workforce benefits from a demonstrable commitment to counter the stigma and discrimination associated with mental illness, and by the provision of a mentally healthy working environment. When stress, personal grievance claims, and labour turnover are reduced, productivity is increased. Non-discriminatory policies provide clear guidance on how to deal with those vulnerable to, or recovering from, mental illness. The ability to be open regarding mental health issues should prevent job insecurity and facilitate the seeking of help. This is the purpose of including mental health in the organisation's overall health and safety policy. Stigmatisation is a significant reason for loss of hope, and relapse. Recruitment and retention of an employee with mental health impairment is endangered by stereotyping, and wrongly assuming the existence of problems only associated with the severest of psychotic illnesses. Stress, anxiety and depression bear no relationship to psychotic illness. It is as misleading to speak collectively of 'mental illness' as it is of 'surgical illness'. There are mild examples of each which are readily treatable. The Royal College of Psychiatrists campaign 'Changing Minds' aims to prevent or modify prejudice in the workplace (RCP, 1998–2003) (see APPENDIX: FURTHER SOURCES OF INFORMATION for contact details).

Prescription drugs and over-the-counter medication

8.16   Prescribed general, psychotropic, and over-the-counter medication (eg antihistamines) can impair workplace performance, both by unwanted effects and by interaction with other substances. Studies of people involved in road traffic accidents confirm that tricyclic antidepressants (TCAs) and benzodiazepines are more likely to be present in the blood of drivers considered to have been responsible for the accident, than in the blood of those who, following assessment, are considered innocent victims.

Appropriately, the Civil Aviation Authority precludes a pilot from flying within three months of taking any antidepressant medication, or within eight hours of consuming alcohol, the so called 'bottle to throttle' obligatory interval. The only 'sleeping pills' (hypnotic) permissable are Zolpidem and

Zopiclone, both of which are short-acting. Transportation and other industries, including the railways, have their own restrictions. Paradoxically, brain surgeons, builders or electricians, to mention just a few, are not so constrained.

Sickness presence, or 'presenteeism', describes the situation when the individual is physically capable of attending the workplace, but cognitive impairment, and/or disorientation, render them ineffective, or even a dangerous liability. Such employees are contravening health and safety legislation, as is the employer whose other employees, contractors, or members of the public may accordingly be at risk. From the point of view of safety, it is academic whether impaired cognitive function, hand-eye co-ordination, or slowed reaction time are due to prescribed medication, alcohol, illicit drugs or substance abuse.

In prescribing psychotropic medication, it is essential to consider the balance between clinical improvement, and the risk of adverse effects in the performance of work, and in the acts of everyday living. Computer programmers can cause economic or administrative chaos, and manual and transportation workers serious accidents, due to impaired psychomotor function in using specific skills (Hindmarch, I, 'Antidepressants, Other Psychotropics and Accident Risk in the Workplace', in 'Workshop on Prescriptive Medicine & Human Performance', pp 5–10, Institute of Petroleum, London, 1999).

The effectiveness in anxiety and depression of any of the antidepressants such – as TCAs, selective serotonin re-uptake inhibitors (SSRIs), selective noradrenaline re-uptake inhibitors (SNRIs) and reversible inhibitors of monoamineoxidaseA (RIMAs) – varies between individuals. However, there are no trials which convincingly demonstrate statistically a superiority of one or other group of antidepressants (Edwards, JG, 'Drug Choice in Depression. Selective Serotonin Reuptake Inhibitors or Tricyclic Antidepressants?', CNS Drugs, 1995 4:141–59; Edwards, JG and Anderson, I, 'Systematic Review and Guide to Selection of Selective Serotonin Reuptake Inhibitors', CNS Drugs, 1999 57: 507–33). Furthermore, idiosyncratic reactions and even some side effects cannot be predicted, although an adverse reaction to one particular antidepressant may be replicated by another drug of the same type. Hindmarch has repeatedly demonstrated a wide range of differences as regards adverse effects on cognitive function and performance. The critical flicker fusion test and choice reaction time, which are measures of cognitive function and psychomotor speed, respectively, were used in Hindmarch's studies. The modes of action of these antidepressants can include serotonergic, noradrenergic, and dopaminergic activity in stabilising and elevating mood, and so improving cognitive function.

Alcohol and illegal drug substances compound the centrally acting effects of concomitant prescribed or over-the-counter medications, and the effect of alcohol in producing a breath alcohol concentration of 80mg% provides a reference point for comparison with the effects of antidepressants.

The term 'behavioural toxicity' is used to describe the adverse effects of any drug on psychomotor performance and cognitive function. Such effects have to be taken into consideration when selecting a drug for a particular patient working in a specific situation.

The effects of a drug on performance relate to the dose, frequency, and timing in which it is used. Both the residual effects of hypnotics, and the continuous effects of antidepressants are important in the context of safety at work. Is it safe to undertake skilled work or to drive the day after taking a hypnotic, or while taking an antidepressant routinely? The absorption, distribution, metabolism and excretion of the parent compound and its active metabolite dictate blood levels and residual daytime impairment. Hypnotics cross the blood-brain barrier easily, making the sedative effect relatively rapid in onset.

Patients must always be given a clear explanation and warning regarding their own legal responsibility when driving on any prescribed medication.

Pharmacology of side effects of antidepressants

8.17   Tricyclic antidepressants such as amitriptyline and dothiepin can have anticholinergic and antihistaminic effects, and cause alpha-adrenergic blockade. The clinical manifestations of these are as follows:

- Anticholinergic effects

  Can cause memory impairment, confusion, dry mouth, constipation and impaired ocular accommodation (focusing difficulty).

- Antihistaminic effects

  Can cause drowsiness, sedation, daytime tiredness, residual hangover and impaired psychomotor speed.

- Alpha-adrenergic block effects

  Can cause hypotension (low blood pressure), impaired balance and inco-ordination.

However, individual susceptibility to these side effects varies widely, some patients being virtually unaffected.

In general, SSRIs, SNRIs and RIMAs cause fewer side effects. It appears that sertraline, paroxetine, citalopram, fluoxetine and venlafaxine have less serious adverse effects on cognitive and psychomotor function. However, a discontinuation syndrome can occur following abrupt withdrawal of all antidepressants, including SSRIs; this occurs more frequently, and is usually more severe, in the case of paroxetine.

Factors affecting the individual

8.18   Factors affecting individual employees include the structure and nature of the organisation, the individual's role, personality, working relationships and career development. Good management identifies specific personality types and plays to their strengths. No matter how sophisticated pre-employment personality assessment may be, the overall aim is to ensure that the individual will be functionally effective in the job for which he or she has been selected. Nevertheless, many personal, domestic and social issues compound workplace stress and are impossible to quantify.

Personality characteristics which are of occupational significance

8.19 Personality encompasses life-long traits which dictate how an individual reacts to a given situation, and how he or she is perceived. It influences the response to occupational stress. Assessment should identify strengths, and the ability to perform as a 'team player', likewise, vulnerabilities. Positive characteristics include integrity, loyalty, mood stability, flexibility, adaptability, self-confidence and esteem, interpersonal skills, energy, motivation, and the ability to be appropriately self-assertive without appearing aggressive. Time management and prioritising abilities are important: the key is managing to control the acceptance of incoming items of work while maintaining optimum productivity.

When a personality trait adversely affects the individual's functional effectiveness, it can constitute a neurosis. The commonest are anxiety, depression and the obsessional states. It is said that up to one-third of all GP attenders have some form of treatable neurotic illness. Epidemiological studies confirm that disorders that are common in the general population are also common in the workplace. Therefore, a proportion of those with neurotic illness will be in employment, although not requiring sickness absence. They may be considered as 'working wounded' and hence have increased vulnerability to workplace stressors.

The *obsessional* personality is extremely thorough, but is slow. Frustration and stress can be caused to other team members, and overall productivity can be impaired. Despite this limitation, attention to detail and the maintenance of high standards are essential in a range of occupations in preventing serious mistakes, or dangerous accidents.

The ability to give oneself 'well dones' without appearing complacent or smug is effective during highly stressful times. The *ultra-sensitive* or *paranoid* personality resents criticism and is often blessed (or cursed) by an elephantine memory. Such people can present a problem, highlighted at the time of job appraisal. The ability to accept both positive and negative feedback is important.

The *cyclothymic* personality, with unpredictable mood swings, can be disconcerting for co-workers due to the uncertainty generated.

Anxiety traits can create the unrealistic impression that the individual is incapable of functioning effectively: his or her assumptions of a negative outcome cause performance anxiety. For example, an excellent airline pilot can experience this prior to simulator and route checks. Such anxiety can also occur in public speaking, the performing arts, academic written, and particularly viva examinations, job interviews, or even when introducing oneself to a group. An inappropriate fear of failure, humiliation and rejection haunts some people. Some self-actualise solely by perceived achievement, and even transient failure can damage already frail self-esteem.

Physical health impairment

8.20   The adverse effect of the onset of physical symptoms is associated with the uncertainty resulting from obligatory medical investigations, which may be followed by the diagnosis of a non life-threatening but chronic condition, with a loss of quality of life in all domains. This increases vulnerability to pre-existing and ongoing work and domestic stress. Despite learning the nature and prognosis of any illness, the patient often has uncertainty regarding its impact on employment: 'Will I still be able to do my job Doctor?' Anxiety and depression may ensue, compounded by the realisation of permanent loss of good health and the difficulty in adapting to the inevitable changes in lifestyle.

The conundrum is whether the degree and duration of anxiety with depression, provoked by the illness, are within normal limits or require treatment. This is typified by musculoskeletal disorders, diabetes, epilepsy and multiple sclerosis: personal health being the individual's most valuable possession.

Physical symptoms relating to psychiatric conditions

8.21   Emotional stress can generate the symptoms of fatigue, dizziness, headache, musculoskeletal pain, and other minor ailments. This assumes clinical significance when such symptoms are perceived by the individual as being due to physical illness. They then present their symptoms to their GP who may set up physical investigations, and so, in turn, they are referred to a consultant. Thus the individual undergoes physical investigations, which inevitably increase anxiety due to the enhanced suspicion of sinister organic disease. This further diverts attention from the underlying psychological causes. Patients often have specific conditions in mind such as cancer, heart disease, AIDS or chronic fatigue syndrome. Of those attending general hospital medical clinics, up to one-fifth are said to have no significant underlying organic disease to account for their symptoms. Hence the importance of direct questioning to identify depression and, or one of the anxiety disorders, be it generalised, panic or phobic disorder. However, Kivimaki, M, et al in a long-term study of 812 employees have shown that those with high job stress have double the risk of cardiovascular mortality ('Work Stress and Risk of Cardiovascular Mortality: Prospective Cohort Study of Industrial Employees', BMJ, Vol 325 857-60, 19 October 2002).

Psychosomatic symptoms

8.22   There are a range of psychosomatic conditions outside the scope of this book, many of which have considerable occupational significance. Untreated occupational mental health problems can trigger or exacerbate insomnia, asthma, migraine, tension headaches, hypertension, irritable bowel syndrome, dermatoses and musculoskeletal pain.

Low-back pain

8.23   It may be that psychological factors generate and perpetuate chronic low-back pain. The sensitisation of heat and touch fibres results in their augmenting pain transmission, resulting in persistent pain which can limit capability for work and daily living. Whereas acute pain responds to minor analgesics, chronic pain may be more resistant. This can result in escalating dosage and the risk of side effects.

Demoralisation and depression may ensue due to impaired mobility, psychosexual adjustment and sleep.

As Waddell ('Recent Developments in Low-Back Pain', ASP Press, 2002) states, the mechanism and management of low-back pain and health service interventions are being challenged. Psychosocial factors are being increasingly recognised. Previously, the biomedical approach assumed organic pathology, without objective evidence, and 'physical' remedies were used. The move to a biopsychosocial human model of pain and disability, was initiated by Waddell ('The Back Pain Revolution', Churchill Livingstone, 1998). Thus, instead of the traditional advice of 'rest until better', maintenance of activity is now recommended and the continuation of normal daily routine. The effectiveness of such an approach is described (Van Tedder et al, 'The Effectiveness of Conservative Treatment of Active/Chronic Low-Back Pain', EMGO Institute, 1999).

Sleep

8.24   Sleep hygiene entails appropriate relaxation – physical, mental and spiritual. Activities which could be contributing to sleep impairment should be avoided later in the day. Therefore, from 6 pm onwards, it is best to avoid distressing telephone calls, writing contentious letters, anger, violent films, TV, or radio, a heavy meal, caffeine, chocolate and alcohol. Frenetic exercising causes arousal due to the outpouring of adrenaline, but a late and leisurely walk is highly beneficial, as is a comfortable bed and room temperature. The maintenance of regular hours for going to bed and rising, even at the weekends, and avoidance of napping during the day facilitates satisfactory sleep.

Post-natal depression and female-specific anxieties

8.25   If she has a partner or a family, a woman may view going out to work as an *additional* job. An otherwise supportive partner may have the knee-jerk response of 'give it up' if she tries to discuss work-related problems, or he may trivialise the necessity for her to work at all. Maternity leave and subsequent return to work can result in an agonising division of loyalty. Inevitably, ambition and career focus become diverted. Whatever her level of seniority and the availability of childcare and domestic help, the maternal instinct may contribute to workplace stress, particularly so for the single mother. The house-husband is a comfortable and reassuring feature of the modern well-adjusted partnership.

In ante-natal classes, although 'baby blues' are explained, there is often an inadequate grasp of the very real clinical entity of post-natal depression, the general prevalence of which is up to 1 in 10 in the absence of any previous psychiatric history or significant obstetric or paediatric complication. However, it is eminently treatable provided that awareness facilitates its early diagnosis. It is important that it is understood and accepted by the partner, and by the extended family. Delayed onset post-natal depression may present following the return to work, inevitably affecting behaviour and performance. It increases vulnerability to workplace stressors. Its identification will be facilitated if it is dealt with in the training programme for occupational health professionals and Human Resources personnel, and is detailed in the company's health policy.

Stress

8.26   Stress is endemic. It is the industrial disease of the twenty-first century. It covers the spectrum from mental health to mental illness. It occurs when external and internal demands exceed the individual's adaptive resources. If prolonged, it may cause psychological and physical impairment. External demands become overwhelming when the individual is incapable of controlling their scope of responsibility, or the flow of work towards them. This can be the result of change in working practices, over or under-load, poor delegation, non-involvement in decision making with failure to empower staff, threat of redundancies causing uncertainty, and the implications for those remaining. Also, stress may be due to, or the perception of, being disliked, victimisation by whistle-blowing, or job insecurity. A project may be passed to a peer co-worker who then completes it successfully, thereby gaining enviable positive feedback. The acquisition of assertive skills can facilitate the handling of such situations. An unexpected adverse job appraisal can predispose to resentment, anger and loss of self-confidence. Potential may be under-used, with boring, repetitive procedures and inadequate feedback. Stress adversely affects health and work performance. Coping with it is essential for health and wellbeing. If ignored, it can predispose to anxiety, depression, domestic and community difficulties, problem drinking and even suicide.

Causes of work-related stress vary with individual organisations: pressure to perform despite excessive work-load, change or uncertainty, long hours, poor ergonomic conditions, competition, or failure to achieve anticipated advancement, also over-promotion with unacceptable responsibility without authority, relocation, local or global commuting, conflict of work with private life, job insecurity, worry about productivity, strained interpersonal relationships, formal complaints, changes exceeding adaptive resources, redundancies, traumatic incidents, such as accidents, illness or death of co-workers. One study (Cooper, C, 'Crisis Talks', *Personnel Today*, 2 October 1997) identified the commonest causes of workplace stress as follows:

- 60% was due to time pressure deadlines;

- 54% was due to work overload;

- 52% was due to the threat of job loss;

- 51% was due to lack of consultation or communication;

- 46% was due to understaffing.

As well as in cardiovascular disease, stress is relevant in the causation of strokes and possibly cancer. It predisposes the individual to musculoskeletal pain, lowers immunity and may result in sickness absence or 'presenteeism'. 'Quick fixes' such as nicotine, caffeine, alcohol or drugs aggravate it. Sickness absence increases when full leave entitlement is not taken because of job insecurity.

The workplace is an integral component of the employee's life and the ideal setting in which to monitor and improve mental health. Personal and wider community lifestyles impact on work. Work-related stress cannot be separated from domestic and community stress. It exerts its adverse effect at personal and organisational levels. An employer's awareness of the employee's non-work-related stressors and problems facilitates good management. Corporate social responsibility is to be encouraged. This is exemplified by the enormously effective welfare support provided to Armed Services families, particularly in unexpected crises, and during unaccompanied postings overseas. Such support would reduce many of the 'ex-patriate' problems experienced in routine company moves abroad, or even within the UK.

Stress management

8.27   Good management of stress entails utilising leisure, friendships and the balancing of occupational and domestic demands. Regular exercise is encouraged, with radical reduction of alcohol, nicotine and caffeine consumption. Team building, teaching of interpersonal skills, assertiveness, and time-management training with ready access to the line manager, constructive positive and negative feedback, and appraisal, with the development of trust, is encouraged. There must be awareness throughout the organisation that stress is recognised.

As dedicated occupational health resources are still so limited, the *usual scenario* is that the GP is consulted for physical symptoms such as headache, musculoskeletal pain, or sleep impairment, when in fact there is an inability to cope with the job. Medication may be prescribed, such as a 'sleeping pill' or antidepressant, and the individual continues at work as 'working wounded' or sickness absence is recommended. The latter is counter-productive if there is no immediate stress management, such as counselling or a daily structured psychotherapeutic programme. Unfortunately, NHS resources rarely allow of immediate access to a counsellor. The patient often refuses such an offer. The vulnerable employee merely ruminates about perceived workload, interpersonal problems, and lack of managerial support with unresolved resentment and anger and increasing apprehension regarding resumption of work. Organisations without counselling resources may be able to buy into local private facilities. Obviously, corporate or individual medical insurance policies should be utilised if available. However, for the majority of small and medium-sized enterprises, this may be perceived as economically unjustifiable. In fact, this is false economy as its personnel constitute an organisation's most valuable asset. As described by R Welch and N Tehrain ('Counselling in the Post Office: Prevention of Mental Ill Health at Work', HMSO, 1992), stress is most effectively managed when there is early intervention by the line manager or Human Resources department staff followed by rapid referral to an occupational health professional, if available. Counselling is then arranged in house, or locally. This is best achieved when the counsellor is familiar with the organisation and the personalities concerned. However, this utopian situation is rarely achieved and sickness absence is certificated as 'stress and anxiety', without further effective intervention. Unfortunately, the patient will then develop an increasingly negative attitude to the employer and begin to hold entrenched views about being incapable of ever returning to work, with ill-health retirement becoming increasingly likely.

Post-traumatic stress disorder

8.28 Post-traumatic stress disorder (PTSD) is a normal mental and physical reaction to an incident, the magnitude of which constitutes a 'near-death' experience, and is for the individual and others, in scope, beyond what could have reasonably been expected. Traumatic events constituting critical incidents include road traffic accidents, safety-critical job accidents, fires, explosions, structural or transportation incidents, robbery and hostage situations. Such trauma can affect victims, co-workers, relatives, Emergency Services, Armed Forces, police, schoolteachers, traffic wardens, social security and healthcare professionals, who are all particularly vulnerable. Following a critical incident, the acute stress reaction may remit spontaneously within a month. Acute onset PTSD may ensue within one–three months after the critical incident, hence awareness of the potential hazards is essential. Debriefing should be available, but only be used when specifically indicated, or requested. Its routine use is strictly contra-indicated, and can actually aggravate the situation. Understandably, some object to 'medicalising' what is a normal reaction to a grossly abnormal situation. Nevertheless, skilled treatment is essential for established PTSD, the onset of which may have been delayed for many years. This situation occurred in 1995, when 50 years after their release, many Far East Prisoners of War presented with PTSD triggered by old newsreels. This could be considered as the responsibility of the organisation, the Ministry of Defence in this case. However, it has to be clarified that PTSD was not recognised as a clinical entity until the early 1980s.

Clinical features

8.29 The symptoms of PTSD include the following:

- hyperarousal such as impaired sleep, irritability, anger, startle response;
- persistent re-experiencing, intrusive rumination, nightmares, or re-living of the experience through illusions, hallucinations or flashbacks;
- avoidance of stimuli connected with the critical incident;
- co-morbid conditions including depression, alcohol, or drug abuse.

Clinical management

8.30 PTSD responds to cognitive behavioural therapy, during which there is active exposure to the incident and avoidance is prevented. The associated depression also responds to cognitive behavioural therapy plus antidepressant medication. The value of eye-movement desensitisation and reprocessing is also becoming increasingly recognised.

Burnout

8.31 This is defined as a syndrome of physical and emotional exhaustion resulting in a negative self-image and attitude to work, with a loss of the ability to relate to co-workers or clients (Webster, L, and Hacket, RK, 'Administration and Policy in Mental Health', Vol 26, No 6, July 1999).

Maslach's 'burnout inventory' identifies three subscales to the condition:

- emotional exhaustion;
- depersonalisation;
- diminished personal accomplishment.

Findings indicate that depersonalisation is specific to the caring services for whom interpersonal relationships are focal. This is particularly worrying, in that the job is to support patients or clients by establishing an effective therapeutic alliance through empathy, sensitivity and mutual respect. Burnout inevitably impairs the quality of care delivered. There is a deterioration of the individual's effectiveness and enthusiasm, ability to utilise skills, and interact, yet to maintain appropriate autonomy.

Organisational systemic issues may impact adversely on the mental health of care workers, and secondarily on that of patients and clients. The individual's confidence in supportive management, with empowerment, reduces the risk of burnout, and facilitates recovery. In the caring professions, particularly in mental health, supervision, monitoring, peer review and appraisal are all crucial in handling the potential intensity of emotional relationships. This is the basis of effective audit and clinical governance, which are now very properly obligatory.

Good leadership promotes effective interaction between mental health care professionals, their patients and clients, and contributes to a positive working environment. It also reduces depersonalisation and emotional exhaustion in staff. These fundamental principles obtain whatever the nature of the operation.

Alcohol and drug abuse

8.32   Both alcohol and drugs act directly on the brain, and have areas of commonality, and difference in their effects. Either can rapidly affect concentration, judgement, behaviour and performance. They impair cognitive function and hand-eye co-ordination, and prolong reaction time. They predispose to impulsive behaviour, with hazards ranging from minor tripping injuries, to dangerous accidents. Behavioural effects can cause difficult interpersonal relationships with co-workers, clients, and in the local community.

Tackling this is beneficial, reducing labour turnover, because functionally-impaired workers are potentially dangerous. Who is at risk? There is no stereotype, but many are in employment. Quite commonly, it is the occasional drinker or drug abuser whose behaviour is unacceptable or who causes an accident: just consider the office Christmas party. As with mental health as a whole, an effective alcohol and drugs policy must apply throughout the workforce, whatever the level of seniority. It raises awareness, and avoids a 'them and us' situation.

Alcohol and drugs policies should be embodied within the organisations overall health and safety policy, recognising that addictive diseases are as much 'illnesses' as are those of the cardio-vascular, respiratory or gastro-intestinal systems. Therefore, the employee deserves the same consideration regarding sickness absence, job security and salary provided that the recommended treatment programme is pursued. This has to be appropriate for the size, structure, and nature of the particular organisation. It is designed to prevent or to reduce to a minimum, the effects of alcohol and drug abuse on the abuser, co-workers, the local community and the environment.

Alcohol and drug policies

8.33   The organisation's alcohol and drug policy should clearly define what is meant by abuse, explaining that both impair health and cognitive function, with psychological and/or physical dependence: hence, there is a need to identify and treat developing habits quickly. The policy encourages self-identification, and confirms confidentiality, the entitlement to sickness absence, and job security, for treatment and rehabilitation purposes, with limited toleration of relapses. It should be clarified that refusal of help and treatment may result in disciplinary action if unsatisfactory behaviour or poor work performance persist. Dismissal may ultimately result. Provision for monitoring requires agreement with unions, or workers' representatives. Police involvement is obligatory for drug trafficking.

It is essential to have links with local NHS community drug and alcohol teams, or private facilities, if corporate medical insurance cover is provided. However, Human Resources or occupational health professionals must always liaise with the GP and the key relative or friend, provided that the employee's formal agreement is obtained.

Screening

8.34

- Screening for alcohol

  Only if agreed with unions or workers representatives, and provided this is clarified in the alcohol policy. Random breath testing may be considered appropriate in specific safety-critical jobs. It is essential in some jobs, and prudent but controversial in others. Each organisation customises its own procedure.

- Screening for drugs

  At pre-employment examination, or randomly for causes such as unacceptable behaviour, after an accident or after a dangerous incident, or if found in possession on site. Routine monitoring is essential during rehabilitation. There must be a reliable and uniform technique for the handling, and analysis of specimens, and written consent must be obtained from the individual. The intention to screen for alcohol and drugs must be clarified at induction, detailed in the alcohol and drugs policy, and reiterated in ongoing health education.

Pre-employment medical examinations

8.35   There are strong arguments for and against initiating pre-employment medical checks. For certain jobs this is mandatory, such as commercial flying where cardio-vascular screening is routine. Specific mental health screening is obligatory only when there is a significant psychiatric history. The validity of the various methods used is questionable (Lucas, G, 'Occupational Aspects of Whole-Person Healthcare', in Christie, MJ, and Mellett, PG (eds), 'Psychosomatic Approach: Contemporary Practice of Whole-Person Care', John Wiley, 1986). More importantly, there is an irrefutable risk of unjustifiable disadvantaging, rejecting, and stigmatising an individual: for instance, this could occur when there has been an acute onset, short-lived depressive episode, resulting from major adversity, in an individual of previously stable personality.

Pre-employment job-orientated examinations to assess *suitability* may be appropriate, however, and in the best interests of other employees, the organisation and productivity. This is to confirm functional effectiveness for the job in question. Is this not merely in keeping with a £35 million footballer being subjected to the most rigorous of medical examinations? Moreover, being too vigorously protective in preventing mental health screening could in fact fuel stigma, however covert, and risk the accusation of positive discrimination, itself being counter-productive. Take the *Employment Protection Act 1975* as an example: this restricted periods of health probation to one year maximum, it previously having been open-ended. An increase in rejection from 17% in 1975 to 46% subsequently was identified in schizophrenic rehabilitees. The adult population prevalence of psychotic illness is 1–3% (Jenkins, R, 'Prevention of Mental Ill Health at Work', HMSO, 1992), but is significantly less in the working population.

Throughout the armed services, irrespective of rank, the annual PULHEEMS examination is mandatory. This categorises every aspect of whole-person health: P denotes physique, U and L limbs, H hearing, E and E eyes, with M and S denoting mental state and stability respectively. According to these categories the serviceman can be restricted to 'home only' duties, or ultimately classified as 'no longer fit for service' – the military equivalent of ill-health retirement.

Prolonged sickness absence

8.36   Undiagnosed work-related stress, anxiety and depression occurs in some 15–30% of the adult population in any one year. This could imply that a similar proportion of workers is being denied, or the worker him or herself is declining, essential assessment and psychotherapeutic input, for stress and anxiety. The refusal of such an offer should be documented. The adverse consequence of such a refusal may become a disciplinary matter if alcohol or drug abuse persists, and behaviour, work performance, or sickness absence continue to be unsatisfactory.

It is said that sickness absence is higher in those workers who do not use up all of their annual leave. Responsible management requires that the full entitlement be taken. Disconcerting, but unconfirmed newspaper claims, have been made that safety-critical transportation industries are even offering to pay overtime to encourage employees to work in their 'holidays'. Contrarywise, misguidedly, some prefer to conceal ill-health by utilising annual leave rather than having sickness absence.

Sickness absence and ill-health retirement

8.37   Prolonged sickness absence can result in ill-health retirement. Initial certification may be continued without sufficient scrutiny. The employee and or employer inappropriately assume that irreversible chronicity has developed, whatever the presenting symptoms. This can create an entrenched attitude in the individual and the key carer so that return to work is no longer an option. This predisposes to premature ill-health retirement, or severance of whatever nature. This is to the disadvantage of the employee and employer, personnel being the organisation's most valuable asset: expensively gained skills, and experience, can be unnecessarily lost.

It is anomalous that retirement on the grounds of *mental* ill-health is even considered before psychiatric assessment has been carried out and treatment instituted. This may include counselling or cognitive behavioural therapy, and psychotropic medication when indicated. These approaches are not mutually exclusive – 'talk for problems, medication for symptoms'. Such early intervention can prevent chronicity and ultimate ill-health retirement. GPs, occupational health professionals, Human Resources department, unions and workers' representatives should all be mindful of the hazards of delay.

Conclusions

8.38   An organisation's health policy should include mental health, alcohol and drug abuse. However, its effectiveness depends on its practical interpretation, and its application throughout the organisation, irrespective of seniority.

The nature and implementation of working practices are rapidly changing and the individual's ability to adapt is crucial. These changes include new technology, increasing use of chemicals in work processes, mechanisation and shift-work practices. Working from home relieves the stress of commuting, but imposes the need for disciplined time-management, and can be isolating: some regret the absence of co-workers, although to others it may be a bonus.

The occupational hazards of the old heavy industries have now been replaced by others, such as deep-sea operations, oil rigs, harmful pathogens, radioactive substances, and waste. Genetic manipulation and computer-based technology have all produced a range of stress-related occupational mental health problems. The workforce as a whole is becoming increasingly aware of personal and community hazards. Work is important in the maintenance of self-esteem, hence the traumatic effects of redundancy. Women who gave it up to rear a family, have a need to return to similar or alternative employment when the children become independent.

Tackling whole-person health facilitates the ability to cope with the inevitable stressors occurring simultaneously in each domain of life. This is relevant in the behaviour and performance of the workforce, and in the productivity of the organisation, whatever its size and the purpose of its operation. Ease of technological communication can be a double-edged sword. Its appropriate use is a skill which must be taught, and customised to specific requirements. However, face-to-face communication remains invaluable, and it is to be encouraged, whenever feasible.

The aim is to put the mental component of health into whole-person health as defined by the World Health Organisation. This ensures awareness, and facilitates self-identification and the request for help, thus achieving effective intervention and proactive strategies by line managers. However, to make it a 'special case', is counter-productive. It must never be suggested that the workplace should be regarded as a large occupational therapy and rehabilitation unit for the psychologically vulnerable. That would constitute unacceptable positive discrimination.

The workplace is a microcosm of the community and an ideal place to be proactive in addressing mental health impairment.

This is the rationale for a comprehensive health policy, including mental health, to ensure awareness and facilitate identification, intervention, supply of appropriate help, monitoring, rehabilitation, and re-entry to the workplace when sickness absence has been required.

9 Personal Protection

Introduction

9.1 Personal protective equipment (PPE) such as safety footwear, safety helmets and respiratory protective equipment (RPE) are widely used in situations where it is not possible to ensure the complete absence of risks in the workplace. Two very different work situations can be identified where personal protection is required:

- that where PPE is worn in case something goes wrong; and

- that where PPE is worn because of continuously present risks.

Examples of the first situations are those in which safety footwear, safety helmets and eye protection are used to protect against unplanned events: no-one would seriously suggest that safety helmets would be a sensible form of protection where heavy items were *continuously* falling on workers' heads. In the second situation, there is a known ongoing potential exposure. Protective clothing, RPE and personal hearing protectors (PHP) are routinely worn in such situations. There are also situations where these latter types of PPE are worn as a back-up to other controls, such as complete containment of a chemical process, in case of failure of the other controls.

The validity of the use of personal protection in the ongoing risk situation must be carefully considered. It is a basic principle of good occupational hygiene that there is a *clear hierarchy of controls*, as follows:

- prevention;

- control at source; and

- PPE.

This control hierarchy is enshrined in both EU and UK legislation. For example, *Article 6* of the European 'Framework' Directive (89/391/EEC) specifies that the employer shall protect his workers on the basis of 'giving collective measures priority over individual protective measures'.

Current HSE guidance on the control of hazards in the workplace is based on a procedure set out in 'COSHH Essentials' (available from HSE Books and on www.hse.gov.uk).

In considering the role of PPE in the workplace it is necessary, therefore, to consider the requirements of the relevant legislation and guidance.

Legal requirements

9.2　The role of PPE in the workplace is very clearly defined in regulations such as the following:

- the *Control of Substances Hazardous to Health Regulations 2002 (SI 2002/2677) (COSHH)*;

- the *Noise at Work Regulations 1989 (SI 1989/1790)*;

- the *Control of Asbestos at Work Regulations 2002 (SI 2002/2675) (CAW)*; and

- the *Control of Lead at Work Regulations 2002 (SI 2002/2676)*.

Note that both the 1999 *COSHH* and 1987 *CAW* regulations have been replaced by new regulations. The specific regulations applying to PPE, however, are not expected to be changed significantly. In all four regulations the hierarchy of control is enshrined in law.

The following regulations also impose specific PPE-related duties:

- the *Construction (Head Protection) Regulations 1989 (SI 1989/2209)*;

- the *Confined Spaces Regulations 1997 (SI 1997/1713)*; and

- the *Personal Protective Equipment at Work Regulations 1992 (SI 1992/2966)*.

Control of Substances Hazardous to Health Regulations 2002

9.3　The requirements of the *Control of Substances Hazardous to Health Regulations 2002 (SI 2002/2677) (COSHH)*, as relevant to PPE, are outlined below.

Regulation 7 – Prevention or control of exposure to substances hazardous to health

9.4　*Regulation 7* provides:

'(1)　Every employer shall ensure that the exposure of his employees to substances hazardous to health is either prevented or, where this is not reasonably practicable, adequately controlled.

(2)　...

(3)　Where it is not reasonably practicable to prevent exposure to a substance hazardous to health, the employer shall comply with his duty of control under paragraph (1) by applying protection measures appropriate to the activity and consistent with the risk assessment, including, in order of priority –

...

(c)   where adequate control of exposure cannot be achieved by other means, the provision of suitable personal protective equipment in addition to the measures required by subparagraphs (a) and (b).

...

(9)   Personal protective equipment provided by an employer in accordance with this regulation shall be suitable for the purpose and shall –

(a)   comply with any provision in the Personal Protective Equipment Regulations 2002 which is applicable to that item of personal protective equipment; or

(b)   in the case of respiratory protective equipment, where no provision referred to in sub-paragraph (a) applies, be of a type approved or shall conform to a standard approved, in either case, by the Executive.

...'

Regulation 8 – Use of control measures etc

9.5   *Regulation 8* provides:

'(1)   Every employer who provides any control measure, other thing or facility in accordance with these Regulations shall take all reasonable steps to ensure that it is properly used or applied as the case may be.

(2)   Every employee shall make full and proper use of any control measure, other thing or facility provided in accordance with these Regulations and, where relevant, shall –

(a)   take all reasonable steps to ensure it is returned after use to any accommodation provided for it; and

(b)   if he discovers a defect therein, report it forthwith to his employer.'

Regulation 9 – Maintenance, examination and testing of control measures

9.6   *Regulation 9* provides:

'(1)   Every employer who provides any control measure to meet the requirements of regulation 7 shall ensure that, where relevant, it is maintained in an efficient state, in efficient working order, in good repair and in a clean condition.

(2) Where engineering controls are provided to meet the requirements of regulation 7, the employer shall ensure that thorough examination and testing of those controls is carried out –

...

(3) Where respiratory protective equipment (other than disposable respiratory protective equipment) is provided to meet the requirements of regulation 7, the employer shall ensure that thorough examination and, where appropriate, testing of that equipment is carried out at suitable intervals.

(4) Every employer shall keep a suitable record of the examinations and tests carried out in accordance with paragraphs (2) and (3) and of repairs carried out as a result of these examinations and tests, and that record or a suitable summary thereof shall be kept available for at least 5 years from the date on which it was made.'

(5) Every employer shall ensure that personal protective equipment, including protective clothing, is:

(a) properly stored in a well-defined place;

(b) checked at suitable intervals; and

(c) when discovered to be defective, repaired or replaced before further use.

(6) Personal protective equipment which may be contaminated by a substance hazardous to health shall be removed on leaving the working area and kept apart from uncontaminated clothing and equipment.

(7) The employer shall ensure that the equipment referred to in paragraph (6) is subsequently decontaminated and cleaned or, if necessary, destroyed.'

Approved Code of Practice relevant to PPE in Regulation 9

9.7   The new Approved Code of Practice has not been published at the time of going to press. However, it is anticipated that specific guidance relevant to PPE will be provided in that section of the new ACOP relevant to *Regulation 9* of *COSHH*. The new ACOP is available from 6 December 2002 from HSE Books – and see www.hse.gov.uk and www.hsedirect.com.

Regulation 12 – Information, instruction and training for persons who may be exposed to substances hazardous to health

9.8   *Regulation 12 provides:*

'(1)   Every employer who undertakes work which is liable to expose an employee to a substance hazardous to health shall provide that employee with suitable and sufficient information, instruction and training.

(2)   Without prejudice to the generality of paragraph (1), the information, instruction and training provided under that paragraph shall include –

(a)   details of the substance hazardous to health to which the employee is liable to be exposed including –

(i)   the names of those substances and the risk which they present to health,

(ii)   any relevant occupational exposure standard, maximum exposure limit or similar occupational exposure limit,

(iii)   access to any relevant safety data sheet, and

(iv)   other legislative provisions which concern the hazardous properties of those substances;

(b)   the significant findings of the risk assessment;

(c)   the appropriate precautions and actions to be taken by the employee in order to safeguard himself and other employees at the workplace;

...'

Approved Code of Practice relevant to PPE in Regulation 12

9.9   The new Approved Code of Practice has not been published at the time of going to press. However, it is anticipated that specific guidance relevant to PPE will be provided in that section of the new ACOP relevant to *Regulation 12* of *COSHH*. The new ACOP is available from 6 December 2002 from HSE Books – and see www.hse.gov.uk and www.hsedirect.com.

Noise at Work Regulations 1989

9.10   The requirements of the *Noise at Work Regulations 1989 (SI 1989/1790)*, as relevant to PPE, are outlined below.

Regulation 7 – Reduction of noise exposure

9.11   *Regulation 7* provides:

> 'Every employer shall, when any of his employees is likely to be exposed to the second action level or above or to the peak action level or above, reduce, so far as is reasonably practicable (other than by the provision of personal ear protectors), the exposure to noise of that employee.'

Regulation 8 – Ear protection

9.12   *Regulation 8* provides:

> '(1)   Every employer shall ensure, so far is as practicable, that when any of his employees are likely to be exposed to the first action level or above in circumstances when the daily personal noise exposure of that employee is likely to be less than 90 dB(A), that employee is provided, at his request, with suitable and efficient personal ear protectors.
>
> (2)   Every employer shall ensure, so far is as practicable, that when any of his employees are likely to be exposed to the second action level or above, or to the peak action level or above, that employee is provided with suitable personal ear protectors which, hen properly worn, can reasonably be expected to keep the risk of damage to that employee's hearing to below that arising from exposure to the second action level, or, as the case may be, to the peak action level.
>
> (3)   Any personal ear protectors provided by virtue of this regulation shall comply with any enactment (whether an Act or instrument) which implements in Great Britain any provision on design or manufacture with respect to health and safety in any relevant Community Directive listed in Schedule 1 to the Personal Protective Equipment at Work Regulations 1992 which is applicable to those ear protectors.'

Regulations 9, 10 and 11

9.13   These regulations impose duties on an employer to designate areas where ear protectors should be worn, to ensure that ear protectors are correctly maintained and that employees are provided information, instruction and training in the use of their personal ear protectors respectively.

The Construction (Head Protection) Regulations 1989

9.14   The *Construction (Head Protection) Regulations 1989 (SI 1989/2209)* apply explicitly to the use of head protection in building operations and works of engineering construction within the meaning of the *Factories Act 1961.*

Regulation 3 – Provision, maintenance and replacement of suitable head protection

9.15   *Regulation 3* provides:

'(1)   Every employer shall provide each of his employees who is at work on operations or works to which these Regulations apply with suitable head protection and shall maintain it and replace it whenever necessary.

(2)   Every self-employed person who is at work on operations or works to which these Regulations apply shall provide himself with suitable head protection and shall maintain it and replace it whenever necessary.

(3)   Any head protection provided by virtue of these Regulations shall comply with any enactment (whether an Act or an instrument) which implements any provision on design or manufacture with respect to health and safety in any relevant Community Directive listed in Schedule 1 to the Personal Protective Equipment at Work Regulations 1992 which is applicable to head protection.

(4)   Before choosing any head protection, an employer or self-employed person shall make an assessment to determine whether it is suitable.

(5)   The assessment required by paragraph (4) of this Regulation shall involve–

(a)   the definition of the characteristics which head protection must have in order to be suitable;

(b)   comparison of the characteristics of the head protection available with the characteristics referred to in sub-paragraph (a) of this paragraph.

(6)   The assessment required by paragraph (4) shall be reviewed if–

(a)   there is reason to suspect that it is no longer valid; or

(b)   there has been a significant change in the work to which it relates, and where as a result of the review changes in the assessment are required, the relevant employer or self-employed person shall make them.

(7) Every employer and self-employed person shall ensure that appropriate accommodation is available for head protection by virtue of these Regulations when it is not being used.'

Regulation 4 – Ensuring suitable head protection is worn

9.16 *Regulation 4* provides:

'(1) Every employer shall ensure, so far as reasonably practicable that each of his employees who is at work on operations or works to which these Regulations apply wears suitable head protection, unless there is no foreseeable risk of injury to his head other than by his falling.

(2) Every employer, self-employed person or employee who has control over any other person who is at work on operations or works to which these Regulations apply shall ensure so far as is reasonably practicable that each such person wears suitable head protection, unless there is no foreseeable risk of injury to that person's head other than by his falling.'

Regulation 5 – Rules and directions

9.17 *Regulation 5* provides:

'(1) The person for the time being having control of a site where operations or works to which these Regulations apply are being carried out may, so far as is necessary to comply with regulation 4 of these Regulations, make rules regulating the wearing of suitable head protection on that site by persons on those operations or works.

(2) Rules made in accordance with paragraph (1) shall be in writing and shall be brought to the notice of persons who may be affected by them.

(3) Every employer may, so far as is necessary to comply with regulation 4(1) of these Regulations, give directions requiring his employees to wear suitable head protection.

(4) Every employer, self-employed person or employee who has control over any other self-employed person may, so far as is necessary to comply with regulation 4(2) of these Regulations, give directions requiring such other self-employed person to wear suitable head protection.'

Regulation 6 – Wearing of suitable head protection

9.18 *Regulation 6* provides:

'(1) Every employee who has been provided with suitable head protection shall wear that head protection when required to do so by rules or directions given under regulation 5 of these Regulations.

(2) Every self-employed person shall wear that head protection when required to do so by rules or directions given under regulation 5 of these Regulations.

(3) Every self-employed person who it at work on operations or works to which these Regulations apply, but who is not under the control of another employer or self-employed person or employee, shall wear suitable head protection unless these is no foreseeable risk of injury to his head other than by his falling.

(4) Every employee or self-employed person who is required to wear suitable head protection by or under these Regulations shall–

    (a) make full and proper use of it; and

    (b) take all reasonable steps to return it to the accommodation provided for it after use.'

Personal Protective Equipment at Work Regulations 1992

9.19 In general, the *Personal Protective Equipment at Work Regulations 1992 (SI 1992/3139)* do not apply where other regulations such as the *Control of Substances Hazardous to Health Regulations 2002 (SI 2002/2677)* or the *Control of Asbestos at Work Regulations 2002 (SI 2002/2675)* apply. However, SI 1992/3139, Reg 5 does apply in such situations:

'(1) Every employer shall ensure that where the presence of more than one risk to health or safety makes it necessary for his employee to wear or use simultaneously more than one item of personal protective equipment, such equipment is compatible and continues to be effective against the risk or risks in question.

(2) Every self-employed person shall ensure that where the presence of more than one risk to health or safety makes it necessary for him to wear or use simultaneously more than one item of personal protective equipment, such equipment is compatible and continues to be effective against the risk or risks in question.'

Confined Spaces Regulations 1997

9.20   These Regulations apply to all work situations covered by the *Health and Safety at Work etc Act 1974*, other than diving operations and work in mines where by virtue of its enclosed nature there is a foreseeable risk or in situations where there may be free-flowing solids such as grain or sand. *Regulation 5* covers emergency arrangements. Paragraph 99 of the Approved Code of Practice (HSE, 1997) addresses the RPE required for such situations, as follows:

> '99 Where respiratory protective equipment (RPE) is provided or used in connection with confined space entry or for emergency or rescue, it should be suitable for the purpose for which it is intended, ie correctly selected and matched both to the job and the wearer. RPE will not normally be suitable unless it is breathing apparatus. For most cases breathing apparatus would provide the standard of protection for entry into confined spaces. Any RPE should comply with the *Personal Protective Equipment (EC Directive) Regulations 1992* (displaying a "CE Mark"), or, where these provisions are not appropriate, be of a standard or to a type approved by HSE.'

Confined space work is a particularly hazardous activity which should be undertaken only by specialists.

Summary and comment on legislation

9.21   From the foregoing, it can be seen that PPE should be used only as a supplement to alternative, preferred, prevention and control techniques. PPE should not be used as the main or sole control technique except in exceptional circumstances, eg in the case of fire-fighters, emergency personnel, workers in confined spaces or in the case of failure situations. An employer should provide supervision to ensure the correct use of PPE and he is legally responsible for the maintenance, examination and testing of PPE. By implication, the employer should appoint a person to be responsible for the management of PPE maintenance. The employer in law can delegate his responsibilities to another; it remains his responsibility, however, to ensure that the person to whom responsibility is delegated is competent to receive such delegation.

Under the *Construction (Head Protection) Regulations 1989 (SI 1989/2209)* suitable head protection should be used on all construction sites unless the only foreseeable hazard is due to persons falling. The specific case of confined space work should be regarded as a specialist activity.

Where PPE is provided as a means of complying with any of the relevant Regulations, it must be EC marked, must be approved by the HSE or must comply with an HSE-approved standard.

Role of personal protection

9.22   In the 'real world', there will be situations where preferred means of completely controlling risks by prevention and control at source are not technically possible and where the use of PPE is unavoidable. Given the legal requirements of regulations such as the *Control of Substances Hazardous to Health Regulations 2002 (SI 2002/2677)*, the *Control of Asbestos at Work Regulations 2002 (SI 2002/2675)* and the *Control of Lead at Work Regulations 2002 (SI 2002/2676) (CLAW)*, the role of PPE should be to provide back-up protection in case of failure of primary controls, to provide protection while implementing alternative preferred controls, to provide protection for non-routine tasks such as emergency maintenance and to supplement inadequate controls where such controls cannot produce a risk-free working environment.

Setting up and running an effective personal protection programme

9.23   To ensure that PPE provides adequate long-term protection, it is necessary to set up a comprehensive programme to ensure that any PPE provided continues to be used correctly and is maintained in an efficient and hygienic condition. The steps required to establish and run an effective PPE programme are summarised below. (For carrying out risk assessments generally, see CHAPTER 10).

Assess risks and identify where control is required

9.24   The essential first step to achieving effective management of safety and health in any workplace is an assessment to identify hazards and quantify any risks. The assessment should identify all unacceptable risks, the individuals at risk and provide the information needed for prevention or control and for selecting adequate and suitable PPE.

Implement all reasonably practicable controls

9.25   If hazardous substances or processes must be used, all reasonably practicable means of reduction of risk at source must be considered before adopting PPE, as required, eg by the *Control of Substances Hazardous to Health Regulations 2002 (SI 2002/2677), Reg 7* (see 9.3).

Identify who needs residual protection

9.26   From the assessment of likely risks and of the effectiveness of any control procedures applied to reduce these risks, all persons still potentially at risk should be identified and the level of residual protection required should be quantified.

Inform wearers of consequences of exposure

9.27 Employees are required to be informed of any risks in their workplace, eg see the *Control of Substances Hazardous to Health Regulations 2002 (SI 2002/2677), Reg 12* (see 9.4). PPE wearers should be made fully aware of the risks to their health and safety in the workplace and the potential consequences if these risks are not adequately controlled. Since many types of PPE are inherently uncomfortable, some wearers may refuse to wear such equipment unless convinced that the imposed discomfort can be justified in terms of reduced risk to themselves.

Select PPE adequate to control residual exposure

9.28 PPE should be selected which reduces all risks to acceptable levels, eg in the case of airborne substances, contaminant levels inside respiratory protective equipment (RPE) facepieces should be reduced to less than 50% of the occupational exposure standard (OEL) or to less than 10% of maximum exposure limit (MEL) or control limits as relevant. PPE should be selected on the basis of demonstrated workplace performance. PPE should not be used if a manufacturer cannot supply workplace data or written assurance as to the level of performance which can realistically be achieved in the workplace.

Involve wearers in PPE selection process

9.29 Wearers should be fully involved in the PPE selection process to ensure that the equipment selected does not impose unacceptable discomfort and to give them a stake in ensuring the programme's overall effectiveness. The importance of such involvement is recognized in *Article 8* of the PPE 'Use' Directive (89/393/EEC), which requires the 'consultation and participation of workers and/or their representatives'.

Match PPE to each individual wearer

9.30 Wearers come in different shapes and sizes. It is therefore essential that each item of PPE is matched to each individual wearer. In addition, given that PPE matched to the wearer may be less uncomfortable than badly matched equipment, the provision of individually matched equipment might encourage regular and correct usage of the PPE.

Some PPE can impose significant stress on the wearer, eg heavy chemical protective suits or breathing apparatus which may weigh up to 18 kg or which requires the wearer to breathe pure oxygen. For such equipment it may be prudent to ensure that only medically fit and suitable persons will be required to wear the equipment.

Carry out objective fit tests of PPE

9.31   The *Control of Asbestos at Work Regulations 2002 (SI 2002/2675)* require that asbestos insulation workers carry out quantitative fit tests of their respiratory protective equipment (RPE). Such tests for other RPE wearers have recently been introduced with the new *Control of Substances Hazardous to Health Regulations 2002*. The results from such tests should not be taken as evidence that the RPE fits the wearer or as any indication of likely protection in workplace.

Ensure that PPE does not create risk

9.32   Some types of PPE can create or exacerbate risks. For example, full-facepiece respirators can affect the wearer's field of vision; personal hearing protectors (PHP) can reduce the ability to hear communication or warning signals or the approach of vehicles; chemical protective clothing can reduce the body's ability to lose metabolic heat, etc. Care should therefore be taken to ensure that any risks likely to be created by the equipment are fully investigated and reduced to acceptable levels. Where some residual risk remains, action should be taken to minimize the risk created by the PPE at source. For example, if personal hearing protectors are used where moving vehicles may be present, the vehicles should be fitted with flashing warning lights so that realization of the approach of the vehicles does not rely on aural warning alone.

If wearers perceive that the consequences of such potential risks are more severe than the risks against which the PPE is provided to protect, they may refuse to wear the PPE.

Ensure PPE are mutually compatible

9.33   Where two or more types of PPE must be worn simultaneously, the different types of PPE may interact to reduce the protection provided by one or both items. For example, for safety helmets worn with full-facepieces, the facepiece can force the safety helmet to tip backwards. Other examples of potentially adverse interactions are respirators worn together with eye protectors where the respirator can prevent the correct fitting of the eye protectors, or eye protectors worn with earmuffs where the legs of the eye protectors can prevent a good seal between the head and the muff. In such situations it is essential that each item of PPE provides the required level of protection without affecting the effectiveness of any other PPE. Care must therefore be taken when selecting PPE for such situations to ensure that all PPE, which may have to be worn together, are mutually compatible.

Train wearers in the correct use of their PPE

9.34 Wearers and their supervisors should be thoroughly trained in how to fit the PPE correctly, how to assess whether the equipment is correctly fitted, how to inspect the PPE to ensure that it has been correctly manufactured and whether reusable equipment has been adequately cleaned and maintained. The potential consequences of PPE failure should be reflected in the thoroughness of the training, ie the greater the risk, the more thorough the training.

Training should cover the correct use of PPE ensembles, eg for respiratory protective equipment (RPE) and protective clothing ensembles, to fit the RPE first, to wear the RPE facepiece or head-harness under the hood of protective clothing and to remove RPE last after completing all required decontamination procedures. Wearers of RPE should be aware that correct fit may depend on there being no facial hair betwee the facepiece and their face and that stubble can be more damaging than a beard. They should therefore be aware that being 'clean-shaven' means having shaved immediately before the start of each period during which RPE might need to be worn. Where possible, the training should involve practical sessions using suitable training tools, eg for RPE, using quantitative fit test equipment to indicate the consequences of facial hair or incorrect fitting.

Supervisors should be trained in how to ensure that wearers are likely to be able to fit their PPE correctly, eg that RPE wearers are clean-shaven or that wearers of personal hearing protectors (PHP) do not have hairstyles which might prevent ear muffs sealing adequately.

Maintenance and inspection staff should be trained in the relevant procedures with particular emphasis being given to ensuring that they are able to carry out such tasks without placing themselves at risk due to contamination on the PPE, eg when cleaning PPE which may be contaminated with substances such as sensitisers or carcinogens.

Minimise wear periods

9.35 Many types of PPE are inherently uncomfortable. Since the acceptability of a given level of discomfort can decrease with increased wear time, it can be important to reduce wear times as far as possible. If it is possible to identify those processes which generate most of the risk it may be possible to achieve adequate reduction of exposure by wearing the PPE only during such processes. However, care must be taken to ensure that contamination of the wearer or PPE in such circumstances does not itself constitute a risk to the wearer.

Supervise wearers to ensure correct use of PPE

9.36 The responsibilities and authority of supervisors in the PPE programme should be specified in their job descriptions. Supervisors should ensure that PPE is correctly worn at all times when required, that wearers are correctly prepared for wearing their PPE, ie are clean shaven for wearing respiratory protective equipment (RPE), and that the necessary personal decontamination procedures are followed. The overall effectiveness of any PPE programme can be critically dependent on the actions of shop-floor supervisors who are close enough to the wearers to actively enforce correct usage of PPE and any other control methods adopted.

Provide suitable storage facilities for PPE

9.37 Where reusable PPE is used, suitable storage facilities should be provided for the clean PPE. Provision of such storage facilities is recommended in some UK guidance, eg guidance on the *Noise at Work Regulations 1989 (SI 1989/1790)* (Health and Safety Commission, 1989).

Maintain PPE in efficient and hygienic condition

9.38 The legal responsibility for maintenance of PPE rests with the employer. Reusable PPE will need to be cleaned, serviced and maintained, both to ensure the ongoing efficiency of the equipment and to ensure that the wearer is not exposed to contamination caused by poorly-cleaned equipment.

Inspect PPE to ensure it is correctly maintained

9.39 The legal responsibility for PPE inspection rests with the employer. It is therefore prudent to maintain records to demonstrate that these duties have been met.

Record usage and maintenance data

9.40   There is no legal duty to record usage and maintenance data. However, such can function as a mechanism of checking if all those who should wear PPE actually do so and to ensure that those who do not are identified so that corrective action can be taken. Keeping inspection records is a statutory duty.

Monitor programme to ensure continuing effectiveness

9.41   It is generally inadequate to put any programme into operation and assume that thereafter it will continue to run smoothly. It is prudent, therefore, to routinely check the operation of the programme, to reinforce training and risk perception and to take any remedial action that may be required.

Provide PPE free of charge

9.42   If the PPE is to be used solely for protection against occupational risks, the equipment must be provided and maintained free of any charge to the wearer.

Types of PPE

9.43   As outlined at 9.1, PPE can be split into two classes:

- PPE primarily intended to protect against unplanned events, such as falling or projected materials; and

- PPE intended to protect against ongoing routine exposures.

The former class includes safety footwear, safety headwear and eye protectors. The protective performance of such PPE can be assumed as long as correctly-fitting PPE has been provided, all types of PPE worn simultaneously have been selected to be compatible and the PPE is worn correctly at all times required. Correct selection and adequate supervision is therefore essential.

The second class of PPE includes respiratory protective equipment (RPE), personal hearing protectors (PHP), protective clothing (PC) and chemical protection gloves. The protective performance of such PPE depends critically on the correct selection and wear and on the ongoing willingness of the employee to wear the equipment correctly at times when required. It can be difficult, therefore, to quantify the actual level of protection provided.

The various limitations and protective performance of RPE, PHP and PC are discussed below.

Respiratory protective equipment

Classes of equipment

9.44   There are two major classes of respiratory protective equipment (RPE): *breathing apparatus* where the wearer is provided with clean breathing gas from a self-contained source, such as a cylinder or a chemical gas producer, or by an umbilical tube from a distant source; and *respirators* or *filter devices* where the breathing gas is obtained by filtering the ambient air in the immediate vicinity of the wearer.

Respirators must not be used in confined spaces unless it has been demonstrated that the air contains sufficient oxygen to support life. The respirator filter may be suitable for particulates only, specified gases or vapours only or a combination of particulates and specified gases or vapours. Filters for gasses or vapours should only be used against the specific gases or vapours identified by the manufacturer or supplier.

There is evidence that the protection provided by conventional RPE may be reduced if wearers sweat heavily. RPE should therefore be selected with care if wearers also need to wear protective clothing which encloses a large proportion of the body surface. In such situations it would be prudent to use only powered or air-fed equipment.

RPE performance – assigned protection factors

9.45   In the UK, RPE is selected on the basis of assigned protection factors (APF) derived from measured performance achieved in real workplaces. The APF is defined as follows:

'[The] level of respiratory protection that can realistically be achieved in the workplace by 95% of adequately trained and supervised wearers using a properly functioning and correctly fitted respiratory protective device' ... (BSI (2001)).

In selecting RPE, the minimum Required APF is calculated as:

$$\text{Required APF} = \frac{\text{Contaminant concentration outside the PPE}}{\text{Permitted concentration in wearer's breathing zone}}$$

For example, select a respirator for use in a workplace in which the airborne concentration of contaminant is 8 mg m^{-3} and the occupational exposure standard (OES) for the contaminant is 0.5 mg m^{-3}, assuming that the concentration in the wearer's breathing zone is to be restricted to 50% of the OES, the minimum Required APF would be:

Required APF = 8/0.25 = 32

For such a workplace, an item of RPE providing an APF of at least 32 could nominally provide adequate protection if the device is matched to the individual wearer, his job and his workplace, is properly fitted and worn and is properly maintained if reusable.

The APF assigned to the different classes of RPE are given in BS 4275 (BSI, 2001) and HSG 53 ('Respiratory Protective Equipment, a Practical Guide for Users', Health and Safety Executive, 1998). Note that only the most up-to-date editions of these references should be used as the current assigned protection factors are substantially lower than the protection factors used in earlier editions.

Maintainance of equipment

9.46   For reusable RPE, it will be necessary to change particulate and gas filters on a regular basis.

Particulate filters

9.47   Particulate filters need to be changed because dust collection can increase airflow resistance, so increasing breathing resistance in unpowered devices or reducing airflow rates in powered devices. For particulate filters which rely on electrostatic properties of the media, the collection of dusts, oils or some organic solvents can cause filter efficiency to fall substantially. Thus, clear written guidance should be sought from the supplier to ensure that the contaminants for which the filter will be used are unlikely to affect filter performance; or to find out when filters should be changed. The efficiency of particulate filters is described using the nomenclature P1, P2 or P3 where 'P' indicates a particulate filter and the number indicates filter efficiency, 1 being the lowest and 3 the highest.

Gas and vapour and combined filters

9.48   Gas and vapour filters need to be changed regularly because the capacity of such filters is finite and exposure to moisture or other contaminants which may be more strongly retained by the filter medium can cause previously retained contaminants to be released into the wearer's breathing gas.

Gas and combined gas and particulate filters are covered by EN 141 and some special filters are covered by EN 371 and EN 372 CEN (1990, 1992a and 1992b). EN 141 has adopted a nomenclature such as 'A2' where the first letter indicates the substances against which the filter should be used and the number indicates the capacity, 1 being the lowest capacity and 3 the highest. Thus an A2 filter is a medium-capacity filter for use against organic contaminants with boiling points higher than 65°C as specified by the manufacturer. The breathing resistance imposed by a gas filter tends to increase with capacity, as does cost. If the filter also provides protection against particulates, the filter nomenclature becomes, for example, 'A2P3', where the 'P3' indicates a high-efficiency particulate filter.

It is not possible to reliably calculate the likely breakthrough time for gas filters in the workplace, even if contaminant concentrations are known, given the complexity of filter chemistry and the possible interactive effects of moisture and other contaminants. Some users who have access to suitable analytical facilities consider it worthwhile to test used filters to determine their residual capacity. This ensures that filter usage is optimised as regards both protective performance and cost.

In all situations where gas filters are to be used, written guidance should be sought from suppliers who should be provided with as much information as possible as regards likely contaminants, contaminant concentrations, any other contaminants likely to be encountered and information on any unusual factors such as unusually high work rates or high ambient temperatures or humidities.

Filters which have previously been exposed to very high gas or vapour contaminant concentrations without breakthrough can release the contaminant on subsequent use. Gas filters should be changed immediately any odour or other subjective effect is detected by the wearer. Such warning effects should be used to supplement a planned filter replacement regimen and should not be relied upon as the indicator of when to change filters since exposure to some materials can cause olfactory fatigue thereby reducing the sensitivity of subjective detection and for some substances the odour or irritation thresholds can be higher than the relevant occupational exposure limits.

As for users of particulate filters, users of gas and vapour filter users should seek clear written guidance from the supplier to ensure both that the correct gas filters are selected and that the filters are changed when necessary.

Conclusions regarding respiratory protective equipment

9.49　RPE depends critically on being correctly selected, correctly worn and correctly maintained. Correctly worn RPE can be uncomfortable and tiring to wear. RPE can work in the real world, but only at very substantially lower levels of performance than indicated by standard laboratory tests. The relatively poor workplace performance of RPE therefore critically underlines the preferred prevention and control techniques outlined in the Control Hierarchy.

Personal hearing protectors

Classes of equipment

9.50   Personal hearing protectors (PHP) are widely used in the UK where noise is likely to cause damage to hearing. Four main different types of equipment are available: ear muffs, ear plugs, semi-aural devices and active noise attenuation devices.

Ear muffs, also called circum-aural devices, fit over the entire ear and are pressed against the sides of the head to prevent or minimise noise leakage between the muff and the head. The muffs may be held in place by a head or neck band or by carriers fitted to a safety helmet. The fit of ear muffs can be severely reduced by spectacle legs, long hair or clothing which interfere with the seal between the muff and the head.

Ear plugs, also called inserts, or ear inserts, fit into the ear canal and are retained in position by friction between the plug and the ear canal. Ear plug performance is critically dependent on correct insertion.

Semi-aural devices are effectively ear plugs which are held in position in the ear canal by a head or neck band.

Active noise attenuation devices are generally ear muffs which contain a microphone and miniature loudspeaker, both of which are connected to an electronic control unit. The microphone senses any noise inside the muff and sends a signal to the electronic unit which generates a signal which is very similar in frequency and level to the noise inside the muff but which is almost exactly 180o out of phase with the noise inside the muff. The noise leaking into the muff is effectively 'cancelled out' by the noise generated by the loudspeaker, ie just as a wave crest in water can be cancelled out by an equal magnitude wave trough.

Active noise attenuation devices are generally very much lighter and less uncomfortable than conventional ear muffs giving similar protection. However, such devices are generally effective only up to about 1 kilohertz. In addition, such devices are relatively expensive, eg about £150 compared to about £10 for conventional ear muffs.

PHP performance – assumed attenuation

9.51   PHP are currently selected on the basis of the performance achieved during standard laboratory tests. The standard laboratory test involves measuring the attenuation provided to a panel of 16 test subjects at defined frequencies, BSI (1995). For each test frequency the *mean* and *standard deviation of attenuations* are calculated. From these figures the *assumed attenuation* is calculated where the assumed attenuation is given by the relevant mean attenuation minus one standard deviation. If it is assumed that the attenuation provided to different wearers is normally distributed, one wearer in six will be afforded less attenuation than given by the mean attenuation minus one standard deviation. That is, only 84% of wearers will be afforded the assumed attenuation. To ensure that at least 95% of wearers are afforded at least the assumed protection, assumed attenuations should be based on mean minus at least 1.7 standard deviations. In its publication 'Reducing Noise at Work' (L108HSE, 1998b) the Health & Safety Executive comments:

> 'In some cases, it is advisable to base ear protection selection on the mean minus two standard deviations, to ensure that the majority are adequately protected, allowing for the imperfect fitting and condition of ear protectors in the working environment.'

That is, the authors of the HSE guidance assume the only reason that PHP performance in the real world may be poorer than in the laboratory is due to imperfect fitting and/or poor condition of the protectors.

However, numerous studies have compared real world and laboratory performance of PHP over the past 25 years or so and have consistently demonstrated that real world performance is substantially poorer than laboratory performance. Various commentators have reported, as follows:

- 'laboratory attenuation should be derated by 60% to rate workplace performance adequately'. (Edwards et al, 'A Field Investigation of Noise Reduction Afforded by Insert-Type Hearing Protectors (Final Report)', NIOSH, 1977);

- 'assumed attenuation should be drastically reduced'. (Alberti, 'Hearing Protectors: Attenuation in Practice and Problems in Fitting', Noise Control Foundation, 1981); and

- 'current predictive values should be reduced by 50%'. (Royster, 'An Evaluation of the Effectiveness of Two Different Insert Types of Ear Protection in Preventing TTS in an Industrial Environment', American Industrial Hygiene Association Journal, 1980).

Further, Lempert and Edwards ('Field Investigations Of Noise Reduction Afforded By Insert-Type Hearing Protectors', American Industrial Hygiene Association Journal, 1983) reported that median attenuations fell from 28 dB in the laboratory to 13 dB in the real world. In a major UK study commissioned by the HSE, Hempstock and Hill ('The attenuation of some hearing protectors as used in the workplace', Annals of Occupational Hygiene, 1990) reported that compared with laboratory test data, real world attenuations, based on mean minus one standard deviation, were 2.5–7.4 dB lower for ear muffs and 6.8–16.1 dB lower for ear plugs. Mean attenuations were lower in the real world than in the laboratory and standard deviations larger.

Berger ('International Review of Field Studies of Hearing Protector Attenuation', Thieme Medical Publishers, Inc, 1996) reviewed the available data on workplace studies covering nine models of insert ear plugs, including one custom-moulded device, one semi-aural device and eight models of ear muffs. These studies covered a total of 2,879 subjects. Of the nine inserts and one semi-aural device evaluated only four devices exhibited any attenuation in the real world at mean minus two standard deviations, the highest attenuation being 8 dB. Overall, the mean attenuation in the real world was effectively zero as against 22 dB in the laboratory. Zero attenuation at mean minus two standard deviation indicates that many wearers will achieve only marginal attenuation. All eight muffs exhibited at least 6 dB assumed attenuation in the real world. However, only three devices provided greater than 10 dB attenuation. The highest attenuation was 13 dB. Overall, the mean assumed attenuation for ear muffs in the real world was c 8 dB compared with 23 dB in the laboratory, ie in-ear noise exposure levels would have been 15 dB higher than expected for about half of the wearers. The Berger review indicates that ear muffs do provide a level of protection, but only at a very substantially lower level than predicted from laboratory test results.

The failure of laboratory tests to adequately indicate the real world performance of all ear plugs tested is unsurprising given that laboratory tests last less than about 30 minutes per fitting and do not include deliberate jaw movement likely to displace plugs (see 9.52), ie the standard laboratory test is an extremely poor simulation of real world conditions.

The extensive PHP field study literature available since the late-1970s clearly demonstrates that selecting PHP on the basis of laboratory attenuation is likely to lead to a significant proportion of PHP wearers achieving less protection than assumed and, thus, incurring avoidable noise-induced hearing loss (see CHAPTER 7). Relevant, well-corroborated information has been available in the scientific literature for well over 15 years, and hence the authors of the current BSI and HSE guidance for PHP, and their organisations, should therefore accept the moral and legal responsibility for all avoidable noise-induced hearing loss due to the provision of incompetent guidance which fails to recognise extensive relevant scientific evidence.

Limitations of ear plugs in use

9.52   The reason for poor ear plug performance is easily demonstrated: place the little finger in the ear canal and chew or speak. The ear canal changes shape and size with movement of the jaw. That is, even if ear plugs are correctly fitted, jaw movement is likely to cause the plug to be ejected from the ear. Abel and Rokas ('The effect of wearing time on hearing protector attenuation', Journal of Otolaryngology, 1986) examined the effects of jaw movement on ear plug attenuation when worn for 60–75 minutes. Little change was observed for foam plugs; pre-moulded silicone plugs exhibited a 6 dB reduction; and self-moulded fibreglass plugs exhibited a 10 dB reduction. That is, correctly fitted ear plugs are likely to lose up to 10 dB attenuation over a period of about one hour. Plugs therefore need to be refitted at least every 30 minutes to maintain attenuation.

To prevent transfer of corrosive, skin-sensitising, irritant, percutaneous uptake or abrasive substances into the ear canal it is essential that the hands are thoroughly decontaminated before refitting plugs. In the food and drug industries, it is essential that the hands are thoroughly washed after removing plugs before handling products. In many work situations ear plugs will therefore be impracticable, even for the few models which exhibit useful attenuation in the real world.

Health surveillance

9.53   As the ultimate object of the *Noise at Work Regulations 1989 (SI 1989/1790)* is to protect hearing, the ultimate test of the effectiveness of PHP is to demonstrate that PHP wearers' hearing is not degrading faster than expected for their age-matched non-noise exposed peers. It has been noted that conventional screening audiometry may be inadequate to detect small changes in hearing ability, Howie ('A specification for audiometric technique in hearing conservation,' Occupational Health Review, 1990). It is suggested, therefore, that the provision of routine high-quality audiometry should be a mandatory duty imposed on all employers who rely on PHP as a means of protecting the hearing of their employees.

Conclusions regarding personal hearing protectors

9.54   From the foregoing, it is recommended that:

- ear plugs should not be used unless the supplier can provide data demonstrating at least 5 dB attenuation in the workplace at mean attenuation minus two standard deviations;

- ear plugs should not be used unless it can be ensured that they can be correctly, safely and hygienically refitted about every 30 minutes;

- ear muffs should be assumed to provide not more than 5 dB attenuation unless relevant data from the real world demonstrate that higher performance can be reliably achieved;

- PHP should be selected only on the basis of workplace data with assumed attenuations based on mean minus two standard deviations; and

- high-performance routine audiometry should be mandatory for all wearers of PHP to ensure that wearers are not suffering from noise-induced hearing loss.

Protective clothing

Classes of equipment

9.55 Protective clothing (PC) is widely used to provide protection against hazardous substances which can cause injury in the following ways:

- by directly damaging the skin, eg chromic acid;

- by penetrating the skin barrier and entering the body, eg isocyanates;

- by contaminating the skin so that if the skin is not adequately decontaminated the substance can be transferred to the hands and either:

  o ingested, eg lead, or

  o can be rendered airborne and inhaled, eg asbestos.

Effective PC therefore has to prevent skin contact by limiting the ingress of contaminants into the space between the body and the clothing.

The protective performance of PC can be limited by penetration or permeation of fabric, seam and fastener and by leakage between the clothing and the wearer's body at openings such as at the neck or wrists. The performance of clean room garments is limited by the same factors.

PC performance

9.56 Howie ('The reality of PPE performance in the workplace', International Occupational Hygiene Association, 1992), found that fabric penetration by respirable asbestos fibres or dusts through cotton, nylon, terylene and spunbonds ranged between 50–80%, was less than 2% for some high performance fabrics and that seam and fastener penetration for some of the high-performance fabrics exceeded 80%. The performance of PC against liquids can depend markedly on the liquid, eg a fabric which allowed 0.3% penetration by water and 9% penetration by xylene. Performance against liquids can also depend on the time of contact with the fabric: the liquid may corrode, dissolve or permeate through the fabric. If PC is likely to be exposed to liquids the user should therefore demand information on fabric performance against the liquids of concern.

Leakage into PC at openings, such as at wrist and neck can limit its performance, eg Ojanen et al, ('Evaluation of the Efficiency and Comfort of Protective Clothing during Herbicide Spraying', Applied Occupational and Environmental Hygiene, 1992) observed leakages up to 33% for garments constructed from fabrics impervious to pesticides, and Fenske et al, ('Occupational Exposure to Fosetyl-Al Fungicide During Spraying of Ornamentals in Greenhouses', Archives of Environmental Contamination and Toxicology, 1987) and van Roouij et al ('Effect of the Reduction of Skin

Contamination on the Internal Dose of Creosote Workers Exposed to Polycyclic Aromatic Hydrocarbons', Scandinavian Journal of Work, Environment and Health, 1993) reported that suit-seal leakage contributed up to about 60% of dermal exposure. Such papers confirm that leakage into protective garments can be a significant route of exposure to hazardous substances.

Determining the protective performance of PC therefore involves knowledge of fabric seam and fastener penetration and suit seal leakage. Lack of knowledge of these factors can prevent determination of the total protective performance.

Risk of heat stress disorders

9.57   The other important characteristic of PC is the thermal consequences of wearing it. Energy for work is derived from food. However, the body is inefficient in converting chemical energy into work. Assuming an average efficiency of 20%, doing 100 W of external work, eg, walking at about 6.5 Kph on the level, requires the metabolic generation of c 500 W of which roughly 400 W is generated as heat. This heat is why we get 'hot' when we undertake physical work.

Under normal circumstances, the body loses heat by humidifying and heating the inhaled air, by convection from uncovered skin, and by sweating – the last being the most important mechanism when working hard or in hot environments. If sweat evaporation is prevented, eg due to enclosing PC, the possible heat loss is substantially reduced. This restriction is exacerbated if the PC is worn together with other PPE such as gloves, respirator or safety helmet.

If the heat loss in insufficient, heat is stored in the body resulting in heat strain with effects ranging from mild discomfort through reduction in cognitive skills to heat cramps, coma and death. Heat strain is usually considered to arise from 'external' sources in high temperatures such as when removing asbestos from live steam pipes. However, heat strain can also arise from 'internal' sources if the body is unable to lose the heat generated by metabolic processes due to wearing well-sealed or thermally insulated PC. Fatal heat strain caused by well-sealed and thermally insulating PC is illustrated by the case of the army trainee diver who died as result of heat strain caused by wearing a diving suit while running over soft sand on a hot day: the diving suit restricted heat loss by preventing sweat evaporation.

Heat strain is a serious potential problem which cannot be ignored if the PC is not itself to lead to increased risk. In some situations, the heat strain risk created by PC itself may be more serious than the risk against which it is intended to protect. Since most PC capable of providing effective protection against airborne substances is unlikely to permit sufficient heat loss to prevent heat strain in other than cool conditions, it may be necessary to limit wear durations to ensure the safety of the wearer. If the reduced wear periods are not acceptable for operational reasons, it may be necessary to use air-fed PC.

Users must therefore demand the information required to ensure that the protective clothing can be used in a given situation to provide adequate protection without causing either excessive discomfort or heat strain. The user should provide the protective clothing supplier with information about the protection required, the wearer's likely work rates, any other items of PPE which will be worn simultaneously with the clothing and information regarding the thermal environment in which the work will be carried out, eg the dry bulb air temperature, the relative humidity and the radiant temperature.

For further discussion of the effects of temperature in the workplace, see CHAPTER 7.

Conclusions regarding protective clothing

9.58 Protective clothing can provide effective protection but to do so without generating unacceptable discomfort or health-threatening heat strain PC must be carefully selected for the hazardous substances likely to be present and correctly matched to the individual wearer, his work and his thermal environment.

Overall summary

9.59 PPE *can* provide effective protection but only if correctly selected, used and maintained. To achieve effective protection, the PPE should be used as only one component of a comprehensive integrated risk control programme and should be selected on the basis of demonstrated workplace performance only. Care should be taken to ensure that PPE does not itself create or exacerbate existing risks such as from moving vehicles in areas where employees are wearing personal hearing protectors (PHP) or where employees are wearing enclosing protective clothing which may cause heat strain.

10 Applying Risk Management and Risk Assessment in Occupational Health

Introduction

10.1 We use the terms 'hazard' and 'risk' in our everyday speech as if they are interchangeable, but in health and safety they have different meanings. A *hazard* is something with the potential to cause harm, but a *risk* arises only when people are exposed to the hazard. So a busy road with a lot of traffic may be a hazard, but it only turns into a risk when you try to walk across it, or drive along it. If you were at the top of a nearby hill, standing in a field watching traffic on the same road it would still be a hazard, but not represent a risk to you at all. In modern health and safety practice everything we do is for the identification of hazards – the potentialities for causing harm – and the evaluation of the risks which can arise.

Making sensible judgements about risk, about how people may be harmed and how serious that harm may be helps us determine what precautions it is appropriate to take. This process is more important in protecting health because many of the hazards are not obvious and the risks that much harder to pin down: it may take years for some agents (eg dust) to cause harm whereas accidents are immediate. Often it is only the risk assessment which raises managers' and staff understanding of the risks in their work and the necessity to take precautions.

It may be argued, with some justification, that success in the management of any enterprise depends in large part on how well risks are managed. These risks may include the reliability of the supply chain – providing the goods and services which the organisation needs to operate – the availability of staff with the necessary competencies, the maintenance of suitable accommodation, access to appropriate finance (and related issues such as currency stability) and many other matters. That this lies at the heart of organisational sustainability is reflected in, for example, the fact that businesses listed on the London Stock Exchange follow the Turnbull Combined Code requirements (see Committee on Corporate Governance, FSA Listing Rules, Gee) to identify their significant risks, to put in place measures to prevent, reduce, mitigate and recover, and to publish the material associated with this process so that shareholders may be reassured. Risk identification, assessment and control forms the core of business risk management, and applies directly to the health and safety of a workforce.

This chapter discusses the legal obligations to engage in the risk management process and the competencies required of those who do so. It also explores the practicalities of occupational health risk assessment. Some tools are provided, such as risk assessment forms and recommendations for record-keeping. There is a statutory obligation for organisations with five or more staff to have written health and safety policies, and these should reflect the commitments not only to prevent accidents but also to protect the health of staff and anyone else who may be affected by the work undertaken.

From hazard identification to health surveillance, whatever is done needs to be properly evaluated, to ensure not only that these health and safety policy commitments are being met, but also that they are adequate to meet the needs of a modern enterprise. Remember above all that the primary purpose of risk assessment is to identify the threats to worker' and other persons' health arising from health hazards at work, and to identify and implement precautions (ie controls) which protect those people from harm.

Finally, two case studies illustrate good and bad practice in this area.

Benefits of a systematic occupational health risk management

10.2   In general terms, risk management is a strategic process which aids and supports decision-making at both strategic and operational levels within an organisation. The more the organisation can improve its understanding and management of the risks likely to affect it the more it will be able to identify opportunities to improve its performance and competitive advantage. It is no different from planning for a football team to do well in the next game: identifying the strengths and weaknesses of both sides enables you to draw up plans which play to your own strengths and to minimise the potential harm arising from the weaknesses.

Protecting worker health is a significant business issue: surveys have shown that sickness absence from the workplace and ill-health early retirements are a major financial burden, estimated at costing over £11 billion a year to UK business ('Healthcare Brief', CBI, December 2001). One startling statistic is that 7% of the working age population in the UK is claiming incapacity benefit; whereas the figure in France, for instance, is 0.3%). Without identifying which elements of work are contributing to ill-health, management is powerless to reduce it, and the key technique available is the process of risk assessment. Managing a complex organisation requires the weaknesses to be identified, and arrangements put in place to either prevent them having a harmful impact at all or to minimise that impact or, at the very least, to allow the organisation to recover rapidly should the harm arise.

In health terms, this type of 'what could go wrong?' forward view is essential, for many health effects are hard to characterise for the following reasons:

- Health can be affected by many factors, both in the workplace and outside (eg is the respiratory complaint the result of breathing in fumes in the workshop, or from helping someone varnish their boat, from smoking, from an infection or from a combination of some or all of these?).

- Ill-health arises partly as a result of an external 'insult' (eg fumes impacting on a body which may be resistant or susceptible to the chemical agent, because of previous exposures or a natural, congenital predisposition).

- Ill-health can arise rapidly (eg from an acute exposure to a highly toxic gas) in the same way that accidents are immediate; but more commonly it takes repeated exposures over long periods to damage lungs, cause musculoskeletal problems or affect hearing.

For these reasons, a systematic, planned approach to identifying risks to health at work is essential if health is to be protected.

What is risk assessment?

10.3   Recently the European Commission published its five-year strategy for health and safety at work, in which it identified that the nature of risks is changing. We have an ageing active population, with consequent pressures to extend working life beyond current retirement ages, and increasing numbers of women working right up to giving birth and returning to work sooner afterwards. We are also witnessing changes in the pressures at work, leading to 'new' issues such as stress, more generally mental ill-health, the recreational use of drugs and other factors.

The target is to move from protecting worker health to promoting wellbeing at work. Hence, the workforce slogan beloved of those wishing to see not just 'presenteeism' (the opposite of absenteeism) but also an increase in productivity, is 'Happy, Healthy and Here'. Risk assessment is the process by which those threats to worker good health which lie within the workplace are identified and evaluated. This enables practical, cost-effective steps to be taken – reducing the harmful impact both in terms of ill-health at work and its impact on effectiveness, and sickness absence.

Legal requirements

10.4   There are many statutory measures which require risk assessments to be conducted on health risks, including:

- The *Health and Safety at Work etc Act 1974, s 2(1)*. It is the duty of every employer to ensure, so far as is reasonably practicable, the health, safety and welfare of his employees (and *section 3* extends this to those at work but not in his employment, and *section 4* to anyone else affected by work carried out under the employer's control). The words 'reasonably practicable' are the key, as they require a judgement to be made as to the quantum of risk to health and safety in order to ascertain what level of preventative action is appropriate. In essence, the only way to demonstrate that what has been done to ensure health and safety at work is 'reasonably practicable' is to have a risk assessment for all but trivial and insignificant risks.

- The *Manual Handling Operations Regulations 1992 (SI 1992/2793)* specifically require the assessment of significant risks arising from manual handling tasks.

- The *Control of Substances Hazardous to Health Regulations 2002 (SI 2002/2677) (COSHH)* require the assessment of risks arising from hazardous substances in the workplace, including both chemical and biological agents.

- The *Control of Asbestos at Work Regulations 2002 (SI 2002/2675)* require the assessment of risk arising from working with or on asbestos-containing materials, and new regulations will require the assessments associated with workplace buildings to be used to develop management plans for safe maintenance.

- The *Control of Lead at Work Regulations 2002 (SI 2002/2676)* require the assessment of risk arising from working with or on lead-containing materials.

- The *Noise at Work Regulations 1989 (SI 1989/1790)* require the assessment of risk arising from significant noise exposures at work.

- The *Health and Safety (Display Screen Equipment) Regulations 1992 (SI 1992/2792)* require the assessment of computer workstations and associated office equipment and environment, in order to identify and control risks which may arise.

- The *Personal Protective Equipment at Work Regulations 1992 (1992/2966)* require the assessment of suitability of the equipment to be provided, essentially linking that supply to the work activity risk assessment which identifies the need for such protective equipment.

- The *Health and Safety (First Aid) Regulations 1981 (1981/917)* set some minimum standards, but also require a formal assessment of first aid needs. The training of first aiders, their numbers and the equipment and the facilities available should all be determined so that they are adequate and appropriate to the risks of injury and ill-health in the workplace. This assessment of first aid requirements will also need to take into account the distance from the workplace to emergency medical services.

- The *Management of Health and Safety at Work Regulations 1999 (SI 1999/3242) (Management Regulations)* essentially acts as a 'catch-all', requiring the assessment of risks which are not formally addressed in other specific regulations and thus applies to risks of psychosocial problems (stress), to heat or cold, to excessive working hours, risks to which young people, pregnant women and other potentially vulnerable or susceptible groups may be exposed and not be adequately protected by the arrangements applicable to all other workers.

In sum, if the work activity engenders a health risk to those carrying it out or others who may be affected by it, and that risk is significant, a written risk assessment is required either under specific regulations or under the *Management Regulations.* This means that if the risk looks as though it may be significant, a risk assessment is needed. If on completion of the assessment the risk is 'downgraded' to trivial, the assessment doesn't need to be recorded and maintained.

There are many other specific regulations which formally required the assessment of risks, such as major hazards, ionising radiation, genetic manipulation, etc. The list provided above addresses only the most common workplace health risks.

Who can undertake health risk assessments?

10.5   The discharge of this legal duty may only be effected by those who are competent. Competence is not just a trait of the individual: it is perfectly proper, and desirable, for teams to be established to conduct risk assessments in complex workplaces. Involving safety representatives or other worker representatives with knowledge of the activities under review is a helpful input into the process. Essentially, competence is about the skill, knowledge and experience which is needed to develop risk assessments which are 'suitable and sufficient', assessments which address the key hazards.

In a very small business the owner/manager is usually in the best position to take on this role. In larger organisations it is common for the senior line managers to take responsibility but to also delegate some of the work to their supervisors with the assistance of safety representatives where they are appointed. In every case, it is necessary to ensure that the managers concerned have competent health and safety assistance, either (and preferably) from internal staff or, failing that, from external consultants. Most large companies and public bodies employ qualified health and safety advisors.

What does 'competence' mean for occupational health risk assessments?

10.6   There isn't a simple definition of 'competence', because the range of risks can vary from the simple and obvious such as protecting the eyes when handling a strong bleach for toilet cleaning to the complex and difficult judgements required to evaluate the significance of exposures to hand-arm vibration. The word 'competent' is used to describe a person and/or a team of people working effectively in concert, in whom there is embodied a level of skill, knowledge and experience which enables suitable decisions and actions to be taken.

The result of the application of this definition is that an understanding of the workplace and the work activities being undertaken are clearly as important as a theoretical knowledge of the principles of effective health and safety management or the clinical issues which may arise from particular health conditions caused or exacerbated by exposure to health risks in the workplace. In order to conduct suitable and sufficient assessments of health risks at work, the people or teams engaged in the task should be able to confirm:

- A basic understanding of the legal framework represented by the *Health and Safety at Work etc Act 1974*, and of the specific regulations which are *relevant* to the activities being undertaken (thus in a quiet office, the *Noise at Work Regulations 1989 (SI 1989/1790)* are not relevant, but the *Control of Substances Hazardous to Health Regulations 2002 (SI 2002/2677)* will apply to cleaning materials and possibly other products in use).

- A basic understanding of the range of controls available which, when properly employed, can protect workers' health; and the strategy for selection, use and maintenance of such controls.

- A basic understanding of the work in which staff are engaged, including 'out-of-normal-hours' maintenance. The risk assessment has to identify all the significant risks, and that depends in turn on an in-depth knowledge of what people are doing and how they do it. Further, the output of a risk assessment ranges from the selection (or endorsement of the existing selection) of suitable controls on work practices to modifications of practices or of equipment – and the selection of such controls will only be practical if it is carried out by people with real competence in that type of work and an understanding of the strengths and limitations of the specific workplace under review.

If risk assessments are incompetently performed, either because they have failed to identify the key risks or have defined precautions which cannot be implemented in practice, they represent a dangerous liability: physically, for the workers engaged in the tasks; and financially for the employer, for whom they increase the risks of people being harmed and of compensation claims being successfully made.

The role of staff

10.7   From the foregoing, it is clear that effective risk assessments depend upon a process which taps into the knowledge of the staff who themselves are directly engaged in the work. Where there are appointed worker representatives, typically trades union appointed safety representatives, there is also an obligation to consult them on the risk assessment process and to a certain extent the outcomes, the risk assessments themselves and how they are to be employed. Thus whether staff are formally entitled to their representatives being invited to participate in risk assessments, or the employer is simply meeting statutory obligations to consult the workforce as a whole, the implication is clear: the workers engaged in the work need to be involved.

Specialist support

10.8   Risk assessments are to be used to manage the whole organisation, define how work is to be undertaken, staff developed and so on. The responsibility for doing this remains with the directors (or trustees) and managers at all levels, but that doesn't mean that the organisation needs to solely rely upon its own in-house expertise. The *Management of Health and Safety at Work Regulations 1999 (SI 1999/3242)* require managers to have access to appropriate support, and whilst there is encouragement to develop expertise within the organisation the complexities of health issues typically require a wide range of specialists. Examples include:

- occupational hygienists, in many ways the health equivalents of safety advisors;

- occupational health nurses, able to generalise from treatment requirements to advise employers on health issues arising within the workforce, including strategies to prevent ill-health;

- occupational physicians, often helping organisations develop comprehensive strategies as well as diagnosing work-related ill-health and defining treatments;

- ergonomists, advising on musculoskeletal and other problems which arise at the person/work interface; and

- toxicologists, industrial psychologists, human resources professionals, ventilation engineers and many others contribute to programmes to tackle chemical risks, stress and many other health issues.

The list extends even to plumbers, ie skilled people crucial to the physical work required to improve welfare facilities.

Figure 1: The risk assessment process

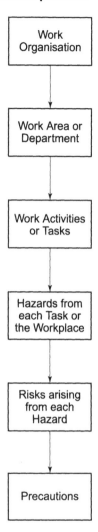

Practical risk assessment for health hazards

10.9   The progression of any risk assessment can be summarised by the following diagram, each stage of which is discussed in the following paragraphs.

The process begins with the identification of hazards to health within the workplace. There are three aspects to be considered:

- Health hazards which are found within the workplace

  These can range from hazardous chemicals (such as those found in the ground of a brownfield site being developed for new housing) to asbestos (perhaps fire protection upstands in the roof space of an office building).

- Health hazards which are brought into the workplace

  These can range from a floor cleaner (the material purchased to strip old polish from the wooden floor in the entrance lobby) to spices (used to manufacture industrial quantities of tandoori chicken for a supermarket cook-chill counter).

- Health hazards which are created in the workplace as a result of the activities carried out there

  These can range from welding fume (generated when welding rods and the substrate metal materials being joined are heated) to the physical stresses and strains on nursing staff (associated with lifting and handling patients).

The other helpful categorisation of health hazards, which should be borne in mind when starting the risk assessment process, is based on the nature of the five types of hazards themselves:

- Chemical hazards, such as acids, alkalis, solvents, fumes, etc which cause harm by:

  o being breathed in (inhalation);

  o entering the body through breaks in the skin or through mucous membranes (which is certainly the case with some materials, such as beryllium, which are able to enter skin cuts);

  o coming into contact with the skin and either damaging the skin directly or being absorbed through the skin to reach a different target organ within the body;

  o being swallowed (ingested), both deliberately but also accidentally from airborne large particles or the hands contaminating the lips and mouth.

  Chemical hazards are discussed in more detail in CHAPTER 6.

- Biological hazards

  Biological hazards such as infectious agents or allergens can be inhaled, ingested or enter skin cuts and through mucous membranes. Sewage and farm workers are at risk from a wide range of human and animal borne agents: the latter are termed 'zoonoses', and the precautions to be taken need to be determined by careful risk assessment of the potential exposures and the nature of the organisms. Peeling Dublin Bay prawns can create an aerosol of material which if breathed in can cause asthma, and again assessment and control are required.

  Biological hazards are discussed in more detail in CHAPTER 5.

- Physical hazards

  Physical hazards such as noise, vibration, extremes of heat or cold and radiation – both ionising (from equipment and the decay of radioactive isotopes) and non-ionising (of which ultra-violet light from the sun is the most common) – should be considered.

  Physical hazards are discussed in more detail in CHAPTER 7.

- Ergonomic hazards

  This loosely describes the interface between our physical bodies and the work we undertake with equipment, machinery, materials in defined environments. When we manage this interface poorly the results can range from minor discomfort to long-term disability as a result of musculoskeletal problems.

  Ergonomic hazards are discussed in more detail in CHAPTER 7.

- Psychological hazards

  Such hazards are becoming increasingly the subject of evaluation and action, as many begin to accept and understand that sickness absence and poor performance is often associated with conditions such as unsustainable stress which can be caused or exacerbated by the workplace arrangements. Bullying, harassment, verbal abuse and even violence at work are all identifiable hazards which require assessment and control.

  Psychological hazards are discussed in more detail in CHAPTER 8.

Stage 1 – Identifying the presence of hazards

10.10   In each work area, for each activity, it is necessary to consider what health hazards may be present or arise. This amounts to no more than asking the questions:

> 'What in the normal course of this work are the potential exposures to one of the five categories of hazard?'

and

> 'What exposures could arise if this work went awry, in ways which could be considered reasonably foreseeable?'

This means checking what dusts, fumes, noise, etc could arise from the work when it is being carried out normally, and the same again during maintenance or other activities which may be considered 'non-standard'. Then you should also consider what could go wrong during the work, in terms of equipment not functioning correctly or other contingencies. As has been indicated above, this can only effectively be concluded in close consultation with staff engaged directly in the work: they will have significant contributions to make in defining both normal and non-standard working, and also in remembering examples of things that have gone wrong in the past.

Given that the first step is the identification of hazards in the working environment and arising from the work it is essential to start with the classification of work activities. In addition, it is necessary to consider the workplace itself, particularly with a view to identifying contamination problems (asbestos in buildings, contaminants in the ground, etc). For a complex workplace, divide it into departments or sections, most usefully along the lines of the line management structure as this is the system that will be used to check the validity of the assessments and to implement any subsequent controls.

Then in each department or section identify all the work activities undertaken covering the maintenance of the premises, the operation of plant and equipment, the staff and the processes they engage in and procedures they follow. Care should be taken to avoid missing key activities which do not form part of the standard '9 to 5'. For example, some years ago a brewery filtered beer into kegs each production day, but on Saturday the production area was subject to cleaning which included replacing the asbestos filters in the core of the filtration unit: an assessment any other day of the week would have missed this potentially hazardous activity.

For each task and activity, it is necessary to think through the hazards which are either intrinsic to the work or which could arise from it. This means thinking about the generation of dusts and fumes, the production of physical hazards such as noise, the nature of the workplace so that extremes of heat and cold are considered, and so on. The identification of hazards can be greatly assisted by looking back at past records: accident reports of back strain injuries or of aggressive behaviour by customers are clear pointers to ergonomic or psychological risks, and the hazards giving rise to those risks should be determined.

Trivial hazards may be discounted (eg risk assessments of inhalation risks from ink toners in laser printers or of the fumes given off by marker pens on white boards need not be documented). The judgements are subjective, but can be discussed and agreed between the competent team members.

Stage 2 – Identifying the controls already in place

10.11   Once the hazards have been listed, it is helpful to identify the precautions which are already in place. To take an example, there is little point assessing the risks associated with the slapdash handling of samples in a pathology laboratory corridor by untrained, unprotected staff when in fact the samples are always handled according to a written audited protocol by trained staff within a secure laboratory, whilst employing appropriate precautions such as protective clothing and hand and face protection.

It is unlikely that many hazards identified will not already be subject to controls which serve to reduce the risks arising, and the risk assessment needs to be of the *residual risk*. The residual risk is judged by looking at the harm which could arise, and the likelihood of that harm arising, despite all the precautions which are already being taken. For instance, if you were evaluating the risks associated with company car driving, and it was company policy that only qualified (licensed) drivers with three years' driving experience be allocated company cars, it would be pointless to try to ascertain the risks of unqualified, inexperienced drivers being handed the keys of an executive saloon. However, assessment of the residual risks might include examination of work schedules which dictate very long working days, bracketed by long car journeys, the dangers associated with travelling and working alone or the use of mobile phones whilst driving.

Stage 3 – Evaluating risk

10.12   As with evaluating hazards, judgement in this area relies upon the skills of the assessor. Factors to be taken into account include:

- Legal

  Many health risks have been effectively assessed by the regulatory authorities, and the scale of risk already determined. For example, action levels have been set for noise exposures; and exposure limits set for a wide range of airborne contaminants, etc.

- Guidance

  Even where there are no formal regulatory risk standards, there are three sources of guidance which should be checked:

  o firstly, the Health & Safety Executive publishes a huge amount of guidance material – some specific to particular hazards (such as asthmagens), some related to particular workplaces (such as motor vehicle repair workshops);

  o secondly, there are trade and other associations which agree standards which, on the basis of 'reasonable practicability', have substantial backing in law (such as the guidance from the Association of the British Pharmaceutical Industry – ABPI – issuing guidance on setting exposure bands for pharmaceutical substances); and

  o thirdly, there are standards set by national and international bodies, such as the BS/EN/ISO standards for equipment and workplace environments.

- Experience

  Despite the often long timescale associated with ill-health compared with accidental injuries, many of the risks which are being assessed will be familiar to an experienced assessor. Such experience provides useful pointers as well as giving employees a degree of confidence in the assessment process.

- Concerns

  Ultimately the assessment of risk is a human judgement, based in part on how acceptable the risks are. It is therefore inevitable that the worries and concerns of the workforce, or the absence of such concerns, will have an impact on the judgement as to the significance of the risk and be reflected in the priorities assigned to the control measures. This is no different to, for instance, public perceptions of the risk of crimes (such as muggings) having a profound influence on policing strategies.

Stage 4 – Categorising risk

10.13 From all the information gathered about the work being undertaken and the hazards present, it is now possible to conduct the risk assessment itself. The decisions to be made are essentially ones of categorisation: by evaluating the criteria, it should be possible to categorise the health risks as either *trivial, tolerable, moderate, substantial* or *intolerable*. The judgment to be made is based on the following criteria which relate to the potential severity of harm, the likelihood of harm and the people likely to be harmed:

- All other factors being equal, something which represents a risk of death or serious permanent harm to health is regarded as being a much higher risk than something which would result in a temporary health effect from which the person concerned fully recovers with no long-term consequences.

- All other factors being equal, something which represents a risk to a person who is vulnerable to harm is regarded as being a much higher risk than that to someone likely to be able to withstand the exposure (for example there is a special duty of care to someone who suffers from asthma if they are exposed to respiratory irritants).

- All other factors being equal, something which represents a risk to a number of people is regarded as being a much higher risk than that which will only harm one individual; and the higher the number potentially affected the higher the risk.

- All other factors being equal, something which represents a risk to members of the public, particularly vulnerable people such as children or older people, is regarded as being a much higher risk than that which only presents a risk to staff . This is partly because the range of controls available cannot usually extend to managing the way in which the non-employees behave, whereas there can be a key control for workers such as the wearing of personal protective equipment.

- All other factors being equal, something which represents a risk which has a great likelihood of actually happening is regarded as being a much higher risk than that which could conceivably occur but is

Table 1: The risk matrix

	Slightly harmful (no health effects or very minor, temporary effects)	*Harmful* (health effects from large, repeated exposures)	*Extremely harmful*
Example effects	Skin on hands reddens in contact with material; effect disappears within minutes of cessation of exposure.	Repeated skin exposure or long single exposures can cause severe skin irritation; in some individuals repeated irritation can lead to dermatitis.	Cancer-causing chemical (carcinogen) capable of being absorbed through the skin.
Highly unlikely	Trivial risk	Tolerable risk	Moderate risk
Unlikely	Tolerable risk	Moderate risk	Substantial risk
Likely	Moderate risk	Substantial risk	Intolerable risk

regarded as being very unlikely. Care must be taken to consider the possibility that some ill-health effects may only arise following many years of exposure.

To make the judgement about the triviality/tolerability/intolerability of the risk, it may be helpful to consider the following matrix, as represented in TABLE 1:

There are three caveats to the above procedures:

● The risk assessments should make sense to the workers, their managers and other stakeholders. If they are uncertain as to the validity of the judgements made, or the practicality of the controls specified, it will be necessary to review the decisions.

● It may prove difficult or impossible to complete the risk assessment without measuring the exposure levels: this often applies to those for which formal standards (statutory, guidance or in-house) have been set. See 10.17 for a discussion of the methods available to complete such assessments.

● Whatever decisions are made during the risk assessment process, particularly for higher risks, it is essential to monitor the implementation of controls and the degree to which they represent adequate protection against ill-health. Such evaluations both initially validate the assessment and also represent a useful mechanism for reviewing and continually improving the precautions.

Stage 5 – Setting priorities

10.14 Once the risks have been evaluated and analysed, it is possible to decide on the appropriate responses, which fall into four basic categories:

- If the risk is trivial, no action is required.

- If the risk is significant, but the existing precautions are adequate then no further action is required other than to document the assessment and ensure that the stated precautions are employed and maintained at all times, and periodically checked and reviewed.

- If the risk is significant and the existing precautions are inadequate, further action is required to improve the protection of health and move this risk into the category above.

- If the risk is significant, and indeed deemed to be intolerable, then

Table 2: Risk levels and action required

Risk level	Action and timescale
Trivial	No action is required, no documentation required (although it may be helpful to avoid others evaluating the same risks without realising they have been categorised as trivial).
Tolerable	No additional controls are required – but care is required to ensure that the existing precautions are maintained, communicated to new workers, subject to periodic monitoring, audit, review. When reviewed, consideration may be given to identifying more cost-effective or improved controls.
Moderate	For such significant risks, efforts should be made to identify more effective precautions which may be implemented in a reasonable timescale, and for which the costs are proportionate to the risks. This is the type of health risk which is likely to require careful exposure monitoring – measuring dust, noise, vibration exposure, etc.
Substantial	This represents a serious health risk, with a high likelihood of permanent health effects arising from the work. If this is planned new work, it should not commence without more effective precautions. If work is already underway, greater precautions are required as a matter of urgency.
Intolerable	Work should not be *started* or *continued* until the risk has been reduced. If the risk cannot be reduced, the work should remain prohibited.

either controls are required to reduce the risk into one of the categories above or the work giving rise to the risk should cease. If the risk is of an acute and immediate effect this will require such work to cease immediately; if the risk is of harm arising in the longer-term as a result of repeated exposures, there may be a longer acceptable timescale for the controls to be introduced, but this will require careful evaluation, documentation and consultation.

Once you have categorised the risks, you may use the following plan to decide on the priorities for implementing precautions, as represented in TABLE 2:

Stage 6 – Taking precautions: exercising control

10.15 The measure of effective risk assessment is the extent to which assessments define suitable precautions to protect health. The control procedures which are identified to reduce risk are the crucial outputs from the assessment process. Controls available range from those which eliminate the risk altogether, to those which reduce it and contain it so that it impinges on fewer people, right down to personal protection for individuals. This is the *hierarchy of controls* into which precautions must be sorted. The preference in managing health risks is, in order:

- To eliminate the risk altogether

    For example, by deciding to change the purchasing instructions so that certain materials arrive to the stores area on pallets for mechanical handling, rather than in smaller packets which have to be carried by the warehouse staff and manually placed on shelves, thus eliminating one of the risks of back-strain injuries.

- To substitute a significant health risk for one which is much lower

    For example, by specifying that for all internal decorations the paint to be used will be water-based, eliminating the organic solvent fumes which are generated by paints containing substances such as toluene and xylene. Substitution in this case effectively eliminates the risk of local staff (typically those engaged in the painting) being exposed to airborne levels of solvent which are harmful both as short term (acute) narcotic agents and which may have longer term effects on the lungs and the central nervous system. Substitution here also eliminates the lower-level but still significant risk that other staff (typically other workers engaged in either the building occupants' normal working in another part of the building, or engaged in other building work associated with a refurbishment) will be adversely affected by the discomfort of smells and health effects such as headaches which can arise from inhaling solvent fumes. Of course, some solvent fumes are also flammable or even explosive in the right airborne concentrations, but water vapour represents a much lower risk all round.

- To use technology to reduce risks

  If the health risk cannot be 'designed out' or 'designed down' to a much lower level, the time has come to limit the risk by making use of technology. This can be the design and installation of local exhaust ventilation to capture wood dust as it is formed by the cutting actions of woodworking machinery in a workshop. Another example is the use of water to create a slurry from dust which would otherwise enter the breathing zone of an operator using a disc cutter to trim tiles, bricks and slabs. Making activities safer by design can involve the moulding of building blocks so that they contain handholds to facilitate safe and easier handling by bricklayers. In a manufacturing environment, the insertion of rubber and spring mounts to machinery will dampen vibration and reduce the noise emissions. Noise exposures can also be reduced by the use of rubber rather than metal crates to catch components at the end of the conveyor belt. In the chemical and pharmaceutical industry any of the feedstock materials can be purchased as a dust-generating powder, or in pellet form which greatly reduces airborne dust. There are innumerable examples which involve design improvements in the work process, the work materials and the work tools.

- To restrict exposure to fewer staff

  Whether or not the work can be made safer, with lower health risks, it is usually possible to restrict exposures to those risks to fewer staff, ie to those directly engaged in the tasks concerned. This may involve restricting certain areas to 'authorised personnel' only, whilst work is going on. For example, this control could apply to painting during redecoration, or the spray application of fire proofing, or noisy work areas segregated from the main workshop by noise insulating barriers. A mixture of containment of a health risk, and restricting those people authorised to enter the containment area will protect everyone not directly engaged in the work itself.

- To restrict individual exposure by increasing numbers of staff involved

  Within a contained area, staff may be exposed to a risk such as noise or airborne dust. In the field of safety, each time anyone is exposed to an injury hazard they suffer an increased risk of actually experiencing the accident and the consequent injury. With health risks there is often a threshold effect, and exposures below the threshold have no adverse consequences. Most people can drink one glass of wine without getting drunk and without their performance being significantly adversely affected. However, if someone drinks a bottle of wine in a short time they will almost certainly appear drunk and, in any event, their perception and reaction times will be drastically affected. So it is with exposures to dust, fumes, noise, vibration and other such hazards to health: a small exposure to all but the most toxic substances, or a short exposure to all but the loudest noises, can be tolerated regularly by our bodies with little or no untoward health effects. This means that one of the precautions available is to 'share' the exposures amongst a group of workers, so that no individual receives a dose liable to harm their health. Managing work schedules so that the noisy work is carried out by a team, with no person doing it for more than a few hours each week, may be managed so that, subject to the intensity and nature of the noise, no-one receives the scale of dose liable to cause noise-induced hearing loss. Similarly burdensome amounts of work may be shared so that no individual works excessively long hours or feels unduly stressed by their workload.

- Increasing personal protection

Finally, if either it is not possible to reduce the health risk to an acceptable level by the techniques described and/or the other controls may need a 'belt and braces' back-up, and/or you need more time to put one or more of the other controls in place (it takes time to source substitute materials, or design and install extract ventilation), then it is permissible to select and supply personal protective equipment, Such equipment includes eye protection, dust masks, hearing defenders and similar items. Their weaknesses are that, at best, they only protect the user and then only to the extent that they are correctly selected and properly used.

Controls available include

10.16

- Chemical risks:

  o choose less toxic or non-toxic materials (water instead of solvent-based);

  o use the material in a form which reduces the risk (pellets instead of powder);

  o use the material in a way which reduces the risk (purchase ready-diluted solution, eliminating handling concentrate and diluting it for use);

  o contain the risk (use fume cabinets or other form of ventilated containment);

  o ensure handling area is well ventilated, to dilute any material in the atmosphere;

  o choose appropriate work methods (sweeping dry dust generates airborne contamination which may be reduced by wet wiping or vacuum cleaning);

  o select and issue appropriate personal protective equipment, and train staff to use it correctly;

○ have contingency arrangements ready (spillage treatment, first aid such as eye wash bottles).

- Biological risks:

  ○ infectious agents should be handled in accordance with a complete protection regime based on the infectivity and the consequence of infection;

  ○ containment, careful handling of material including waste disposal, design of work to minimise risk of personal contamination, use of protective clothing and equipment;

  ○ evaluate infection risks to determine immunological status required (immunisation is appropriate for certain risks);

  ○ ensure staff are well trained in the risks, and suitable precautions and how to implement them;

  ○ for biological agents which can cause sensitisation, the precautions associated with effective control of airborne contamination (chemical) should be applied rigorously coupled with routine health checks (health surveillance).

- Physical risks:

  ○ noise can often be reduced at source, by careful design of equipment and processes: techniques include decoupling noisy equipment from the floor with resilient noise and vibration dampening mounts, and the installation of silencers in air ducts;

  ○ where noise has been reduced by application of noise reduction techniques, careful maintenance regimes are required as poorly-maintained equipment typically generates more noise;

  ○ noise exposures can be reduced by containing noise in acoustically-designed chambers, and by using sound-absorbent materials to reduce reverberation;

  ○ vibration exposures from hand tools can be reduced by keeping the tools sharp, well-maintained and designed with handles which reduce the transmission of vibration to the hands.

- Ergonomic risks:

  ○ some physical work (lifting and handling) can be eliminated be effective job design;

  ○ the provision of aids which include hoists, trolleys, etc can greatly reduce the load on individuals;

  ○ the working environment can be designed to reduce potential adverse impact – from the careful design of workstations to lighting and access routes.

Monitoring health risk exposures

10.17 There are five main reasons to measure a health risk and its effects:

- To ascertain whether or not there is a significant risk: measuring airborne dust, fumes, noise and vibration exposures for example. This type of monitoring forms an element of the risk assessment process.

- To ascertain whether or not the controls in place are adequate and functioning correctly: for example, measuring the level of airborne dust where dust extraction equipment is in place. This type of monitoring can be repeated periodically as a way of checking that the controls remain effective.

- To measure individual exposures, in order to confirm compliance with statutory or other exposure limits.

- To evaluate the personal uptake of a contaminant in the working environment by biological monitoring, for example solvents may be detected and measured on the exhaled breath and/or analytes in the urine of exposed workers.

- Health surveillance doesn't directly measure exposures to risks, but instead looks to detect the early signs and symptoms arising from such exposures (such surveillance is appropriate either for certain materials designated by the *Control of Substances Hazardous to Health Regulations 2002 (SI 2002/2677)*, eg vinyl chloride monomer; or where there is an identifiable disease or adverse reaction related to exposure, where exposure levels make such reactions likely, and there are valid techniques for detecting indications of such an effect).

The techniques to be employed are specific to the nature of the hazard, but the common themes are that competent people need to make use of calibrated equipment, and that samples should be taken so that the data generated is representative of the worker exposures.

Recording risk assessments

10.18 There are many risk assessment forms in use across the UK, and the following is provided as an example which may be amended and modified to suit particular circumstances.

Keeping health risk assessment records

10.19 Risk assessment records should be maintained so that they can be easily accessed and used during the work to which they apply. They also

Figure 2: Sample risk assessment form

Health Risk Assessment								
Department/work area				Date of assessment				
Risk assessor				Checked by				
Work activity	Task	Hazard to health	Risk to health	Current precautions	Residual risk			Action required to improve control
					Trivial	Moderate	Substantial	Intolerable	

should be used to review training arrangements, and when considering changes in work practices or the working environment. There are a few basic rules but the rest depends on the organisation: computerised records are acceptable, as are paper files:

- all risks which are greater than trivial should be subject to written risk assessments;

- all written risk assessments should be kept until they are superseded;

- when work practices, materials, published standards or anything else changes, the relevant risk assessments should be reviewed;

- even if no change has apparently occurred, it is sensible to review risk assessments periodically, and the periodicity should reflect the degree of risk; and

- if personal exposure data has been gathered as part of the risk assessment process, this data should be kept for 40 years.

Review and audit

10.20   Risk assessments are designed to be guides for action, defining the controls required to protect health and the arrangements for the effective maintenance of those controls. Such documents should be subject to two types of regular checking, with a periodicity which reflects the seriousness of the risks themselves:

- the assessments themselves should be reviewed, to ensure that they correctly characterise the work, the hazards intrinsic to that work, the risks arising from exposure to the hazards and the precautions which are required. The review, in other words, is into the *validity* of the assessments; and

- the audit process is a way of evaluating how effectively the precautions defined in assessments are being applied. The audit, in other words, checks on the *implementation* of the assessments.

Much of health risk management is based on the management cycle:

Plan ➜ Do ➜ Check ➜ Act

Risk assessments are the plans for healthy working, implementing the plans is the next step, followed by checks on their implementation and effectiveness, completed by acting on the findings of those checks.

Case studies

10.21

Case study 1 – the bad company

The health and safety policy was just a 'safety policy', the health issues which arose in the engineering workshops were not reflected in either the top-level policy or the day-to-day procedures. Although later it became apparent that the shop floor workers and their safety representative knew about some of the safety issues, they had never been consulted.

Problems came to light when a small group of staff developed skin irritations. It began with one lathe operative, who assumed it was a personal health matter and nothing to do with anyone else. Later, when two of his colleagues complained about the same problem, it was identified as probably work-related. A link was made to the smell they had been complaining of from the cutting fluids reservoir. It had become contaminated with a bacterial growth, and as well as the smell had developed some ingredients to which several of the exposed workers had become sensitised.

The Health & Safety Executive were called in, and it was immediately obvious that health issues had not been included in any of the risk reviews: for instance, eye protection from metal swarf had been called for in previous risk assessments, but noise, oil mist, skin contamination, manual handling and various other health issues had not been considered.

The company was served a prohibition notice on the cutting fluid, which had to be replaced by a new system for disinfection with alternative biocides. The result was interesting, in that the new system meant that the cutting fluid lasted longer, saving the company money: bad health was also bad business. An improvement notice was served to force an updating of the risk assessments, so that they properly reflected the health risks associated with engineering work.

From the company's point of view, however, being *forced* to carry out the improvements meant that it did not receive any credit from the workforce.

Case study 2 – the good company

The tunnelling company was commissioned to drive a new roadway for many hundreds of metres underground, a large bored tunnel to be constructed using the most modern techniques. From the outset there was a clear focus on the health issues which could arise, reflected in a health and safety policy statement which discussed health and expressed a commitment to protect the workforce. A qualified and experienced health and safety advisor was appointed, with access to sources of occupational health support.

The design process was set up so that each element of the tunnel was subject to review, seeking to establish the nature of the health risks which could arise and the alternatives which were available. For example, many tunnels have been built with workers operating inside compressed air chambers (the pressure maintains the integrity of the tunnel face until permanent supports and water barriers are installed), but this creates the risk of developing compression sickness and poses problems if emergency assistance is required. The tunnel in question was built using a tunnel boring machine which was set up to be maintained at normal pressures; thus, the pressurised head did not need operators to work within it, as it was controlled from outside. In order to document the risks, the methods for elimination and reduction and the issues which needed to be communicated to the work teams and their managers, a risk register was created and used throughout the design phase.

Staff engaged to carry out the work were given pre-employment health checks, to ensure fitness for the work, and the opportunity taken to give them a detailed, personal health briefing. This was then supplemented by regular 'toolbox talks' on various health aspects. These were also used as an opportunity to consult staff on the arrangements for their health protection. The welfare facilities provided on site were specified with reference to the risk assessments, with a hand cleaning system which included skin emollients, showers and a general divide between 'clean' and 'dirty' to minimise the risk of contamination between personal clothing and that being taken off site. Tools selected for hand work, which was minimised but could not be eliminated by the design, were selected partly against vibration criteria and each was tagged with the maximum usage per day to assist in the programme to reduce the risk of hand arm vibration syndrome.

Once work got underway, tests were conducted to monitor air quality in the tunnel as boring progressed. Other tests evaluated noise and vibration exposures. The monitoring was conducted by qualified occupational hygienists, seeking to supplement and confirm the

(cont'd)

information used to develop the risk assessments. In the light of the data, some of the preliminary risk assessments were amended and updated.

As part of the multi-faceted approach, in addition to pre-employment health checks targeting general fitness, a health surveillance programme was put in place. Workers exposed to dermatitic agents, the use of vibrating tools, heavy manual work or other significant health risks were subject to regular health checks. In each case, as with the design, training and planning aspects of health protection, each element of the health check was determined by reference to the risk assessments. As a result of all the efforts, these regular health checks carried out by occupational health nurses under the direction of a qualified occupational health physician confirmed that the risk management process was indeed protecting health.

11   Using External Expertise

Introduction

11.1   Very few organisations can claim to have all of the expertise they need to cover every business contingency in-house: there are times when any organisation needs to obtain expert help from outside. This may be for IT, for legal advice, for taxation advice, or more technical matters such as designing interior lighting or servicing the air-conditioning system. Whatever the need, employing an outside 'consultant' can be expensive and to get best value for money you have to be sure that the need is real, that the question you want answered is properly thought through, and that you choose a consultant who has the right qualifications, experience and knowledge to be able to provide the advice you need. This is no different in occupational health. If you have an employee health problem and you do not have access to occupational health advice within the organisation you may want to get an external opinion. You will need to apply the same criteria for engaging the help of any other consultants.

Is the need a real one?

11.2   What is the problem? You may have an employee who is having a considerable amount of time off through sickness absence and you want advice on whether the medical condition has been caused by work (there may be potential for litigation if that is the case), and you want advice on if, and when, the person is likely to be fully fit for work again. There is little doubt in a case such as this that you need expert advice from an occupational health professional who can investigate the medical condition and provide advice on possible work-related causes and prospects for return to work, or the alternative of ill-health retirement. Whether or not you need to buy in that advice depends on whether you have an occupational health nurse or doctor contracted to your organisation. If not then you will have to engage the help of an external consultant.

Sometimes the need is not so clear cut. You may have had a visit from the Health & Safety Executive (HSE) Inspector who has advised that you need to undertake a risk assessment of your manual handling operations. Manual handling is a common activity within the organisation so there is likely to be a need for repeated assessments and to keep the assessment under review. You have a number of health and safety assistants but none of them have been trained to undertake manual handling assessments. In this case, it may be much better to train one or two people from within the organisation rather than buying in someone from outside (see 11.5).

Carefully consider the questions you want answered

11.3   If you decide you need to engage the help of an external consultant you will need to provide a carefully thought out brief or scope of work. Money is often wasted, and good will destroyed, by the consultant and the client having different perceptions of what was required. The following scenario serves as an example.

Company A thought it had a sick building syndrome problem because a number of staff were complaining of headache and fatigue. The popular view among staff was that it was caused by a lack of fresh air and that the air conditioning was faulty. The company decided it should engage the help of a consultant and because it had become a common view that it was caused by the air conditioning, the expert that was called in was an air conditioning engineer. The brief he was given was to check the performance of the air conditioning unit and to check the air exchange rate. This may have been *a* question but it wasn't *the* question that needed asking. The relevant questions were whether the complaint rate of headache and fatigue were significant and, if so, what was causing them? The air conditioning was found to be working well so the expensive checks on its performance proved unnecessary and did not contribute to an understanding of what was causing the problem. Had the question been better formulated a consultant with broad experience of investigating building-related illness would have found, as proved to be the case, that it was glare and poor lighting that was causing the problem.

Similar issues can also arise when asking an occupational physician for a medical opinion on a member of staff. What you want from the doctor must be carefully thought through before you refer the employee. The doctor should be given a written note on the background to the case and what questions you want answered. For example, your referral letter may say Mr X has had a history of sickness absence and give details of the frequency and length of sick leave and the reasons given on the sickness certificates. The questions you want answered are:

- are the reasons for Mr X's sickness history genuine?;

- what is the prognosis for his recovery, and is he likely to return to reasonable fitness for work?; and

- with an eye to the *Disability Discrimination Act 1995*, is there a possibility of return to work but with restrictions?

Do not ask the doctor for information on the employee's medical condition or other information which is medically 'in confidence' because the doctor will be unable to disclose that (without the individual's consent). Asking questions that are likely to breach medical confidentiality is a frequent cause of discontent between managers and occupational health professionals.

Choose a consultant who has the right experience for the job

11.4 This is often the most difficult part of the decision process. The question of who is right for the job depends first of all on defining what work you want undertaken (see 11.3). Whoever you choose must be 'competent' to undertake the work you have defined. It is not only in the interests of your organisation to get the best possible advice but there is a legal obligation to ensure that anyone providing health and safety advice is competent. The *Management of Health and Safety at Work Regulations 1999 (SI 1999/3242), Reg 7* says that competence means having sufficient training and experience or knowledge and other qualities to enable the competent person to properly to assist in undertaking the measures required. The associated Approved Code of Practice (L21, HSE, 2000) provides further advice on competence. It says that competence does not necessarily depend on the possession of particular skills or qualifications. Competence requires the following:

- an understanding of the relevant current best practice;

- an awareness of the limitations of one's own experience and knowledge; and

- the willingness and ability to supplement existing experience and knowledge when necessary, by obtaining external help and advice.

In choosing a consultant therefore, it is necessary to ensure that the person you engage is 'competent' to undertake the work you expect of him or her. From the meaning of competence discussed above it follows that it does not necessarily mean *qualifications*. Someone with a formal qualification in, say, occupational hygiene, may not have the necessary experience or be adequately equipped to carry out a noise survey. In choosing the consultant it is necessary to ask the appropriate questions about experience in undertaking the type of work you want to have done. It is quite in order to ask what other work of a similar nature the consultant has undertaken in the past. For major pieces of work or advice that may have serious implications for the organisation (potential litigation, for example), it is common practice to ask for anonymised examples of reports that the consultant has produced for other organisations. At the very least, it is now usual to ask to see the consultant's CV before engaging him/her and to keep a copy of the CV with any reports the consultant produces for you. In that way, if ever the question of competence was challenged, you would have evidence that you took all reasonable steps to check that the consultant was suitably knowledgeable and experienced to carry out the work.

In-house versus external assistance

11.5 A question often arises as to whether it is better to buy in external assistance or to try to provide the occupational health support you need from within the organisation. The answer to this question depends on a number of factors.

The size of the organisation

11.6   Does the amount of occupational health support needed financially justify the appointment of an in-house occupational health specialist (an occupational health nurse for example)? If it does then decisions have to be made about how much, and what mix of, expertise is required.

The nature of the organisation

11.7   Is the work of such a nature that it regularly exposes people to chemical, physical or biological hazards? If so, the need for regular surveillance and expert preventative planning may require some regular in-house specialist support. The size of the organisation and the number of employees exposed will determine the amount of support required.

The occasional need

11.8   Many organisations, especially those in low-risk environments, do not see the need for in-house provision of occupational health expertise. Quite justifiably, there is often no need for regular advice or support on occupational health matters. All organisations need help from time to time, however, and they should have access to an occupational health provider for advice on the occasional one-off medical or other occupational health problem. Nearly always this is support for the Personnel or Human Resources department to provide an opinion on an individual employment health issue. It is a good idea, therefore, for the Personnel department to locate, and perhaps retain, an experienced occupational health provider for the occasional ad-hoc advice and support (see 11.11 *et seq*).

Legal requirements

11.9   In some jobs there is a statutory requirement for medical fitness for work or for routine medical surveillance. This exists, for example, where staff are working with ionising radiation and are 'classified' because of their possible level of exposure or where employees are working with lead, asbestos or in compressed air or diving. Under the relevant regulations pertaining to these jobs, there is a legal requirement for an employment medical advisor (an HSE doctor) or an 'appointed' doctor to ensure medical fitness for work. An appointed or approved doctor is one appointed or approved by the HSE for carrying out the medical provision of the relevant legislation. If you think you may have a need for statutory medicals under such regulations you should seek advice from the local HSE Employment

Medical Advisor who will, if necessary, put you in touch with a suitably qualified doctor who will then need to be appointed for your purposes.

Many organisations employ drivers either because driving is the job itself or because there is a need to drive as part of the work. Drivers of passenger carrying vehicles require a PCV licence and those driving large goods vehicles require an LGV licence, both of which have certain requirements for medical fitness to drive. All company drivers, however, should comply with the medical standards for driving contained within the *Road Traffic Act 1988*.

In some organisations there is a quasi-legal need for medical fitness to be approved. In the railway industry for example, the legal requirement under the *Railways (Safety Critical Work) Regulations 1994 (SI 1994/299)*, is for the employer to ensure that any of his employees who will be engaged on safety critical work are 'competent and fit to undertake the work'. It is the railway industry's own safety guidelines which specify the medical standards for fitness to work on the railways ('Safety Requirements for Track Safety: Medical and Alcohol and Drug Screening and Certification, RT/LS/S/018 June 2000, Appendix A. Minimum Medical Fitness Standards for Personal Track Safety, Railtrack, 2000). Similarly in the offshore industry it is the Industry's own medical standards for fitness to work which determine the need for medical assessments to be carried out ('Guidelines for medical aspects of fitness for offshore work', Issue number 4, UK Offshore Operators' Association, 2000).

In these and in a few other areas, such as the employment of commercial pilots and merchant seamen, there is a medical standard to be met, which will require some form of medical examination or assessment usually carried out by a suitably experienced doctor. Unless you have an in-house medical advisor, it will be necessary to buy in the medical opinion necessary to meet these legal or quasi-legal requirements.

Routine occupational health management

11.10 There are many tasks that relate to employee health that an organisation has to perform on a regular basis and keep up-to-date. These usually relate to assessment for health-related risks, for example under the following regulations:

- the *Health and Safety (Display Screen Equipment) Regulations 1992 (SI 1992/2792)*;

- the *Manual Handling Operations Regulations 1992 (SI 1992/2793)*;

- the *Control of Substances Hazardous to Health Regulations 2002 (SI 2002/2677) (COSHH)*;

- the *Noise at Work Regulations 1989 (SI 1989/1790)*; and

- the *Management of Health and Safety at Work Regulations 1999 (Management Regulations) (SI 1999/3242)*.

The *Management Regulations, Reg 7(8)* states that where there is a competent person in the employer's employment, that person shall be appointed to assist in the provision of health and safety measures 'in preference to a competent person not in his employment'. The reason why it is preferable to have someone from within the organisation is that it is more likely that the person will understand the culture and structure of the organisation and also that there will be a greater sense of ownership of the assessment and any shortcomings it might reveal. It is preferable, therefore, to train someone (or several people) from within the organisation to carry out the regular non-specialist occupational health tasks (such as risk assessments). Remember, however, that trained health and safety assistants must be 'competent' and they should recognise the limits of their own ability and experience. Their work may need to be supplemented by expertise bought in to provide, for example, specialist noise assessments, vibration exposure assessments, health surveillance or chemical monitoring.

Where to get occupational health advice

11.11 Competent occupational health advice is not in great supply in the UK and you have to look carefully for the type of help you need and the level of expertise appropriate to the nature of the question you have determined. There are a number of options as to how you might be able to find the help you want.

Direct employment

11.12 You could, for example, directly employ an occupational health nurse or doctor either on a full-time or part-time basis. As mentioned, above the justification for doing this will depend on the size of the organisation, the nature of the hazards to which employees are exposed and the number of people exposed to these hazards.

Agencies

11.13 Occupational health nurses are the only occupational health professionals that can be supplied from an agency. If you have determined that you need specialist occupational health advice and you engage an occupational health nurse through an agency, make sure the nurse is on the specialist register of the Nursing and Midwifery Council (see 11.20). Also having determined what you want from the nurse make sure that he or she is *competent* to provide the specific services you need.

Specialist service provider

11.14 Occupational health can be bought from a specialist service provider. Local NHS trusts (through NHS Plus – see 3.27), some of the health insurance companies, university departments specialising in occupational health, private occupational health companies and a few 'group' occupational health services can provide occupational health services on a fee-paying basis. A service provider will normally have the advantage over agency staff of being properly equipped for occupational health investigations (for lung function tests and hearing tests, for example), and will usually have their own clinic for investigations. Many will also have portable equipment for use on the client's premises where this is feasible.

Sharing a service with others

11.15 You could share a service with other local employers. Ask around to see if there is a large local organisation with it's own occupational health service which you might be able to buy in to. For small companies, another way of sharing is to see if other local businesses would like to share the cost of employing an occupational health nurse. This is likely to be more cost effective than buying on a regular basis from an agency. One company will need to take the lead and employ the nurse and have a service agreement and agreement on cost sharing with the others.

Local general practice

11.16 Many organisations buy medical expertise from the local general practice. Some GP's will have a qualification in occupational medicine (such as the Associateship in the Faculty of Occupational Medicine (AFOM) or the Diploma in Occupational Medicine) but many will have no specialist knowledge of occupational or employment health issues. Some GP's will have taken a Faculty of Occupational Medicine (nine-day) course in occupational medicine. Although this shows that the GP has an interest in occupational health, it is not evidence of a specialist knowledge of occupational medicine. Some aspects of an occupational health service can be competently provided by a GP without specialist training. Many routine examinations, such as lung function tests, skin examinations, general fitness for work examinations, or treatments such as travel vaccinations, can be carried out by a GP. There will, however, sometimes be the need for advice from someone with experience and specialist training in occupational medicine. In that case you will need to seek the help of an Accredited Specialist in Occupational Medicine (see 11.19).

Some general practices and primary care groups will provide the services of a practice nurse. However, most practice nurses will not be experienced or qualified in occupational health and, again, you will need to be sure that the nurse has the experience and 'competence' to carry out the work you require.

HSE appointed doctor

11.17   If your work requires medical examinations by a doctor appointed or approved for the purposes by the HSE, you should seek advice from the Employment Medical Advisory Service (see 3.31 and 11.9).

Health and safety professionals

11.18   It is important to understand what qualifications and what checks on professional registrations are appropriate for the main professional groups that provide occupational health support.

Occupational physician

11.19   Occupational physicians apply their medical knowledge and skills to work-related causes of illness and disease. Occupational physicians should have the ability to interface effectively with management to advise managers on the medical aspects of employment, including fitness to work, sickness absence, return to work and rehabilitation and ill-health retirement. Many occupational physicians will also have additional specific expertise in areas such as occupational psychology, industrial physiology, toxicology, ergonomics, public health medicine and epidemiology, and will be able to provide expert medical advice in these fields. If you have a specific problem which needs advice from an occupational physician it may be necessary to seek someone with special interests and expertise in the appropriate speciality.

Occupational physicians are medical practitioners on the register of the General Medical Council (GMC) but, in addition, they hold a qualification in occupational medicine with the Faculty of Occupational Medicine (FOM) of the Royal College of Physicians.

To train as an accredited specialist in occupational medicine, a doctor must first of all undertake a programme of study and examination to acquire the Associateship of the Faculty of Occupational Medicine (AFOM). Some doctors will not proceed further than this and will practice occupational medicine with an AFOM, but they will not be regarded as accredited specialists. Membership or Fellowship of the Faculty of Occupational Medicine (MFOM or FFOM) may be obtained after a further period of study and research, and this will afford a doctor consultant status and will allow him or her to be on the specialist register of the GMC as an Accredited Specialist in Occupational Medicine. The Faculty of Occupational Medicine also awards a Diploma in Occupational Medicine which is a generalist qualification intended for doctors working part-time in general practice or hospital medicine and part-time in occupational health. Holders of the Diploma are not accredited specialists. The general registration of doctors and their inclusion on the specialist register can be checked with the Registration Department of the General Medical Council – for contact details, see APPENDIX: FURTHER SOURCES OF INFORMATION.

When engaging a doctor you should ask to see their GMC certificate of registration and hold a copy of this on file. In addition to checking professional credentials it is also advisable to take up references from recent or current employers.

The Faculty of Occupational Medicine can advise on relevant qualifications; whereas the Society of Occupational Medicine can advise in the location of a suitable physician (for contact details of both bodies, see APPENDIX: FURTHER SOURCES OF INFORMATION).

Occupational health nurse

11.20 Occupational health nurses are trained to extend their nursing knowledge and skills to the workplace. Their work involves advising management on work-related health risks and in advising management on means of controlling health risks and in dealing with the employment issues arising from ill-health.

Occupational health nurses will have qualified as registered nurses and then gone on to specialise in occupational health nursing. Evidence of their specialism, and current registration to practice is held on the specialist register of the Nursing and Midwifery Council (NMC). The title of 'nurse' is protected by law and the NMC defines an occupational health nurse as 'a registered nurse with a recognised qualification in occupational health nursing recorded on the register'. Qualifications for occupational health nursing are:

- the Occupational Health Nursing Certificate (OHNC);

- a Postgraduate Diploma; or

- a Degree in Occupational Health Nursing; and

- additionally, some occupational health nurses will have gone on to do a Masters Degree (MSc) in Occupational Health.

If you intend to use the services of an occupational health nurse you should seek evidence and confirmation of their qualifications from the NMC's Registration Confirmation Service.

In addition to checking professional credentials it is advisable to take up references from other recent or current employers of the occupational health nurse. If you are engaging the services of an occupational health nurse through an agency, ask to see the agency's check on the nurse's professional registration.

Many nurses working in industry have no qualifications in occupational health nursing. Sometimes such nurses (quite legally) call themselves 'industrial nurses'. The question of whether you employ a qualified occupational health nurse involves again the consideration of competence. Employers have to be careful not to place duties on the 'company nurse' which might contravene the meaning of competence under the *Management of Health and Safety at Work Regulations 1999 (SI 1999/3242)*. A general nurse without specific training or experience in work-related health problems may not have the competence to recognise the causes of occupational illness or be able to provide management with competent advice on how to deal with individual cases.

For contact details, see APPENDIX: FURTHER SOURCES OF INFORMATION.

Occupational hygienist

11.21   Occupational hygienists specialise in the measurement of chemical and physical hazards in the workplace. Measurement of noise, vibration, dust, fumes, temperature, lighting etc, is sometimes necessary in order to undertake an adequate risk assessment. The occupational hygienist also advises on control measures and personal protective equipment. Where there is exposure to chemicals which have a maximum exposure limit (MEL), an occupational hygienist may be needed to periodically check that any statutory limits on exposure are not being exceeded and to ensure that control measures are adequate to minimise the risk. Occupational hygienists normally support the role of the occupational health team but in a small organisation, without other occupational health personnel, they may report their findings and recommendations directly to management.

The qualifications and examination of occupational hygienists in the UK is controlled by the British Institute of Occupational Hygienists (BIOH). Occupational Hygienists practice with five different levels of professional qualification:

- Certificates of Proficiency

  These are evidence that the hygienist has taken and passed individual modules of training in specific areas of asbestos work approved by the BIOH.

- Occupational Hygiene Modules

  Occupational hygienists may have taken and passed individual modules in a variety of subject areas. These include hazardous substances, noise and vibration, the thermal environment and non-ionising radiation, and ergonomics. Holding one of these modules is evidence of a qualification approved by the BIOH in that subject area, but not evidence of any broader level of training in occupational hygiene.

- Certificate of Competence (in an individual subject)

  A certificate of competence is evidence of a level of competence in a specified subject area. The certificate is gained only after passing both a written examination and oral examination.

- Certificate of Operational Competence in Occupational Hygiene

  This qualification is held by hygienists who have responsibility within the profession for surveys of the working environment. The examination consists of a Part 1 (core) which is obtained by a number of routes, including acquiring a number of Occupational Hygiene modules; and a Part 2 which is an oral examination.

- The Diploma of Professional Competence in Occupational Hygiene

  This qualification is held by occupational hygienists who have been required to accept professional responsibility for all aspects of an occupational hygiene programme for at least five years. It is usually gained by passing a number of written examinations and an oral examination.

There are other variations by which someone will have gained experience and qualification as an occupational hygienist or will be able to show qualification in a specific subject area. Although no longer available, some occupational hygienists may hold the Preliminary Certificate (PCert) in a specified subject area. These have been replaced in recent years by the Occupational Hygiene modules (see above). Occupational hygienists may also have entered the profession by obtaining a BSc and/or MSc and may have then obtained exemptions from the routes described above to achieve Diploma status. From January 2002, the BIOH has modified its modular scheme.

The Grade of Membership of the BIOH is a key indicator of the professional recognition of the hygienist:

- Fellow

  This is awarded to those who can demonstrate seniority in the field of occupational hygiene and have made a distinct contribution to the profession.

- Member

  This is open to those who are holders of the Diploma of Professional Competence in Occupational Hygiene.

- Specialist Member

  This is open to those who have experience at an advanced level in specialist aspects of occupational hygiene such as occupational health, toxicology, etc.

- Licentiate

   This is open to holders of the Certificate of Operational Competence in Occupational Hygiene.

- Graduate

   This is open to those with an Honours or Postgraduate Degree in Occupational Hygiene or equivalent.

The qualifications held by occupational hygienists can therefore be extremely varied and as with other professions supporting occupational health practice, it is important to be sure that you are engaging a hygienists who is *competent* to undertake to work you need. Ask to see the hygienist's CV, which should tell you what qualifications he/she holds and how recently these were obtained, and should also detail experience of undertaking similar work. Since January 2000 the BIOH has operated an optional continuing professional development (CPD) scheme. Participants in the CPD scheme can call themselves 'registered occupational hygienists' and use the designation ROH after their name. Participation in the CPD scheme is evidence of the hygienist's willingness to demonstrate that he/she is keeping up to date with current practice.

Currently there are two bodies of which occupational hygienists may be members. The British Occupational Hygiene Society (BOHS) and the British Institute of Occupational Hygiene (BIOHS). The BOHS is a learned society and membership is open to anyone with an interest in the working environment. Membership of the BOHS does not imply any particular qualification in occupational hygiene. After January 2003, the two bodies will merge under the title of the BOHS. Within the new BOHS there will be a Faculty of Occupational Hygiene which will assume the responsibility for professional qualifications.

For contact details, see APPENDIX: FURTHER SOURCES OF INFORMATION.

Ergonomist

11.22   The work of ergonomists concerns the matching of work and work environment to the abilities of the people undertaking that work. Ergonomists are concerned with the design of work systems to minimise the demands made on workers and designing workplaces and workstations to match the physical and mental attributes of people at work.

Ergonomics advice is usually sought to ensure that physically or mentally demanding work does not exceed the limitations of the human body. Determination of safe lifting limits, the design, dimensions and layout of computer workstations and the design of systems of work are examples of how applying ergonomic principles can help reduce the risk of occupational ill-health. The risk of musculoskeletal injury and stress-related disorders can be reduced by ensuring good ergonomic design of the workplace and the system of working. Ergonomics is best applied preventatively at the design stage of a new process or when new equipment and furniture is being procured. However, ergonomists are often employed to troubleshoot a particular problem and to advise on modifications to the work and working environment in order to reduce the risk after a problem has become apparent.

Ergonomists usually have backgrounds as psychologists, physiologists, physiotherapists or engineers and may have moved into ergonomics by experience or may have taken a Masters (MSc) in Ergonomics or Health Ergonomics. The question of competence is again important and should be taken into account when commissioning work from an ergonomist. The Ergonomics Society has a list of members but this is not a guarantee of competence in a particular field of ergonomics.

For contact details, see APPENDIX: FURTHER SOURCES OF INFORMATION.

Physiotherapist and chiropractor

11.23 Physiotherapists and chiropractors can provide therapies, which both prevent and treat a wide range of musculoskeletal disorders. Physiotherapists and chiropractors are trained to treat disorders of the musculoskeletal system by a variety of manipulative and physical methods. Some organisations employ practitioners to treat early symptoms of musculoskeletal disorder in sedentary workers and in those with more physically demanding jobs where there is a risk of musculoskeletal disorder. Sometimes chiropractors and physiotherapist are employed to advise on design of workplaces and methods of working to avoid musculoskeletal injury. If such advice is being sought you should make sure that the practitioner has experience of workplace issues and preferably has some training in ergonomics principles.

Although chiropractors use different manipulative techniques they have the same aim as physiotherapists in treating musculoskeletal disorders. Chiropractors also claim to treat some organic disorders (eg migraine) by chiropractic techniques.

For contact details, see APPENDIX: FURTHER SOURCES OF INFORMATION.

Appendix
Further Sources of Information

General health and safety

Baxter, PJ et al (eds), *Hunter's Diseases of Occupations* (9th edition, 2000), Hodder Arnold

Butterworths, *Employment Law Handbook* (9th edition), LexisNexis Butterworths Tolley

Chartered Institute of Personnel Development, *Employee Absence Survey 2002* (2002), CIPD

Cox, R et al (eds), *Fitness for Work – The Medical Aspects* (3rd edition), Oxford Medical Publications

Department for Work and Pensions, *A Guide to Registered General Practitioners – Advice to patients regarding fitness for work*, DWP (available at http://www.dwp.gov.uk/medical/medicalib204/index.htm)

Department of Environment, Transport and Regions, *Revitalising Health and Safety: Strategy Statement* (June 2000), DETR

Department of Health and Department of Social Security, *Staying Fit for Work: a report of a conference on 8th March 2001, sponsored by the Department of Health and the Department of Social Security and supported by the Health & Safety Executive* (2001) (available through the SignUp website, http://www.signupweb.net/)

Faculty of Occupational Medicine, *Good Medical Practice For Occupational Physicians*, FOM

Faculty of Occupational Medicine, *Guidance on Ethics for Occupational Health Physicians* (5th edition), FOM

General Medical Council, *Guidance on Good Practice*, GMC

Health & Safety Commission, *Securing Health Together: A long-term occupational health strategy for England, Scotland and Wales* (2000) MISC 225, HSE Books

Health & Safety Executive, *Management of Health and Safety at Work Regulations 1999: Approved Code of Practice and Guidance* (2000), L21, HSE Books

Health & Safety Executive, *Preventing Asthma at Work: How to control respiratory sensitisers* (1994), HSE Books

Health & Safety Executive, *RIDDOR explained: The Reporting of Injuries,*

Diseases and Dangerous Occurrences Regulations 1995 (2000), HSE31 (rev1), HSE Books

Health & Safety Executive, *Successful Health and Safety Management* (2nd edition, 1997), HSE Books

Health & Safety Executive, *Workplace (Health Safety and Welfare) Regulations 1992: Approved Code of Practice* (1992), L24, HSE Books

Kloss, D, *A Servant with two Masters* (2001), Occupational Health Review 90, pp 26–30

Mason and McCall Smith, *The Law and Medical Ethics* (6th edition, October 2002), LexisNexis Butterworths Tolley

Nursing and Midwifery Council, *Code of Professional Conduct 2002*, NMC

Occupational Health Advisory Committee, *Report and Recommendations On Improving Access to Occupational Health Support* (2000), OHAC/HSC

Peacock, N and Foster, C, *Clinical Confidentiality* (October 2000), Monitor Press

Whitaker, S, *Ethics and ethical dilemmas in Occupational Health* (2001) Occupational Health Review 89, 13–15

Statutory materials

- Health and Safety at Work etc Act 1974 (as amended), HMSO

- Management of Health and Safety at Work Regulations 1999 (SI 1999/3242), HMSO

- Reporting of Injuries, Diseases and Dangerous Occurrences Regulations 1995 (SI 1995/3163), HMSO

- Workplace (Health Safety and Welfare) Regulations 1992 (SI 1992/3004), HMSO

Addresses

Health & Safety Executive Books
PO Box 1999
Sudbury
Suffolk
CO10 2WA
tel: 01787 881165
fax: 01787 313995
website: http://www.hsebooks.co.uk/

The Stationery Office
PO Box 29
Norwich
NR3 1GN
tel: 0870 600 5522
fax: 0870 600 5533
website: http://www.hmso.gov.uk/

The Professional Organisations in Occupational Safety and Health

The Professional Organisations in Occupational Safety and Health (POOSH) exists to promote the continuous improvement of the practice of occupational safety and health through education, communication and the encouragement of co-operation between all persons and agencies involved in the provision of a healthy and safe working environment.

At present the following organisations are represented on POOSH:

Organisation	Web address
Association of Occupational Health Nurse Practitioners (UK)	www.lj-riseborough.freeserve.co.uk
British Institute of Occupational Hygienists	www.bioh.org/
British Occupational Hygiene Society	www.bohs.org/
Chartered Institute of Environmental Health	www.cieh.org.uk/
The Ergonomics Society	www.ergonomics.org.uk/
Faculty of Occupational Medicine	www.facoccmed.ac.uk/index.htm
International Institute of Risk and Safety Management	www.iirsm.org/
Institute of Risk Management	www.theirm.org/
Institution of Occupational Safety and Health	www.iosh.co.uk/index.cfm
Royal Society for the Promotion of Health	www.rsph.org
Royal Society of Chemistry	www.rsc.org/
The Safety and Reliability Society	www.sars.u-net.com/

Society of Occupational Health Nursing	www.data.rcn.org.uk/services/ profess/forums/employ.htm
The Society of Occupational Medicine	www.som.org.uk

Ergonomics

Dul, J and Weerdmeester, B, *Ergonomics for Beginners* (2001), Taylor and Francis

Health & Safety Executive, *Upper Limb Disorders in the Workplace* (2002), HSG60 (rev), HSE Books

Statutory materials

- Health and Safety (Display Screen Equipment) Regulations 1992 (SI 1992/2792), HMSO

- Manual Handling Operations Regulations 1992 (SI 1992/2793), HMSO

Addresses

Association of Chartered Physiotherapists in Occupational Health
PO Box 121
London
E17
website: www.acpoh.co.uk

British Association of Occupational Therapists
College of Occupational Therapists
106–114 Borough High Street
London
SE1 1LB
tel: 020 7357 6480
fax: 020 7480 2299

British Chiropractic Association
Blagrave House
17 Blagrave Street
Reading
RG1 1QB
tel: 0118 950 5950
fax: 0118 958 8946

Chartered Society of Physiotherapists
14 Bedford Row
London
WC1R 4ED
tel: 020 7306 6666
fax: 020 7306 6611
website: http://www.csp.org.uk/

The Ergonomics Society
Devonshire House
Devonshire Square
Loughborough
LE11 3DW
tel: 01509 234904
fax: 01509 235666
e-mail: ergsoc@ergonomics.org.uk

(The Ergonomics Society is an international organisation for professionals using knowledge of human abilities and limitations to design and build for comfort, efficiency, productivity and safety.)

Health and medical information

Baxter, PJ et al (eds), *Hunter's Diseases of Occupations* (9th edition, 2000), Hodder Arnold

Rom, WN (ed), *Environmental and Occupational Health* (2nd edition), Little, Brown and Company

Addresses

Faculty of Occupational Medicine of the Royal College of Physicians
6 St Andrew's Place
Regent's Park
London
NW1 4LB
tel: 020 7317 5890
fax: 020 7317 5899

(The Faculty was set up in 1978 to provide a professional and academic body empowered to develop and maintain high standards of training, competence and professional integrity in occupational medicine.)

General Medical Council – Registration Department
178 Great Portland Street
London
W1N 6JE
tel: 020 7915 3630
fax: 020 7915 3558

NHS Plus *see* USEFUL WEB ADDRESSES *below*

Nursing and Midwifery Council
23 Portland Place
London
W1B 1PZ
tel: 020 7637 7181
website: www.nmc-uk.org

For the Registration Department, tel: 020 7333 9333

(The Nursing and Midwifery Council is the largest regulatory body for health professionals. Its remit is to protect the public through setting and monitoring standards, and to deal with those who fail to meet the standards.)

Society of Occupational Health Nursing – Royal College of Nursing
20 Cavendish Square
London
W1G 0RN
tel: 0845 772 6100

Society of Occupational Medicine
6 St Andrew's Place
Regent's Park
London
NW1 4LB
tel: 020 7486 2641
fax: 020 7486 0028
e-mail: admin@som.org.uk

(SOM is concerned with, the protection of the health of people in the workplace, the prevention of occupational injuries and disease and related environmental issues.)

Biological hazards

Advisory Committee on Dangerous Pathogens, *Protection against blood-borne infections in the workplace: HIV and Hepatitis* (1995), HMSO

Dawood, R, *Traveller's Health – How to stay healthy abroad* (1999), Oxford University Press

Department of Health, *Health advice for travellers* (1997), DOH

Department of Health, *Health information for overseas travellers* (2001), DOH

Department of Health, *Information for Undertakers: Infectious Diseases* (1988), PL/CMO(88)7, DOH

Health & Safety Commission, *Categorisation of Biological Agents according to Hazard and Categories of Containment*, Advisory Committee on Dangerous Pathogens/HSC, HSE Books

Health & Safety Commission, *General Control of Substances Hazardous to Health Approved Code of Practice, Carcinogens Approved Code of Practice and Biological Agents Approved Code of Practice* (1999), L5 HSE Books

Health & Safety Commission, *Legionnaires' disease; the control of legionella bacteria in water systems, Approved Code of Practice* (2000), HSE Books

Health & Safety Commission, *Working safely with research animals* (1997), Advisory Committee on Dangerous Pathogens/HSC, HSE Books

Health & Safety Executive, *Five steps to risk assessment* (2002), IND163(Rev1), HSE Books

Health & Safety Executive, *Blood-borne viruses in the workplace: Guidance for employers and employees* (2001), HSE Books

Health & Safety Executive, *Common zoonoses in agriculture* (2002), Agricultural information sheet No 2 (rev), HSE books

Health & Safety Executive, *Anthrax* (1997), HSG174, HSE Books

Health & Safety Executive, *Cattle associated Leptospirosis and human health* (1997), HSE Books

Health & Safety Executive, *Leptospirosis* (1996), IND(G)84L, HSE Books

Health & Safety Executive, *Protection of workers & general public during the development of contaminated land* (1991) HSG66, HSE Books

Health & Safety Executive, *The Occupational Zoonoses* (1993), HSE Books

Health Services Advisory Committee, *Safe disposal of clinical waste* (2nd edition, 1999), HSE Books

Health Services Advisory Committee, *Safe working and the prevention of infection in clinical laboratories* (1991), HMSO

Health Services Advisory Committee, *Safe working and the prevention of infection in the mortuary and post mortem room* (1991), HMSO

Addresses

British Institute of Occupational Hygienists
Suite 2, Georgian House
Great Northern Road
Derby
DE1 1LT
tel: 01332 298087
fax 01332 298099
e-mail: admin@bioh.org

(BIOH is a professional organisation that exists to promote occupational hygiene and to regulate its professional practice. Membership is qualification dependent.)

British Occupational Hygiene Society
Suite 2, Georgian House
Great Northern Road
Derby
DE1 1LT
tel: 01332 298101
fax: 01332 298099
e-mail: admin@bohs.org

(BOHS is a learned society, for the development of members, working towards securing health in the workplace. Membership is open to all those with an interest in occupational hygiene. Note: The BOHS and the BIOH will merge on 1 January 2003 under the title British Occupational Hygiene Society.)

Chartered Institute of Environmental Health
Chadwick Court
15 Hatfields
London
SE1 8DJ
tel: 020 7928 6006
fax: 020 7827 5866
e-mail: info@cieh.org

Chemical hazards

Budavari, S, *The Merck Index* (12 edition, 1996), Merck & Co Inc

Clayton, GD and Clayton, FE (eds), *Patty's Industrial Hygiene and Toxicology*, Vol ll, Part A, Chapter 1, 'Industrial Toxicology: Retrospect and Prospect' (Zapp, JA and Doull, J) (1993), John Wiley & Sons

Commission of the European Communities, Directive 67/548/EEC (*on the approximation of laws, regulations and administrative provisions relating to the classification, packaging and labelling of dangerous substances*, 27 June 1967)

Commission of the European Communites, Directive 90/394/EEC (*on the protection of workers from the risks related to exposure to carcinogens at work*, 28 June 1990)

Fenske, RA, Hamburger, SJ and Guyton, CL (1987) *Occupational Exposure to Fosetyl-Al Fungicide During Spraying of Ornamentals in Greenhouses* (1987), Archives of Environmental Contamination and Toxicology, Vol 16: 615–621

Health & Safety Commission, *Approved Supply List: Information approved for the classification and labelling of substances and preparations dangerous for supply* (7th edition), 2002b, L 129, HSE Books

Health & Safety Commission, *Chemicals (Hazard Information and Packaging for Supply) Regulations 2002*, 2002a, HSE Books

Health & Safety Commission, *Control of Asbestos at Work Regulations,* 1998a, HSE Books

Health & Safety Commission, *Control of Lead at Work Regulations,* 1998b, HSE Books

Health & Safety Commission, *Control of Substances Hazardous to Health Regulations 1999* (1999), HSE Books

Health & Safety Commission, *General Control of Substances Hazardous to Health Approved Code of Practice, Carcinogens Approved Code of Practice and Biological Agents Approved Code of Practice* (1999), L5, HSE Books

Health & Safety Commission, *Safety data sheets for substances and preparations dangerous for supply: Approved Code of Practice* (2nd edition, 1996), L 62, HSE Books

Health & Safety Commission, *Supplement to the third edition of the Approved Supply List* (1997), L100, HSE Books

Health & Safety Executive, *Assessing and managing risks at work from skin exposure to chemical agents* (2001), HSG 205, HSE Books

Health & Safety Executive, *Cost and effectiveness of chemical protective gloves in the workplace* (2001), HSG 206, HSE Books

Health & Safety Executive, *Occupational Exposure Limits 2002* (2002), EH 40, HSE Books

Health & Safety Executive, *Solder Fume and You* (1997), IND(G) 248L, HSE Books

Lewis, RJ, *Sax's Dangerous Properties of Industrial Materials* (9th edition, 1996), Van Nostrand Reinhold

National Institute for Occupational Safety and Health, *Pocket guide to chemical hazards* (1997), NIOSH, US Department of Health and Human Services, Washington DC

Zapp, JA and Doull, J *see* Clayton et al (eds) *above*

Statutory materials

- Control of Asbestos at Work Regulations 1987 (SI 1987/2115), HMSO

- Control of Asbestos at Work (Amendment) Regulations 1998 (SI 1998/3235), HMSO

- Control of Asbestos at Work Regulations 2002 (SI 2002/2675), HMSO

- Control of Lead at Work Regulations 2002 (SI 2002/2676), HMSO

- Control of Substances Hazardous to Health Regulations 2002 (SI 2002/2677), HMSO

Addresses

For the British Institute of Occupational Hygienists and the British Occupational Hygiene Society *see* BIOLOGICAL HAZARDS *above*

Physical hazards

American Conference of Industrial Hygienists, *Threshold Limit Values for 1994–95* (1994), ACIH Cincinnati

Baxter, PJ et al (eds), *Hunter's Diseases of Occupations*, Chapter 15, 'Heat and Cold' (Oakley, EHN) (9th edition, 2000), Hodder Arnold

British Occupational Hygiene Society, *The Thermal Environment* (1990), BOHS Technical Guide No 8, Science Reviews, Leeds

British Standards Institute, *Ergonomic requirements for office work with visual display terminals (VDTs) –Guidance on the work environment* (2000), BS EN ISO 9241(6), BSI

Chartered Institution of Building Services Engineers, *Code for Lighting* (2002), CIBSE (available on CD ROM)

Commission of the European Communities, *Communication from the Commission on the Precautionary Principle* (2000), Brussels (COM (2000) 1 02.02.2000)

Commission of the European Communities, Council Directive 2002/44/EC (*on the minimum health and safety requirements regarding the exposure of workers to the risks arising from physical agents (vibration)*, 25 June 2002)

Health & Safety Commission, *Noise at Work Regulations 1989* (1989), HSE Books

Health & Safety Executive, *Hand Arm Vibration* (2001), HS(G) 88 (reprinted with amendments 2001), HSE Books

Health & Safety Executive, *Health Risk from Hand Arm Vibration – Advice for Employers* (1998), IND(G) 175 (rev1), HSE Books

Health & Safety Executive, *How to Deal with Sick Building Syndrome – Guidance for employers, building owners and building managers*, HSG 132, HSE Books

Health & Safety Executive, *Lighting at Work* (1998), HS(G)38, HSE Books

Health & Safety Executive, *Reducing Noise at Work*, 1998b, L108, HSE Books

Health & Safety Executive, *Sick Building Syndrome: A Review of the Evidence on Causes and Solutions* (1992), Contract Report No 42/1992, HSE Books

Health & Safety Executive, *Vibration Solutions: Practical Ways to Reduce the Risk of Hand Arm Vibration* (1997), HSG170, HSE Books

Health & Safety Executive, *Work With Ionising Radiation: The Ionising Radiation Regulations: Approved Code of Practice and Guidance*, L121, HSE Books

Independent Expert Committee on Mobile Phones, *Mobile Phones and Health* (the Stewart Report) (May 2000) IECMP, available from the National Radiological Protection Board

International Organisation for Standardisation, *Hot Environments – Estimation of the Heat Stress on a Working Man, Based on the WBGT-index* (1982, revised 1989), ISO 7243, BSI

International Commission on Non-Ionising Radiation Protection, *Guidelines for limiting exposure to time-varying electric, magnetic and electromagnetic fields (up to 300 GHz)* (1998), Health Phys. 74 No 4 494–522.

National Radiological Protection Board, *Board Statement: Advice on the 1998 ICNIRP Guidelines for Limiting Exposure to Time-varying Electric, Magnetic and Electromagnetic Fields (up to 300GHz)* (1999), Vol 10 No 2, NRPB

National Radiological Protection Board, *Board Statement on Restrictions on Human Exposure to Static and Time Varying Electromagnetic Fields and Radiation* (1993), Vol 4 No 5, NRPB

Oakley, EHN *see* Baxter, PJ et al (eds) *above*

Railtrack, *Safety Requirements for Track Safety: Medical & Alcohol & Drug Screening & Certification*, 'Appendix A: Minimum Medical Fitness Standards for Personal Track Safety' (June 2000), RT/LS/S/018, Railtrack

Siple, PA and Passell, CP, *Dry atmospheric cooling in sub-freezing temperatures* (1945), Proc.Am.Phil.Soc. 89:177–199

UK Offshore Operators Association, *Guidelines for medical aspects of fitness for offshore work* (2000), Issue number 4, UKOOA

Statutory materials

- Diving at Work Regulations 1997 (SI 1997/2776), HMSO

- Ionising Radiations Regulations 1999 (SI 1999/3232), HMSO

- Noise at Work Regulations 1989 (SI 1989/1790), HMSO

- Provision and Use of Work Equipment Regulations 1998 (SI 1998/2306), HMSO

- Railways (Safety Critical Work) Regulations 1994 (SI 1994/299), HMSO

- Work in Compressed Air Regulations 1996 (SI 1996/1656), HMSO

Addresses

The British Occupational Hygiene Society and the British Institute of Occupational Hygienists *see* CHEMICAL HAZARDS *above*

Chartered Institution of Building Services Engineers
222 Balham High Road
Balham
London
SW12 9BS

National Radiological Protection Board
Cilton
Didcot
OX11 0RQ

Mental health

Cooper, C, *Crisis Talks* (1997), Personnel Today, 2nd October 29–32

Edwards, JG, *Drug Choice in Depression: Selective Serotonin Reuptake Inhibitors or Tricyclic Antidepressants?* (1995), CNS Drugs 4:141–59

Edwards, JG and Anderson, I, *Systematic Review and Guide to Selection of Selective Serotonin Reuptake Inhibitors* (1999), CNS Drugs 57:507–33

EU Statistics Office, EUROSTAT Ill Health Module Labour Force Survey (1998/99)

Gramberadina, MA (ed), *An updated review: Refresher Course Syllabus, 'Recent Developments in Low-Back Pain'* (Waddell, G) (2002), ASP Press, Seattle

Health & Safety Executive, *Occupational health provision at work* (1993), Contract Research Report 57, HSE Books

Health & Safety Executive, *Scale of occupational stress – A further analysis of the impact of demographic factors and type of job* (2000), Contract Research Report 311, HSE Books

Health & Safety Executive, *Scale of occupational stress: The Bristol health at work study* (2000), Contract Research Report 265, HSE Books

Health & Safety Executive, *Stress at Work – A Guide for Employers* (1995)

Health & Safety Executive, *Survey of work related illness* (1990), HSE Books

Health & Safety Executive, *Survey of work related illness* (1995), HSE Books

Hindmarch, I, *Antidepressants, Other Psychotropics and Accident Risk in the Workplace*, in *Workshop on Prescriptive Medicine & Human Performance* (1998), Institute of Petroleum, London

Jenkins, R, *Prevention of Mental Ill Health at Work*, 'Prevalence of Mental Illness in the Workplace' (1992), HMSO

Kivimaki, M, et al, *Work Stress and Risk of Cardiovascular Mortality: Prospective Cohort Study of Industrial Employees*, BMJ, 325:857–860

Kloss, D, *Occupational Health Law* (3rd edition, 1998), Blackwell Science

Lloyd, GC, *Davidson's Principles and Practice of Medicine* (8th edition, 1999) Churchill Livingstone

Lucas, G, *Mental Health at Work* (1989) 97 Employment Gazette 637–676

Lucas, G, *Occupational Aspects of Whole-Person Healthcare*, in Christie, MJ, and Mellett, PG (eds), *Psychosomatic Approach: Contemporary Practice of Whole-Person Care* (1986), John Wiley

Maslach, Jackson and Leiter, *Burnout Inventory* (1996)

Quine, L, *Workplace Bullying in NHS Community Trusts: Staff Questionnaire Survey* (1999), BMJ, 318:228-232

Royal College of Psychiatrists, *Changing Minds* (1998–2003)

Smith, Brice, Collins, Matthews and McNamara, *The scale of occupational stress: A further analysis of the impact of demographic factors and type of job* (2000), Centre for Occupational and Health Psychology, School of Psychology, Cardiff University, ISBN 0 7176 1910 9, HSE Books

Van Tedder et al, *The Effectiveness of Conservative Treatment of Active/Chronic Low-Back Pain* (1999), EMGO Institute, Amsterdam

Waddell, G, *The Back Pain Revolution* (1998), Churchill Livingstone

Waddell, G *see also* Gramberadina, MA (ed) *above*

WBCSD, *Stakeholder Dialogue on Corporate Social Responsibility* (1998), 6–8 September 1998

Webster, L and Hacket, RK, *Administration and Policy in Mental Health* (1999), Vol 26, No 6 July

Welch, R and Tehrain, N, *Counselling in the Post Office: Prevention of Mental Ill Health at Work* (1992), HMSO

World Health Organisation, *Health aspects of wellbeing in working places: report of a WHO working group* (1980), Prague, 18–20 September 1979, Copenhagen: WHO (Euroreports & Studies 31 1980)

Statutory materials

- Disability Discrimination Act 1995, HMSO

- Management of Health and Safety at Work Regulations 1999 (SI 1999/3242), HMSO

Addresses

British Association of Counselling and Psychotherapy
1 Regent Place
Rugby
CV21 2PJ
tel: 0870 443 5252
e-mail: bac@bac.co.uk

Royal College of Psychiatrists
17 Belgrave Square
London
SW1X 8PG
tel: 020 7235 2351
fax: 020 7245 1231
e-mail: rcpsych@rcpsych.ac.uk

Personal protection

Abel, S and Rokas, D, *The effect of wearing time on hearing protector attenuation* (1986), Journal of Otolaryngology, Vol 15(5) 293–297

Alberti, PW, Riko, K and Abel, S *see* Royster, LH et al (eds)

Axlesson, A, Borchgrevink, H, Hamernik, RP, Hellstrom, P, Henderson, D, and Salvi, RJ (eds), *International Review of Field Studies of Hearing Protector Attenuation*, 'Scientific Basis of Noise-Induced Hearing Loss' (Berger, EH, Franks, JR and Lindgren, F) (1996), 361–377, Thieme Medical Publishers, Inc, New York

Berger, EH, Franks, JR and Lindgren, F *see* Axlesson, A et al (eds)

British Standards Institute, *Acoustics – Hearing Protectors* (1995), BS EN 24869-1, BSI

British Standards Institute, *Guide to implementing an effective respiratory protective device programme*, (2001), BS 4275, BSI

Comité Européen de Normalisation, *Respiratory Protective Devices – AX Gas Filters and Combined Filters Against Low Boiling Organic Compounds – Requirements, Testing, Marking* (1992), EN 371:1992, CEN, Brussels

Comité Européen de Normalisation, *Respiratory Protective Devices – Gas Filters and Combined Filters –Requirements, Testing, Marking* (1990), EN 141:1990, CEN, Brussels

Comité Européen de Normalisation, *Respiratory Protective Devices – SX Gas Filters and Combined Filters Against Specific Named Compounds – Requirements, Testing, Marking* (1992), EN 372:1992, CEN, Brussels

Commission of the European Communities, Directive 89/391/EEC (*on the introduction of measures to encourage improvements in the safety and health of workers at work*, 12 June 1989)

Commission of the European Communities, Directive 89/393/EEC (*on the minimum health and safety requirements for the use by workers of personal protective equipment at the workplace,* Third individual directive within the meaning of Article 16(1) of Directive, 30 November 1989)

Commission of the European Communities, Directive 89/686/EEC (*on the approximation of the laws of the member states relating to personal protective equipment,* 21 December 1989)

Department of Trade and Industry, *Personal Protective Equipment (EC Directive) Regulations 1992* (1992), HMSO

Edwards, RG, Hauser, WP, Moiseev, NA, Broderson, AB and Green, WW, *A Field Investigation of Noise Reduction Afforded by Insert-Type Hearing Protectors (Final Report)* (1977), NIOSH, Cincinnati, Ohio

Health & Safety Commission, *Construction (Head Protection) Regulations 1989* (1989), HMSO

Health & Safety Commission, *Control of Substances Hazardous to Health Regulations 1999* (1999), HSE Books

Health & Safety Commission, *Draft Approved Code of Practice for the Control of Carcinogenic Substances* (1988), HMSO

Health & Safety Commission, *General Control of Substances Hazardous to Health Approved Code of Practice, Carcinogens Approved Code of Practice and Biological Agents Approved Code of Practice* (1999), L5, HSE Books

Health & Safety Commission, *Health and Safety at Work etc Act 1974* (1974), HMSO

Health & Safety Commission, *Noise at Work Regulations 1989* (1989), HSE Books

Health & Safety Commission, *Personal Protective Equipment at Work Regulations 1992* (1992), HMSO

Health & Safety Commission, *Safe Work in Confined Spaces: Approved Code of Practice for The Confined Spaces Regulations 1997* (1997), L101, HSE Books

Health & Safety Executive, *Respiratory Protective Equipment, a Practical Guide for Users* (1998), Health and Safety Series Booklet (1998a) HSG 53, HSE Books

Health & Safety Executive, *Reducing Noise at Work* (1998), L108, HSE Books

Hempstock, TI and Hill, E, *The attenuation of some hearing protectors as used in the workplace* (1990), Annals of Occupational Hygiene, Vol 34(5), 453–470

Howie, RM, *A specification for audiometric technique in hearing conservation* (1990), Occupational Health Review, June/July, 21–23.

Howie, RM, *The reality of PPE performance in the workplace* (1992), Proceedings of the First International Scientific Conference, Brussels, International Occupational Hygiene Association, Derby

Lempert, BL and Edwards, RG, *Field Investigations Of Noise Reduction Afforded By Insert-Type Hearing Protectors* (1983), American Industrial Hygiene Association Journal, Vol 44: 894–902

Ojanen, K, Sarantila, R, Klen, T, Lotjonen, A and Kangas, J, *Evaluation of the Efficiency and Comfort of Protective Clothing during Herbicide Spraying* (1992), Applied Occupational and Environmental Hygiene, Vol 7: 815–819

van-Roouij, GM, van-Lieshout, EMA, Bodelier-Bade, MM and Jongeneelen, FJ, *Effect of the Reduction of Skin Contamination on the Internal Dose of Creosote Workers Exposed to Polycyclic Aromatic Hydrocarbons* (1993), Scandinavian Journal of Work, Environment and Health, Vol 19(3) 200–207.

Royster, LH, *An Evaluation of the Effectiveness of Two Different Insert Types of Ear Protection in Preventing TTS in an Industrial Environment* (1980), American Industrial Hygiene Association Journal, Vol 41: 161–169

Royster, LH, Hart, FD, and Stewart, ND (eds) *Proceedings of the 1981 National Conference on Noise Control Engineering, Raleigh, North Carolina, 8–10 June 1981,* 'Hearing Protectors: Attenuation in Practice and Problems in Fitting' (Alberti, PW, Riko, K and Abel, S) (1981), Noise-Con 81 137–140, Noise Control Foundation, New York

Statutory materials

- Confined Spaces Regulations 1997 (SI 1997/1713), HMSO

- Construction (Head Protection) Regulations 1989 (SI 1989/2209), HMSO

- Control of Substances Hazardous to Health Regulations 2002 (SI 2002/2677), HMSO

- Noise at Work Regulations 1989 (SI 1989/1790), HMSO

- Personal Protective Equipment at Work Regulations 1992 (SI 1992/2966), HMSO

- Personal Protective Equipment (EC Directive) Regulations 1992 (SI 1992/3139), HMSO

Useful web addresses

Web address	Organisation
1. General health and safety	
www.hse.gov.uk/hsehome.htm	The Health & Safety Executive (HSE) website home page.
http://www.hsebooks.co.uk/homepage.html	HSE Books catalogue of publications. *(cont'd)*

www.hmso.gov.uk	Her Majesty's Stationery Office. Full text of UK Acts of Parliament since 1988 and statutory instruments since 1987.
www.hsedirect.com	A site offering facility to download HSE documents, legislation etc, but you will need a subscription or pay for day ticket.
http://europe.osha.eu.int	The European Occupational Health and Safety Agency Website. Set up by the EU to provide the public and professionals with information on health and safety matters.
www.ccohs.ca	A collaborative site between the EU and the Canadian Centre for Occupational Health.
www.uksafety.net/	Site for searching for safety consultants and products and services. Orientated more towards safety than health.
www.info4education.com	An invaluable site with full texts of all UK legislation, HSE leaflets, guidances, approved codes of practice, British Standards etc, but needs a subscription.
www.tuc.org.uk/	A helpful site from the TUC offering information on occupational health and safety matters as they affect workers.
www.safetynews.co.uk	Health and safety information on a wide range of topics. Freely available and contains a very comprehensive set of links to other health and safety sites.
www.eurofound.ie	The European Foundation for the Improvement of Living and Working Conditions.
www.icoh.org.sg/	International Commission for Occupational Health (ICOH) website. Contains it's own useful information and provides links to other occupational health sites.

www.ilo.org/public/english/ protection/safework/cis/ index.htm	The International Labour Organisation's (ILO), Occupational Safety and Health Information Centre
www.who.int/peh/ Occupational_health/ occindex.html	The World Health Organisation (WHO) website with a gateway to many useful Occupational Health sites worldwide.
www.cdc.gov/niosh/about. html	The (United States) National Institute for Occupational Safety and Health. A huge resource of occupational health Information
www.healthandsafety managment.co.uk	Jordan' health and safety management site providing health and safety managers with up to date news.
www.maybo.com	Maybo Limited are conflict management specialists who have direct experience of advising high-profile organisations on how to manage workplace violence and conflict.
www.osh.net	A useful entry point to wide range of health and safety information.
2. *Ergonomics*	
www.ergonomics.org.uk	The Ergonomics Society website.
www.backpain.org	A source of information on back pain and back care.
http://ergo.human.cornell.edu	A gateway site to a wide range of useful ergonomics information.
www.mmm.com/cws/selfhelp/ introto.html	3M's site practical information site on office ergonomics.
3. *Health and medical information*	
http://www.nhsplus.nhs.uk/	NHS Plus is a network of NHS occupational health departments across England, supplying quality services to non-NHS employers. NHS Plus offers support to industry, commerce, and the public sector, with a focus on small and medium-sized enterprises. *(cont'd)*

305

www.vh.org	The Virtual Hospital from University of Iowa. Information on a wide range of illness but not all occupationally related.
www.netdoctor.co.uk	Explains many common illnesses and contains an extensive medicines database.
http://www.doh.gov.uk/traveladvice/	The Department of Health site for travel medical advice.
http://www.nlm.nih.gov/medlineplus/	One of the gateways to access MEDLINE, an extensive bibliographic database of medical literature. Payment usually necessary to download original papers.
4. Mental health and stress	
http://www.stress.org/	An American site dealing with stress issues. Contains pages on job stress.
www.suzylamplugh.org/index.htm	The Suzy Lamplugh Trust's site providing information on personal safety, violence and bullying at work and stress.
http://www.healthatwork.org.uk/work/mental.asp	Provided by Greater Glasgow NHS Board's Health Promotion Department. Site deals with mental health at work issues including stress.
5. Chemical safety	
http://msds.pdc.cornell.edu/msdssrch.asp	Cornell University's searchable material safety data sheets. Searchable and very useful.
http://www.coshh-essentials.org.uk/Home.asp	A resource from HSE in collaboration with the TUC and CBI to help undertake a COSHH assessment.
http://physchem.ox.ac.uk/MSDS/	Chemical safety database form Oxford University.

Table of Cases

A-G's Reference (No 2 of 1999) [2000] 2 Cr App R 207,
   [2000] 3 All ER 182 — 2.7
Clark v TDG Ltd t/a Novacold [1999] IRLR 318 — 2.33
College of Ripon & York St John (Appellants) v Hobbs
   (respondent) [2002] IRLR 185 — 2.31
Commission of the European Communities v United Kingdom
   [1994] ECR I-02435 (joint judgment for Cases C-382/92 and
   C-383/92) — 4.35
East Lindsay District Council v Daubney [1977] IRLR 188 — 2.19
Hardman (Mrs JB) v Mallon (Miss M) (t/a Orchard Lodge
   Nursing Home) [2002] IRLR 516 — 2.1
Heinz (HJ) v Kenrick [2000] IRLR 144 — 2.33
Holmes v Whittington & Porter Ltd unreported — 2.21
International Sports Co Ltd v Thomson [1980] IRLR 340 — 2.17, 2.18
Kenny v Hampshire Constabulary [1999] IRLR 76 — 2.33
Lynock v Cereal Packaging Ltd [1988] IRLR 510 — 2.17, 2.18
Morgan v University of Staffordshire [2002] IRLR 190 — 2.35
Mountenay v Bernard Mathews plc (1994) 5 Med LR 293 — 2.12
Nahhas v Pier House (Cheyne Walk) Management Ltd and
   Another, The Times, 10 February 1984 — 2.13
O'Brien v The Prudential Assurance Co Ltd [1979] IRLR 140 — 2.14
R v Swan Hunter Shipbuilders Ltd and Telemeter Installations
   Ltd [1981] IRLR 403 — 2.2
Rugamer (Appellant) v Sony Music Entertainment UK Ltd
   (Respondents); McNicol (Appellant) v Balfour Beatty Rail
   Maintenance Ltd (Respondents) [2001] IRLR 644 — 2.31
Spencer v Paragon Wallpapers [1976] IRLR 376 — 2.19
Surry Police v Marshall (2002) EAT/774/01 — 2.9
Sutherland (Chairman of The Governors of St Thomas Becket
   RC High School) (Defendant/Appellant) v Hatton (Claimant/
   Respondent); Somerset County Council (Defendants/Appellants)
   v Barber (Claimant/Respondent); Sandwell Metropolitan Borough
   Council (Defendants/Appellants) v Jones (Claimant/Respondent)
   Baker Refractories Ltd (Defendants/Appellants) v Bishop
   (Claimant/Respondent) [2002] IRLR 263 — 2.35
Tarasoff v Regents of the University of California, 551 P 2d
   334 (Cal 1976) — 2.34
W v Egdell [1990] 1 All ER 835 — 2.34
Walker v Northumberland County Council [1995] IRLR 35 — 8.6
Walpole v Rolls Royce Ltd [1980] IRLR 343 — 2.17, 2.18
Walton v TAC Construction Materials Ltd [1987] IRLR 351 — 2.14
Young v The Post Office [2002] IRLR 660 — 2.30

Table of Statutes

Access to Health Records Act
1990   3.23

Access to Medical Reports Act
1988   3.23

Data Protection Act 1998 2.10, 2.26
   s 2(e)   2.10

Disability Discrimination Act
1995   2.11, 2.21, 2.22,
2.31, 2.33, 2.35,
3.12, 8.8, 11.3
   s 5(1)–(3)   2.33
   s 6(2)–(4), (6)   2.33
   Sch 1 para 4   2.11, 2.32

Employment Protection Act 1975
  8.34

Employment Rights Act 1996
  4.35
   s 98(1)(b)   2.18
   (2)(a), (3)   2.20

Factories Act 1961   4.4, 9.14

Food Safety Act 1990   5.38

Health and Safety at Work etc Act
1974   1.1, 2.7, 3.28,
4.26, 5.3, 6.2,
9.20, 10.6
   s 2   2.1, 2.2, 3.28,
7.5, 7.76
   (1)   1.1, 2.2, 7.24,
7.62, 10.4
   (2)   7.24
    (c)   1.10
   (3)   1.8
   (4)   4.35
   s 3   3.28, 10.4
   s 4   10.4
   s 6   3.28, 6.3
   (1)   6.3
   ss 7, 8   4.35

Human Rights Act 1998
   s 8(1)–(2)   2.34

Radioactive Substances Act 1993
  7.79

Regulation of Investigatory
Powers Act 2000   2.26

Road Traffic Act 1988   4.8, 11.9
   Pt I   8.12

Table of Statutory Instruments

Chemicals (Hazard Information
and Packaging for Supply)
Regulations 2002
(SI 2002 No 1689)   6.2, 6.4, 6.13,
6.15, 6.17, 6.20
Reg 2   6.5
Reg 3   6.6
Reg 4   6.7
Reg 5   6.8
Reg 8   6.9
Sch 2   6.7, 6.10
Sch 3   6.11
Sch 4   6.8
Confined Spaces Regulations
1997
(SI 1997 No 1713)   9.2, 9.20
Reg 5   9.20
Construction (Head Protection)
Regulations 1989
(SI 1989 No 2209)   9.2, 9.14, 9.21
Reg 3   9.15
Reg 4   9.16
Reg 5   9.17
Reg 6   9.18
Control of Asbestos at Work
Regulations 2002
(SI 2002 No 2675)   9.2, 9.19, 9.22,
9.31, 10.4
Control of Lead at Work
Regulations 2002
(SI 2002 No 2676)   9.2, 9.22, 10.4
Control of Substances Hazardous
to Health Regulations 2002
(SI 2002 No 2677)   4.26, 5.1–5.3,
5.15, 6.1, 9.2, 9.3, 9.19, 9.22, 10.4,
10.6, 10.17, 11.10
Reg 6   5.2
Reg 7   9.4, 9.25
Reg 8   5.2, 9.5
Reg 9   5.2, 9.6, 9.7
Reg 11   5.2, 5.15, 5.20, 5.24
Reg 12   5.2, 9.8, 9.9, 9.27

Health and Safety (Consultation
with Employees) Regulations
1996 (SI 1996 No 1513)   4.35
Health and Safety (Display
Screen Equipment) Regulations
1992 (SI 1992 No 2792)   3.4, 3.8,
3.34, 7.24, 7.56, 7.58, 10.4, 11.10
Sch 3   7.30
(e), (g)   7.24
Health and Safety (First Aid)
Regulations 1981
(SI 1981 No 917) 4.4, 4.5, 4.8, 10.4
Reg 2   4.4
Reg 3(1), (2)   4.4
Reg 4   4.4
Ionising Radiation (Medical
Exposure) Regulations 2000
(SI 2000 No 1059)   7.79
Ionising Radiations Regulations
1999
(SI 1999 No 3232) 7.79–7.81, 7.83
Regs 2, 13   7.81
Management of Health and Safety
at Work Regulations 1999
(SI 1999 No 3242)   4.5, 4.26, 4.27,
4.35, 5.3, 7.5, 7.7, 7.14, 7.18, 7.21
7.21, 7.24, 7.56, 7.62, 7.63, 8.7,
10.4, 10.8, 11.10, 11.20
Reg 3   2.2, 7.12, 7.62, 7.76
(1)   2.37
(6)   7.62
Reg 7   7.62, 11.4
(8)   11.10
Reg 16   2.1
Manual Handling Operations
Regulations 1992
(SI 1992 No 2793)   3.8, 7.56, 7.58,
10.4, 11.10
Medicines (Administration of
Radioactive Substances)
(Amendment) Regulations 1995
(SI 1995 No 2147)   7.79

Noise at Work Regulations 1989
(SI 1989 No 1790)   7.5–7.7, 9.2,
          9.10, 9.53, 10.4, 10.6, 11.10
     Reg 7   9.11
     Reg 8   9.12
     Regs 9–11   9.13
Notification of New Substances
     Regulations 1993
     (SI 1993 No 3050)   6.7
Personal Protective Equipment at
     Work Regulations 1992
     (SI 1992 No 2966)   7.56, 9.2, 9.4,
          9.19, 10.4
     Reg 5   9.19
     Sch 1   9.12, 9.15
Personal Protective Equipment
     (EC Directive) Regulations 1992
     (SI 1992 No 3139)   9.20
Provision and Use of Work
     Equipment Regulations 1998
     (SI 1998 No 2306)   7.30, 7.56
     Reg 13   7.24
     Reg 21   7.30
Public Health (Infectious
     Diseases) Regulations 1988
     (SI 1988 No 1546)   5.5
Radiation (Emergency
     Preparedness and Public
     Information) Regulations 2001

(SI 2001 No 2975)   7.83
Radioactive Material (Road
     Transport) Regulations 2002
     (SI 2002 No 1093)   7.79
Railways (Safety Critical Work)
     Regulations 1994
     (SI 1994 No 299)   11.9
Reporting of Injuries, Diseases
     and Dangerous Occurrences
     Regulations 1995
     (SI 1995 No 3163)   2.2, 2.3, 2.5,
          2.37, 3.32, 4.25, 5.16, 7.14
     Sch 2   2.4
     Sch 3   2.4, 2.6, 5.4
Safety Representatives and Safety
     Committees Regulations 1977
     (SI 1977 No 500)   4.35
Telecommunications (Lawful
     Business Practice) (Interception
     of Communications)
     Regulations 2000
     (SI 2000 No 2699)   2.26
Workplace (Health, Safety and
     Welfare) Regulations 1992
     (SI 1992 No 3004) 7.24, 7.30, 7.62
     Regs 5, 6   7.62
     Reg 7   7.24, 7.62
     Reg 8   7.30, 7.62
     Regs 9, 10   7.62

Table of European Legislation

Council Directive 67/548/EEC
(on the approximation of laws, regulations and administrative provisions relating to the classification, packaging and labelling of dangerous substances, 27 June 1967)   6.4

Council Directive 89/391/EEC
(on the introduction of measures to encourage improvements in the safety and health of workers at work, 12 June 1989)
Article 6   9.1

Council Directive 89/393/EEC
(on the minimum health and safety requirements for the use by workers of personal protective equipment at the work-

place, third individual Directive within the meaning of Article 16(1) of Directive, 30 November 1989)
Article 8   9.29

Council Directive 90/394/EEC
(on the protection of workers from the risks related to exposure to carcinogens at work, 28 June 1990)   6.19

Council Directive 2002/44/EC
(on the minimum health and safety requirements regarding the exposure of workers to the risks arising from physical agents (vibration), 25 June 2002)
7.12–7.14

Index

A

Absence. *See* Sickness absence
Active noise attenuation devices
    9.50
Agencies   11.13
AIDs   5.18
Air conditioning   11.3
Air velocity   7.16, 7.23
Alcohol abuse   8.16, 8.32–8.34
Animals   5.21–5.25
Antidepressants   8.16–8.17
Anxiety   8.4, 8.18, 8.19
Approved Codes of Practice
    9.7–9.8, 9.21
Approved Supply List   6.12–6.20
Armed forces   8.35
Asbestos   9.31, 9.56
ASHRAE Thermal Comfort Scale
    7.25
Associateship of the Faculty of
    Occupational Medicine   11.19
Asthma   1.4, 5.8, 5.16
Audiometry   7.7
Audits   1.20

B

Back disorders   7.33, 8.23
Bakeries, risk assessment in   5.16
Behavioural toxicity   8.16
Benchmarking   4.2
Beta-napthylamine   6.1
Bilharziasis   5.36
Biological hazards   5.1–5.38, 10.9
Blanching   7.10
Blood borne viruses   5.17–5.20, 5.31
Blood tests   5.24
Bovine spongiform encephalopathy
    5.22
Breaks   7.41
British Institute of Occupational
    Hygiene   3.11, 11.21
Bulb temperatures   7.16, 7.23
Bullying   2.36, 8.10
Burnout   8.31
Butanone   6.16

C

Cable bugs   7.69
Carcinogens   6.1, 6.17, 6.19–6.20
Case conferences   4.24
Case management   4.23–4.24
Case studies   3.33–3.34
Certificates of first aid competence
    4.4
Chemical Abstract Service   6.16
Chemicals   4.26, 5.14, 6.1–6.20,
    10.9, 10.16
Chiropractors   11.23
Cholera   5.34
Chronium compounds   6.19
Clients   4.2
Clinical management   8.12
Clothier Report   2.9
Clothing   7.16, 7.23, 7.51, 9.55–9.58
Cold environment, working in
    7.20–7.23, 7.49
Colour   7.28
Communication, importance of   3.33
Confidentiality   2.34, 3.21–3.24, 6.15
Confined spaces   9.20
Conflicts of interest   1.8
Conjunctivitis   5.8
Consent forms   2.23
Construction workers   5.25
Consultants   11.4
Control of substances hazardous to
    health   5.2, 9.4–9.8, 9.31
Corporate manslaughter   2.7
Corporate social responsibility   8.10
Counsellors   3.15, 8.11, 8.27
Criminal offences   1.4, 2.6–2.7, 6.20
Customers   4.2
Cyclothymic personalities   8.19

D

Damages   1.4
Dangerous substances and
    preparations, classification of
    6.7, 6.10–6.12, 6.19, 6.20
Data protection   2.10
Deafness   7.4–7.7

Deaths in service 4.34
Definition of employee health 1.1–1.10
Definition of health 1.3
Definition of occupational health 1.3
Dengue 5.36
Depression 2.32, 3.33, 8.3, 8.16, 8.20, 8.23, 8.25
Dermatitis 1.2, 7.55, 7.68
Design 3.13, 7.41–7.43, 7.58, 10.22
Destigmatisation 8.15
Detectives, use of private 2.26
Diptheria 5.36
Disability discrimination 2.31–2.33
  depression 2.32, 3.33
  disability, definition of 2.31
  employer responsibility 2.33
  guidance 2.32
  mental health 8.14
  psychosomatic conditions 2.31
  reasonable adjustments 2.11, 2.21, 2.33, 4.11
  recruitment 2.11
  sickness absence, long-term 2.21
  stress 2.35
Disciplinary procedure 2.24, 2.27–2.29, 4.11, 4.13
Diseases, reporting 2.5
Dismissal 2.14, 2.18, 2.20, 2.36, 4.11
Display screen equipment 7.24, 7.28, 7.30, 7.55, 7.66–7.68
Doctors. See also General practitioners, Occupational physicians 3.9, 11.9
Drivers 11.9
Drug abuse 8.16, 8.32–8.34
Drugs, prescription 8.16–8.17

E

Ear muffs 9.50, 9.51
Ear plugs 9.50, 9.51–9.52
Ear protection 9.12–9.13, 9.50–9.54
EC law
  carcinogens 6.19
  chemical hazards 6.4, 6.19
  personal protective equipment 9.1
  risk assessment 10.3
  safety representatives 4.35
  vibration 7.12

Electromagnetic radiation 7.72–7.76
Emergencies 7.83–7.86
Employment Medical Advisory Service 3.31
Endotoxins 5.11
Enforcement 3.28–3.32
  Employment Medical Advisory Service 3.31
  entry, powers of 3.28
  first aid 4.4
  food preparation 3.28
  Health and Safety Executive, role of 3.28
  improvement notices 3.29
  inspectors, role of 3.28
  local authorities, role of 3.28
  notices 1.4, 3.30
  prohibition notices 3.30
  reporting 3.32
Entry, powers of 3.28
Environmental health officers 1.4
Epileptic seizures 7.55
Equipment. See also Personal protective equipment 7.24, 7.29, 7.42
Ergonomics 3.13, 7.31–7.58, 10.9, 10.16, 11.22
Erythema 7.68
Ethical practice 3.26
Ethyl methy ketone 6.16
European Inventory of Commercial Chemical Substances 6.16
European Union. See EC law
Exhaustion 8.31
External expertise 4.4, 7.81, 11.1–11.23
External health teams 3.7
Extrinsic allergic alveolitis 5.9, 5.10
Eyestrain 7.29

F

Facial dermatitis 7.55
Faculty of Occupational Medicine 2.1
Fainting 7.17
Family, right to respect for the 2.34
Filters 9.44, 9.47–9.48
Fines 1.4
First aid 4.4–4.10
Fitness for work 1.9–1.10, 3.19
Fluorescent lights 7.29

Food heath 3.28, 5.37–5.38
Force 7.39

G

Gas and vapour filters 9.48
General Medical Council 2.1
General practitioners 2.22, 3.9, 4.23, 8.10, 11.2
Glare 7.28, 7.30
Gram-negative bacteria 5.11

H

Hand-arm vibration 7.8–7.10, 7.14, 7.48
Hand-held tools 7.8, 7.42, 7.48
Harassment 2.36
Head protection 9.15–9.18
Health and safety, meaning of 1.2
Health and Safety Executive 1.4, 11.2
  doctors appointed by 11.17
  Employment Medical Advisory Service 3.31
  enforcement 3.28, 4.4
  inspectors 3.28
  measurement 4.3
  mental disabilities 8.3
  reporting 5.4
Health questionnaires 2.9, 3.24
Health records 2.9, 3.23, 5.24
Health surveillance 4.32–4.34
  biological hazards 5.2
  covert 2.24, 2.26
  deaths in service 4.34
  external agencies 11.5–11.10
  individual health status 4.33
  ionising radiation 7.82
  malingerers 2.24, 2.26
  medical retirements 4.33
  noise 7.7
  personal hearing protectors 9.53
  risk assessment 10.1, 10.18
  stress 8.5
  vibration 7.14
  zoonoses 5.24
Hearing loss 7.4–7.7, 7.47
Heat stress disorders 7.17–7.19, 9.57
Heat stroke 7.17

Height of work surface 7.44
Hepatitis 5.18, 5.20, 5.31
HIV 5.18
Home and work, interaction between 1.6
Home, right to respect for the 2.34
Home visits 2.34
Hot environments, working in 7.16
Human factors specialists 3.13
Human Rights Act 1998 2.34
Humidifiers 5.10
Humidity 7.16, 7.23, 7.24, 7.71
Hypersensitivity pneumonitis 5.10
Hypothermia 7.20

I

Identification doctrine 2.7
Identification of hazards 4.27
Illuminance 7.28, 7.29, 7.30
Immunisation 5.26, 5.29–5.31, 5.33–5.35
Improvement notices 1.4, 3.29
Incident Contact Centre 2.6
Individual health status 4.33
Industrial nurses 11.20
Infectious diseases, notification of 5.5
Ingestion 6.1
Inhalation 6.1, 6.17
In-house teams 3.8, 11.5–11.10
Inspections of personal protective equipment 9.39
Inspectors, role of 3.28
Instructions 9.8
Insulation 7.16
International Commission on Non-Ionising Radiation Protection 7.77
Ionising radiation 7.78–7.86
Irritants 5.7, 5.14

L

Labelling 6.10
Laboratory tests 9.51, 9.56
Layout of workstations 7.46
Leakages 9.56
Legionella 5.12, 5.13
Light 7.26–7.30, 7.50, 7.65
Local authorities 3.28

Long-term or acute sickness absence
2.19–2.22, 4.13
Lower limb disorders 7.35
Lying, disciplinary procedures for
2.14

M

Maintenance 9.6, 9.15, 9.34,
9.38–9.40, 9.46–9.48
Malaria 5.32
Malingerers 2.23–2.29
Managers and occupational health
practitioners, relationship
between 3.25
Managing occupational health
3.1–3.34
aims and objectives 3.1
ethical practice 3.26
morale 3.3
process of 3.3
productivity 3.3
risk assessment 3.3
small and medium-sized
enterprises 3.2
stress 8.27
support, kinds of 3.4
Manual handling 7.54
Marketing 4.2
Measurement 4.3, 4.14–4.22, 4.24
Medical assessments 1.7, 2.9, 2.21,
8.35
Medical certificates 3.33
Medical evidence, conflicting 2.18,
2.21
Medline 6.20
Meningitis 5.36
Mental health 8.1–8.36
Medical reports, consent of
employees and 2.23
Merck Index 6.1, 6.16
Metal working fluids 5.10
Micro shocks 7.70
Mixtures 6.5
Mobile phones 7.75
Monitoring hazards and ill-health
4.26–4.31
Mood swings 8.19
Musculoskeletal disorders
7.32–7.56, 8.3,
11.22–11.23

N

National Arrangements for
Incidents Involving
Radioactivity 7.85
National Institute for Occupational
Safety and Health (USA) 6.19
National Radiological Protection
Board 7.77, 7.81
Negligence 1.4, 2.13
Neurosis 8.19
NHS Plus standards 3.27
Noise 7.2–7.7, 7.47, 9.10–9.13
Non-ionising radiation 7.72–7.76
Nurses
agencies 11.8
code of professional conduct 2.1
industrial 11.20
Nursing and Midwifery Council
2.1, 3.10, 11.20
qualifications 11.20
referrals to 3.16–3.20, 3.33
title of nurse 11.20
training 3.10, 11.20

O

Obsessional personalities 8.19
Occupational diseases 1.6
Occupational health and safety 1.2
Occupational health nurses 11.20
Occupational health teams 3.6–3.8,
3.21–3.24
Occupational hygienists 3.11, 11.21
Occupational physicians 3.16–3.20,
3.25, 3.33, 11.19
Occupational health service 4.23
Occupational health systems
4.1–4.37
Occupational therapists 3.12
Off site, working 4.7
Over the counter medication
8.16–8.17

P

Pacing 7.41
Packaging 6.10
Paints 6.17, 6.16
Paranoid personalities 8.19
Performance management systems
4.2

Personal hearing protectors
9.50–9.54
Personal protective equipment 7.51,
9.1–9.59
Approved Code of Practice
9.8, 9.21
asbestos 9.31
clothing 9.55–9.58
compatibility of, ensuring 9.33
confined spaces 9.20
consequences of exposure,
informing wearers of 9.27
EC law 9.1
head protection 9.15–9.18
hierarchy of control 9.1
inspection 9.39
maintenance 9.15, 9.34, 9.38–9.40
match to wearer 9.30
monitoring 9.41
noise 9.10–9.13
occupational hygienists 11.21
personal hearing protectors
9.50–9.54
reasonably practicable controls,
implementing 9.52
record usage 9.40
residual exposure, select
equipment adequate to 9.28
residual protection, identification
of people who need 9.26
respiratory 9.20, 9.34, 9.44–9.49
risk, creating 9.32
risk assessment 9.24, 10.15
selection, involve wearers in 9.29
setting up and running effective
programmes 9.23–9.42
storage 9.37
supervision 9.36
training 9.34
types of 9.43–9.58
wear periods, minimizing 9.35
Personality characteristics 8.19
Personality tests 4.12
Physical hazards
7.1–7.86, 10.9, 10.16
Physical work environment
7.47–7.51
Physiotherapists 3.14, 11.23
Pilots 8.16
Polio 5.30
Post-natal depression 8.25

Post-traumatic stress disorder
8.27–8.30
Posture 7.38
Precautionary principle 7.75
Precautions
biological hazards 5.13
blood borne viruses 5.19, 5.20
food borne diseases 5.37
legionella 5.12
malaria 5.32
risk assessment 10.1, 10.6, 10.15
sick building syndrome 7.63
skin disorders 5.15
travellers' diseases 5.32, 5.36
zoonoses 5.21, 5.25
**Pre-employment health
questionnaires** 2.9, 3.24
**Pre-employment medical
assessments** 1.7, 2.9, 8.35
Pregnant workers 2.1, 7.82, 8.25
Preparations 6.5
Prescription drugs 8.16–8.17
Print 6.16
Private life, right to respect for 2.34
Products 4.2
**Professional advisers,
confidentiality and** 3.21
Professional bodies 2.1
Professional resources 4.1
Prohibition notices 3.30
Proprietary products 6.18
Prosecutions, register of 1.4
Psychiatrists 8.8
Psychological effects 7.3, 7.5, 7.15,
7.52–7.53, 10.9
Psychosomatic conditions 2.31,
8.22–8.23
Psychotherapy 8.12

R

Radiant heat/cold 7.16, 7.23
Radiation 7.55
Railways 11.9
Reasonable adjustments 2.11, 2.21,
2.33, 4.11
Reasonably practicable 2.2, 2.7, 9.52
Record-keeping 4.20, 4.22, 4.24,
4.33
Recovery 4.30
Recruitment 2.8–2.14

Referrals, making 3.16–3.20, 3.33,
4.13, 4.20, 4.24,
4.33
Rehabilitation 8.12
Repetition 7.40
Repetitive strain injuries 3.34, 7.34
Replies to referrals 3.20
Reporting
  criminal offences 2.6
  definition 2.4
  diseases, reportable 2.5
  enforcement 3.32
  Health and Safety Executive 5.4
  Incident Contact Centre 2.6
  industrially linked diseases 2.4
  major injuries 2.4
  minor injuries 2.4
  notification, method of 2.6
  responsibility for 3.32
  risk assessment 2.5, 4.25, 10.18,
10.19
  sickness absence 8.37
  statutory duties 2.3–2.6
  vibration 7.14
  violence 2.36, 4.25
Reputation 1.4
Resources 4.3
Respiratory disorders 5.7–5.13
Respiratory protective equipment
9.20, 9.34,
9.44–9.49
Rest 7.19, 7.41
Retirement 4.33, 8.37
Return to work, managing 2.30
Rhinitis 5.8
Risk assessment 1.7, 7.57–7.58,
10.1–10.22
  asthma 5.16
  audits 10.20
  bakeries 5.16
  biological hazards 5.2–5.3, 5.13,
10.9, 10.16
  blood borne viruses
5.17, 5.19–5.20
  case studies 10.21–10.22
  categorising risk 4.31, 10.13
  checklist 7.58
  chemical hazards 6.1, 6.12, 6.20,
10.9, 10.16
  cold 7.21–7.22
  competence 10.5–10.6

  construction workers 5.25
  control of substances hazardous to
    health 5.2
  controls 4.29, 10.11, 10.15, 10.16
  definition 10.3
  design 7.58, 10.22
  EC law 10.3
  ergonomics 7.57–7.58, 10.9, 10.16
  first aid 4.5–4.8
  food borne diseases 5.37
  food health 5.38
  hazards, meaning of 10.1
  health surveillance 10.1, 10.18
  heat stress disorder 7.18–7.19
  identifying hazards 10.10
  ionising radiation 7.79–7.80, 7.82
  legal requirements 10.4
  managing occupational health 3.3
  mental health 8.7
  monitoring hazards and ill-health
4.28, 10.17
  musculoskeletal disorders 7.56
  noise 7.6
  non-ionising radiation 7.76
  occupational hygienists 3.11, 11.21
  personal protective equipment
9.24, 10.15
  persons who can undertake 10.5
  physical hazards 10.9, 10.16
  precautions 10.1, 10.6, 10.15
  pregnancy 2.1
  priorities, setting 10.14
  psychological hazards 10.9
  recording 10.18, 10.19
  reporting 2.5, 4.25
  reviews 10.20
  risk management 1.7, 1.10, 2.2, 10.1
  safety representatives 10.7
  sewage treatment 5.20
  sick building syndrome 7.62–7.65
  sickness absence, costs of 10.2
  skin disorders 5.15–5.16
  specialist support 10.8, 10.21
  staff, role of 10.7
  surveys 7.57
  technology, use of 10.15
  temperature 7.18–7.21, 7.24–7.25
  travellers' health 5.26, 5.36
  vibration 7.12
  violence 2.37
  zoonoses 5.21, 5.23, 5.25

Routine occupational health
  management   11.10

S

Safety, health and   1.2
Safety committees   4.36
Safety data sheets
      6.8, 6.14, 6.17, 6.20
Safety representatives   4.35, 10.7
Sample consent forms   2.23
Sax's Dangerous Products   6.16
Screening   1.9, 7.14, 8.34
Seizures   7.55
Self-certification   2.25
Sensitisers   1.2, 5.7–5.8, 5.14
Service organisations,
  characteristics of   4.2
Service users   4.2
Services, types of   3.5
Setting up systems   4.3
Sewage treatment   5.20
Sharing external services   11.15
Short-term absence   2.15–2.18, 4.11,
  4.13
Sick building syndrome   7.59–7.65,
  11.3
Sick pay schemes   2.25, 4.12, 4.13
Sickness absence   4.11–4.14
  age   4.12
  benefits of reducing   4.11
  case conferences   4.24
  case study   4.11
  checklist   3.16
  contributory factors   4.12
  costs of   10.2
  disability discrimination   4.11
  disciplinary procedure   2.28–2.29
  frequency distribution   4.20
  guidance, standard sickness   2.25
  impact of   1.4
  incidence, notion of   4.15, 4.24
  investigations   4.13
  measurement   4.14–4.22, 4.24
  mental health   8.3, 8.11, 8.12,
    8.36–8.37
  patterns of   4.13
  percentage working time lost   4.21,
    4.24
  personality tests   4.12
  population at risk   4.19

prevalence   4.15, 4.18, 4.24
record-keeping
      4.20, 4.22, 4.24, 4.33
referrals   3.16, 3.33, 4.20
reports   4.24, 4.33
retirement   8.37
risk assessment   10.2
self-certification   2.25
severity   4.17, 4.24
sickness absence   8.36
size of work groups   4.12
spells per person, mean
  number of   4.16
women   4.12
working conditions   4.12
Sickness presence   8.16
Side-effects of prescription drugs
      8.17
Sitting versus standing   7.45
Skin disorders   1.2, 5.6, 5.14–5.16,
  6.1, 7.55, 7.68
Sleep   8.24
Solutions   6.5
Sound   7.2–7.7
Specialist support   10.8, 10.21, 11.14
Standards   3.27, 7.2–7.7, 7.14, 7.47
Static electricity   7.66–7.71
Statutory duties   2.1–2.6
Stigma of mental disabilities   8.8
Stress   1.6, 2.35, 8.2, 8.3,
  8.26–8.31, 8.38
age and sex-related distribution
      8.5
  burnout   8.31
  causes of   8.26
  counselling   8.27
  definition   8.2
  disability discrimination   2.35
  ergonomics   7.35
  exhaustion   8.31
  foreseeability   2.35
  guidance   2.35
  health surveillance   8.5
  heat   7.17–7.18
  legal requirements   8.6
  management   8.26
  noise   7.3
  physical symptoms   8.21
  post-traumatic stress disorder
        8.28–8.30
Support   1.5, 1.8, 3.4

T

Task designs 7.41
Task lights 7.28
Technology, use of 10.15
Temperature 7.15–7.25, 7.49
Testing 4.12, 6.1–6.2, 9.6, 9.51, 9.56
Tetanus 5.28
Thermal comfort 7.23, 7.24–7.25
Tick-borne encephalitis 5.36
Training
 control of substances hazardous
  to health 9.8
 emergencies 7.86
 first aid 4.4–4.6
 ionising radiation 7.86
 mental health 8.14
 nurses 3.10
 occupational health nurses 11.20
 occupational health physicians
  11.19
 personal protective equipment
  9.34
Transport 4.7
Travellers' health 5.26–5.37
Tuberculosis 5.33
Typhoid 5.28

U

Upper limb disorders 7.34

V

Vapour filters 9.48
Ventilation 7.65
Vibration 7.8–7.14, 7.48

Vibration white finger 7.10
Violence 2.36, 4.25, 2.37
Visual discomfort 7.55
Visual display units 7.24, 7.28, 7.30,
 7.55, 7.66–7.68

W

Warnings 2.12, 2.17
Whole-body vibration 7.8–7.9, 7.11,
 7.14, 7.48
Wind chill 7.22
Work surface height 7.44
Working conditions 4.12
Workload 3.34, 7.16
Workplace environment 7.59–7.65
Work-related upper limb disorders
 7.34
Workstations
 assessment 3.34
 design 3.13, 7.43
 layouts 7.46
 repetitive strain injuries 3.34
 work surface height 7.44
World Health Organisation 8.1, 8.38

X

X-rays 7.78

Y

Yellow fever 5.35

Z

Zoonoses 5.21–5.25